RADIATION TOXICITY: A PRACTICAL GUIDE

Cancer Treatment and Research

Steven T. Rosen, M.D., *Series Editor*

Sugarbaker, P. (ed.): *Peritoneal Carcinomatosis: Principles of Management.* 1995. ISBN 0-7923-3727-1.
Dickson, R.B., Lippman, M.E. (eds): *Mammary Tumor Cell Cycle, Differentiation and Metastasis.* 1995. ISBN 0-7923-3905-3.
Freireich, E.J., Kantarjian, H. (eds): *Molecular Genetics and Therapy of Leukemia.* 1995. ISBN 0-7923-3912-6.
Cabanillas, F., Rodriguez, M.A. (eds): *Advances in Lymphoma Research.* 1996. ISBN 0-7923-3929-0.
Miller, A.B. (ed.): *Advances in Cancer Screening.* 1996. ISBN 0-7923-4019-1.
Hait, W.N. (ed.): *Drug Resistance.* 1996. ISBN 0-7923-4022-1.
Pienta, K.J. (ed.): *Diagnosis and Treatment of Genitourinary Malignancies.* 1996. ISBN 0-7923-4164-3.
Arnold, A.J. (ed.): *Endocrine Neoplasms.* 1997. ISBN 0-7923-4354-9.
Pollock, R.E. (ed.) *Surgical Oncology.* 1997. ISBN 0-7923-9900-5.
Verweij, J., Pinedo, H.M., Suit, H.D. (eds): *Soft Tissue Sarcomas: Present Achievements and Future Prospects.* 1997. ISBN 0-7923-9913-7.
Walterhouse, D.O., Cohn, S.L. (eds): *Diagnostic and Therapeutic Advances in Pediatric Oncology.* 1997. ISBN 0-7923-9978-1.
Mittal, B.B., Purdy, J.A., Ang, K.K. (eds): *Radiation Therapy.* 1998. ISBN 0-7923-9981-1.
Foon, K.A., Muss, H.B. (eds): *Biological and Hormonal Therapies of Cancer.* 1998. ISBN 0-7923-9997-8.
Ozols, R.F. (ed.): *Gynecologic Oncology.* 1998. ISBN 0-7923-8070-3.
Noskin, G.A. (ed.): *Management of Infectious Complications in Cancer Patients.* 1998. ISBN 0-7923-8150-5.
Bennett, C.L. (ed.): *Cancer Policy.* 1998. ISBN 0-7923-8203-X.
Benson, A.B. (ed.): *Gastrointestinal Oncology.* 1998. ISBN 0-7923-8205-6.
Tallman, M.S., Gordon, L.I. (eds): *Diagnostic and Therapeutic Advances in Hematologic Malignancies.* 1998. ISBN 0-7923-8206-4.
von Gunten, C.F. (ed.): *Palliative Care and Rehabilitation of Cancer Patients.* 1999. ISBN 0-7923-8525-X.
Burt, R.K., Brush, M.M. (eds): *Advances in Allogeneic Hematopoietic Stem Cell Transplantation.* 1999. ISBN 0-7923-7714-1.
Angelos, P. (ed.): *Ethical Issues in Cancer Patient Care* 2000. ISBN 0-7923-7726-5.
Gradishar, W.J., Wood, W.C. (eds): *Advances in Breast Cancer Management.* 2000. ISBN 0-7923-7890-3.
Sparano, Joseph, A. (ed.): *HIV & HTLV-I Associated Malignancies.* 2001. ISBN 0-7923-7220-4.
Ettinger, David, S. (ed.): *Thoracic Oncology.* 2001. ISBN 0-7923-7248-4.
Bergan, Raymond, C. (ed.): *Cancer Chemoprevention.* 2001. ISBN 0-7923-7259-X.
Raza, A., Mundle, S.D. (eds): *Myelodysplastic Syndromes & Secondary Acute Myelogenous Leukemia* 2001. ISBN: 0-7923-7396.
Talamonti, Marks, S. (ed.): *Liver Directed Therapy for Primary and Metastatic Liver Tumors.* 2001. ISBN 0-7923-7523-8.
Stack, M.S., Fishman, D.A. (eds): *Ovarian Cancer.* 2001. ISBN 0-7923-7530-0.
Bashey, A., Ball, E.D. (eds): *Non-Myeloablative Allogeneic Transplantation.* 2002. ISBN 0-7923-7646-3.
Leong, Stanley, P.L. (ed.): *Atlas of Selective Sentinel Lymphadenectomy for Melanoma, Breast Cancer and Colon Cancer.* 2002. ISBN 1-4020-7013-6.
Andersson, B., Murray, D. (eds): *Clinically Relevant Resistance in Cancer Chemotherapy.* 2002. ISBN 1-4020-7200-7.
Beam, C. (ed.): *Biostatistical Applications in Cancer Research.* 2002. ISBN 1-4020-7226-0.
Brockstein, B., Masters, G. (eds): *Head and Neck Cancer.* 2003. ISBN 1-4020-7336-4.
Frank, D.A. (ed.): *Signal Transduction in Cancer.* 2003. ISBN 1-4020-7340-2.
Figlin, Robert, A. (ed.): *Kidney Cancer.* 2003. ISBN 1-4020-7457-3.
Kirsch, Matthias, Black, Peter McL. (ed.): *Angiogenesis in Brain Tumors.* 2003. ISBN 1-4020-7704-1.
Keller, E.T., Chung, L.W.K. (eds): *The Biology of Skeletal Metastases.* 2004. ISBN 1-4020-7749-1.
Kumar, Rakesh (ed.): *Molecular Targeting and Signal Transduction.* 2004. ISBN 1-4020-7822-6.
Verweij, J., Pinedo, H.M. (eds): *Targeting Treatment of Soft Tissue Sarcomas.* 2004. ISBN 1-4020-7808-0.
Finn, W.G., Peterson, L.C. (eds): *Hematopathology in Oncology.* 2004. ISBN 1-4020-7919-2.
Farid, N. (ed.): *Molecular Basis of Thyroid Cancer.* 2004. ISBN 1-4020-8106-5.
Khleif, S. (ed.): *Tumor Immunology and Cancer Vaccines.* 2004. ISBN 1-4020-8119-7.
Balducci, L., Extermann, M. (eds): *Biological Basis of Geriatric Oncology.* 2004. ISBN
Abrey, L.E., Chamberlain, M.C., Engelhard, H.H. (eds): *Leptomeningeal Metastases.* 2005. ISBN 0-387-24198-1.
Platanias, L.C. (ed.): *Cytokines and Cancer.* 2005. ISBN 0-387-24360-7.
Leong, Stanley P.L., Kitagawa, Y., Kitajima, M. (eds): *Selective Sentinel Lymphadenectomy for Human Solid Cancer.* 2005. ISBN 0-387-23603-1.
Small, Jr. W., Woloschak, G. (eds): *Radiation Toxicity: A Practical Guide.* 2005. ISBN 1-4020-8053-0.

RADIATION TOXICITY: A PRACTICAL GUIDE

Edited by
WILLIAM SMALL, JR., MD
Robert H. Lurie Comprehensive Cancer Center
Northwestern University Medical School
Northwestern Memorial Hospital
Chicago, IL

GAYLE E. WOLOSCHAK, PhD
Robert H. Lurie Comprehensive Cancer Center
Northwestern University
Feinberg School of Medicine
Chicago, IL

Springer

William Small, Jr.
Northwestern Memorial Hospital
Galter LC 178
251 East Huron
Chicago, IL 60611
USA
w-small@northwestern.edu

Gayle E. Woloschak
Department of Radiology
Northwestern University Feinberg School of Medicine
303 East Chicago Avenue, Ward 13-002
Chicago, IL 60611
USA
g-woloschak@northwestern.edu

Library of Congress Cataloging-in-Publication Data

Radiation Toxicity: a practical guide / edited by William Small, Jr., Gayle E. Woloschak.
p. ; cm. – (Cancer treatment and research ; 128)
Includes index.
ISBN-10: 1-4020-8053-0 e-ISBN-10: 0-387-25354-8
ISBN-13: 978-1402-08053-1 e-ISBN-13: 978-0387-25354-1
1. Cancer—Radiotherapy—Complications. 2. Radiation—Toxicology. 3. Radiation tolerance. I. Small, William. II. Woloschak, Gayle E. III. Cancer treatment and research; v. 128.
[DNLM: 1. Neoplasms—radiotherapy. 2. Radiation Injuries. 3. Radiation Tolerance.
QZ269 R1286 2005]
RC271.R3R3335 2005
616.99'40642—dc22

2005046421

Printed in the United States of America.

9 8 7 6 5 4 3 2 1 SPIN 11054047

springeronline.com

To my mother's battles with cancer that inspire me daily.
To my patients' courage and trust that I never take for granted.
To my residents' desire to learn.
Most of all, to Julie, Christina and Rebecca, without their support this would not have been possible.

William Small Jr., M.D.

To the residents in our program who have kept me sharp over the years.

Gayle Woloschak, Ph.D.

CONTENTS

LIST OF CONTRIBUTORS

Johanna C. Bendell, MD, Assistant Professor, Division of Oncology and Transplantation, Duke University Medical Center, Durham, NC

Angel I. Blanco, MD, Assistant Professor, Department of Radiation Oncology, The University of Texas M.D. Anderson Cancer Center, Houston, TX

Jeffrey Bradley, MD, Assistant Professor, Department of Radiation Oncology, Alvin J. Siteman Cancer Center, Washington University School of Medicine, St. Louis, MO

Linda Casey, MS, ARNP, AOCN, James A. Haley VA Medical Center, Tampa, FL

Clifford Chao, MD, Department of Radiation Oncology, The University of Texas M.D. Anderson Cancer Center, Houston, TX

Mark A. Engleman, MD, Chief Resident, Radiation Oncology, Robert H. Lurie Comprehensive Cancer Center Northwestern University Medical School, Chicago, IL

Kathryn McConnell Greven, MD, Professor of Radiation Oncology, Department of Radiation Oncology, Comprehensive Cancer Center of Wake Forest University School of Medicine, Winston Salem, NC

Michael C. Joiner, PhD, Professor, Department of Radiation Oncology, Karmanos Cancer Institute and Wayne State University, Detroit, MI

Benjamin Movsas, MD, Chair, Department of Radiation Oncology, Henry Ford Hospital, Detroit, MI

Tatjana Paunesku, PhD, Research Assistant Professor, Department of Radiology, Feinberg School of Medicine, Northwestern University, Chicago, IL

Mike E. Robbins, PhD, Professor and Section Head, Radiation Biology, Department of Radiation Oncology, Brain Tumor Center of Excellence, Comprehensive Cancer Center of Wake Forest University School of Medicine, Winston-Salem, NC

Edward G. Shaw, MD, Department of Radiation Oncology, Brain Tumor Center of Excellence, Comprehensive Cancer Center of Wake Forest University School of Medicine, Winston-Salem, NC

William Small, Jr., MD, Associate Professor of Clinical Radiology, Division of Radiation Oncology, Robert H. Lurie Comprehensive Cancer Center Northwestern University Medical School, Northwestern Memorial Hospital, Chicago, IL

Andy Trotti, MD, Director, Radiation Oncology Clinical Research, H. Lee Moffitt Cancer Center, Tampa, FL

Julia White, MD, Associate Professor, Department of Radiation Oncology, Medical College of Wisconsin, Milwaukee, WI

Christopher Willet, MD, Professor and Chair, Department of Radiation Oncology, Duke University Medical Center, Durham, NC

Gayle E. Woloschak, PhD, Professor of Radiology, Robert H. Lurie Comprehensive Cancer Center Northwestern University, Feinberg School of Medicine, Chicago, IL

Gloria Wood, RN, BSN, Radiation Therapy, H. Lee Moffitt Cancer Center, Tampa, FL

RADIATION TOXICITY: A PRACTICAL GUIDE

INTRODUCTION

WILLIAM SMALL JR., M.D.
GAYLE WOLOSCHAK, Ph.D.

The Robert H. Lurie Comprehensive Cancer Center, Northwestern University Medical School, Chicago, IL.

Since the discovery of radium by the Curies,[1] radiotherapy has offered incalculable benefits for cancer patients. Radiation is used in a wide variety of tumors for both curative and palliative indications. Advances in treatment delivery, diagnostic imaging, and treatment planning systems have improved tumor control and, in many cases, reduced toxicity.

A. ANTICIPATED APPROACHES TO REDUCTION OF TISSUE TOXICITY BY RADIATION

Despite these advances, radiation toxicity remains a major obstacle to effective therapy. In fact, the dose of radiotherapy that can be administered is often limited by the toxic effects of the therapy. For example, in the treatment of cervical cancer, there is good evidence of a dose–response for both the control of disease[2] and the risk of toxicity.[3] This dose–response relationship has also been observed in prostate cancer.[4,5] The ability to target radiotherapy and avoid normal tissue outside the planned radiotherapy field has been dramatically improved with the development of conformal radiotherapy and intensity-modulated radiation therapy. Future developments in these areas will no doubt further enhance the risk-benefit ratio of treatment.

Another approach that is likely to significantly reduce normal tissue toxicity is the rising use of diagnostic imaging and treatment delivery. Image-guided radiation therapies that are currently being developed will allow for simultaneous imaging of the tumor and treatment of the tumor in an individual. This will permit individualized care such that the tumor will be treated while the normal tissue will be spared as much as possible by actually visualizing the treatment area during the delivery of therapy. This will allow for a reduction in planning target volumes now added to the target to account for set up errors and internal organ motion.

Finally, special emphasis is being placed on understanding why some individuals have different levels of radiation toxicity than others. Once these markers have been identified, it may be possible to predict which patients are likely to have normal tissue toxicity complications from radiation exposure. For example, it is now known that expression of TGF-beta is associated with the development of lung fibrosis following radiation exposure.[6] Characterization of the molecular basis of this response may lead to the establishment of particular genotypes or polymorphisms in the TGF-beta gene or its promoter that are predictable of a fibrotic response in a patient. Identification of such patients who are at-risk for fibrosis development and those who are not could permit dose escalation in selected patients who are not likely to develop fibrosis. The extension of this to other types of radiation toxicities and other genes might eventually lead to the profiling of each patient for susceptibilities and treatment planning based on expected radiation responses.

B. ACUTE AND LONG-TERM TOXICITY

Radiotherapy toxicity is generally separated into acute toxicity and long-term toxicity. Acute toxicity occurs during or shortly after the radiotherapy whereas long-term toxicity can manifest itself months to years after the completion of the treatment. Both acute and long-term toxicities show a dose-threshold and therefore fit into the realm of deterministic responses to radiation (as opposed to cancer development which is considered a stochastic response with no threshold).

It is generally accepted that acute toxicity occurs by direct cytotoxicity to rapidly proliferating normal tissue cells. The exact etiology behind long-term radiotherapy toxicity is somewhat a matter of controversy. The two major theories are (1) that long-term toxicity is caused by the depletion of slowly proliferating stem cells and (2) that long-term damage is related to damage to the vasculature. In actuality, the exact etiology is probably much more complex than our current level of understanding permits, involving depletion of stem cells, changes in vasculature, and alterations in cellular factors including cytokines, small molecular mediators, and others.

As advances in treatment modalities are made, more focus is shifting to a close examination of quality-of-life issues. They are particularly relevant to radiation therapy since the consequences of toxicity can be debilitating and dramatically affect bodily function. Even when disease is controlled, the short- and long-term effects of radiotherapy can have a significant impact on the quality-of-life. Patients who receive curative radiotherapy for head and neck cancers are often left with a dry mouth and consequently have great difficulty in eating and swallowing. Patients who receive pelvic radiotherapy will in many instances be left with sexual difficulties.

The purpose of this book is to provide a framework for considering normal toxicities when using radiotherapy for cancer treatment. While long-term toxicities often cannot be reversed, approaches have been developed that will permit a reasonable quality of life. Considerations to be made in treatment decisions, approaches to alleviate some consequences of tissue toxicity, and other similar matters are all discussed in the chapters that follow. It is hoped that this will be a guide to the Radiation Oncologist, Medical Oncologist, Oncology Nurses, Radiation Therapists, and all who are involved in treatment of patients with radiation.

REFERENCES

1. Curie, P, MP Curie, and Bemont G. 1898. Sur une novellle substance fortement radioactive comntenue dans la penchblende (presented by M. Bequerel). Compt Rend Acad Sci (Paris) **127:**1215–1217.
2. Perez, CA, PW Grigsby, KSC Chao, et al. 1998. Tumor size, irradiation dose and long-term outcome of carcinoma of the uterine cervix. Int J Radiol Onocol Biol Phys **44:**855–866.
3. Lanciano, RM, K Martz, GS Montana, et al. 1992. Influence of age, prior abdominal surgery, fraction size and dose on complications after radiation therapy for squamous cell carcinoma of the uterine cervix. Cancer **69:**2124–2130.
4. Pollack, A, GK Zagars, G Starkschal, et al. 2002. Prostate cancer radiation dose response: results of the M.D. Anderson phase III randomized trial. Int J Radiol Onocol Biol Phys **53:**1097–1105.
5. Zelefsky, MJ, D Cowen, Z Fuks, et al. 1999. Long term tolerance of high-dose three-dimensional radiotherapy in patients with localized prostate cancer. Cancer **85:**2460–2468.
6. Rodemann, HP and M Bamberg. 1995. Cellular basis of radiation-induced fibrosis. Radiother Oncol **35:**83–90.

1. The Management of Radiation-Induced Brain Injury

EDWARD G. SHAW, M.D. AND MIKE E. ROBBINS, Ph.D.

Comprehensive Cancer Center of Wake Forest University School of Medicine, Winston-Salem, NC

INTRODUCTION

Neoplasms of the central nervous system (CNS) are a pathologically diverse group of benign and malignant tumors for which a variety of management strategies, including observation, surgery, radiation therapy, and/or chemotherapy, are employed. Shown in Table 1 are the usual radiation doses used to treat primary and metastatic brain and spinal cord tumors, which span a broad range of total doses and doses per fraction. Regardless of the type of CNS tumor treated, what usually limits the dose of radiation that can be utilized, and therefore what typically determines the local control and cure rate of that tumor, are the tolerance doses of the adjacent or underlying normal tissues in and around the CNS. This chapter will outline the biologic and clinical principles of CNS radiation tolerance and the management of radiation-induced CNS injury.

A. PATHOGENESIS OF RADIATION-INDUCED CNS INJURY

A1. Classical Model of Parenchymal or Vascular Target Cells

Vascular abnormalities and demyelination are the predominant histological changes seen in radiation-induced CNS injury. Classically, late delayed injury was viewed as due solely to a reduction in the number of surviving clonogens of either parenchymal, i.e., oligodendrocyte,[5] or vascular, i.e., endothelial,[6] target cell populations leading to white matter necrosis.

Table 1. Radiation treatment recommendations for primary central nervous system tumors

Pathologic type	Gross tumor volume (GTV)	Clinical tumor volume	Total dose (Gy)/ number of fractions
Glioblastoma (WHO IV) anaplastic astrocytoma (WHO III)*			60/30 or 64.8/36
Initial field	Edema and enhancing tumor	GTV + 2–3 cm margin	46/23 or 50.4/28
Boost field	Enhancing tumor	GTV + 2–2.5 cm margin	14/7 or 14.4/8
Astrocytoma (WHO II)†,‡	Edema (and enhancing tumor if present)	GTV + 1–2 cm margin‡	50.4/28 to 59.4/33
Pilocytic Astrocytoma (WHO I)	Enhancing tumor	GTV + 1–2 cm margin‡	50.4/28 to 55.8/31
Meningioma¶	Enhancing tumor	GTV + 1–2 cm margin‡	50.4/28 to 59.4/33
Medulloblastoma and anaplastic ependymoma			55.2/34 to 55.8/35
Initial volume	Entire brain and spine	GTV + 1–2 cm margin§	30.6/17 to 36/24
Boost volume	Enhancing tumor	GTV + 1–2 cm margin	19.8/11 to 25.2/14
Ependymoma	Enhancing tumor	GTV + 1–2 cm margin‡	50.4/28 to 59.4/33

* For anaplastic astrocytomas that are non-enhancing, plan similarly to a low-grade diffuse astrocytoma.
† Most astrocytomas (WHO I) are non-enhancing. The tumor (i.e., edema) is best seen on the T2-weighted MRI. If there is enhancing tumor, plan similarly to a glioblastoma multiforme.
‡ Reduce to a 1-cm margin after 50.4 Gy if total dose exceeds 50.4 Gy.
¶ Malignant meningiomas should be planned similarly to glioblastoma multiforme. For meningeal hemangiopericytoma, the CTV should include the GTV + 2–3 cm margin.
§ Margin at skull base should be about 1 cm, including cribiform plate. Margin on spinal canal should be 1.5–2 cm except inferior border of lower spine field, which should be at bottom of S3.
Data from Levin et al.,[1] Scally et al.,[2] Kun,[3] and Halperin et al.[4]

Vascular Hypothesis

Proponents of the vascular hypothesis argue that vascular damage leads to ischemia with secondary white matter necrosis. In support of this hypothesis is the large amount of data describing radiation-induced vascular changes including vessel wall thickening, vessel dilation, and endothelial cell nuclear enlargement.[6–8] Quantitative studies in the irradiated rat brain have noted time- and dose-related reductions in the number of endothelial cell nuclei and blood vessels prior to the development of necrosis.[8] Further, recent boron neutron capture studies in which radiation was delivered essentially to the vasculature alone still led to the development of white matter necrosis.[9] In contrast, radiation-induced necrosis has been reported in the absence of vascular changes.[7] Moreover, while the vascular hypothesis argues that ischemia is responsible for white matter necrosis, the most sensitive component of the CNS to oxygen deprivation, the neuron, is located in the gray matter, a relatively radioresistant region. Thus, it seems unlikely that radiation injury is due solely to damage to the vasculature alone.

Parenchymal Hypothesis

The parenchymal hypothesis for radiation-induced CNS injury focuses on the oligodendrocyte, required for the formation of myelin sheaths. The key cell for the generation of mature oligodendrocytes is the oligodendrocyte type 2 astrocyte (O-2A) progenitor cell.[10] Irradiation results in the loss of reproductive capacity of the O-2A progenitor cells in the rat CNS.[11,12] It is hypothesized that radiation induces loss of O2-A progenitor cells, leading to a failure to replace oligodendrocytes and demyelination. However, a mechanistic link between loss of oligodendrocytes and demyelination has yet to be established. Further, while the kinetics of oligodendrocytes is consistent with the early transient demyelination seen in the early delayed reactions, it is inconsistent with the late onset of white matter necrosis.[13] Thus, it is unlikely that loss of O2-A progenitor cells and oligodendrocytes alone can lead to late radiation injury.

Recent findings suggest that the classic model of parenchymal or vascular target cells is oversimplistic. Pathophysiological data from a variety of late responding tissues, including the CNS, indicate that the expression of radiation-induced normal tissue injury involves complex and dynamic interactions between several cell types within a particular organ.[7,14,15] In the brain, these include not only the oligodendrocytes and endothelial cells, but also the astrocytes, microglia, and neurons. These now are viewed not as *passive* bystanders, merely dying as they attempt to divide, but rather as *active* participants in an orchestrated, yet limited, response to injury.[16] This new paradigm offers an exciting new approach to radiation-induced normal tissue morbidity, i.e., the possibility that radiation injury can be modulated by the application of therapies directed at altering steps in the cascade of events leading to the clinical expression of normal tissue injury. Since such a cascade of events does not occur in tumors, where direct clonogenic cell kill predominates, such treatments should not negatively impact antitumor efficacy.

A2. Astrocytes

Astrocytes make up approximately 50% of the glial cell population in the brain, and are up to 10 times more numerous than neurons in the mammalian CNS.[17] Once viewed as playing a mere supportive role in the CNS, astrocytes are now recognized as a heterogeneous class of cells with many important and diverse functions in the normal CNS.[18] Astrocytes secrete a variety of cytokines, proteases, and growth factors that regulate the response of the vasculature, neurons, and oligodendrocyte lineage in the normal CNS.[19,20] Recent data suggest that hippocampal astrocytes are capable of regulating neurogenesis by instructing the stem cells to adopt a neuronal fate.[20] In addition, astrocytes assume a critical role in the reaction of the CNS to various forms of injury, including radiation, and are vital for the protection of endothelial cells, oligodendrocytes, and neurons from oxidative stress.[21] In response to injury, astrocytes exhibit two common reactions, a relatively acute cellular swelling and a more chronic hypertrophy–hyperplasia. Of note, time- and dose-dependent increases in astrocyte number have been observed in the irradiated rat and mouse brain.[6,8,22] In addition to increased cell number, an increase in GFAP staining intensity indicative of reactive astrocytes has been observed.[22] However, the precise pathogenic mechanism(s) impacted by the astrocyte in radiation-induced CNS injury remains unknown.

A3. Microglia

Microglia contribute approximately 10% of the total glial cell population in the adult CNS.[23] Microglia respond to virtually any, even minor pathological event in the CNS, and in most pathological settings are assisted by infiltrating macrophages.[24] Upon activation, they can proliferate, phagocytose, and enhance or exacerbate injury through the production of reactive oxygen species, lipid metabolites, and hydrolytic enzymes.[24] Irradiation of the CNS has been shown to result in increased numbers of microglia in areas of tissue injury, and can occur during the latent period before the clinical expression of injury.[22,25] Thus, microglia may play a role in determining the severity of radiation-induced injury in the CNS.

A4. Neurons

In view of the classic model of radiation-induced normal tissue injury, where DNA damage and loss of slowly turning over stem cell populations led to late effects, the non-proliferating neuron was thought to be radioresistant and a non-participant in radiation-induced CNS injury. Recent data documenting chronic and progressive cognitive dysfunction in both children[26–28] and adults[29–31] following whole brain or large field irradiation have suggested that neurons are indeed sensitive to radiation. Moreover, in vivo and in vitro experimental studies have shown radiation-induced changes in hippocampal cellular activity, synaptic efficiency and spike generation,[32,33] and in neuronal gene expression.[34] Thus, it seems likely that radiation-induced alterations in neuron function play a role in the development and progression of radiation-induced CNS injury. An additional and important component of radiation injury is the relatively recent observation that irradiation can inhibit hippocampal neurogenesis.

A5. Neural Stem Cells/Neurogenesis

The hippocampus is central to short-term declarative memory and spatial information processing. It consists of the dentate gyrus, CA3 and CA1 regions. The dentate gyrus represents a highly dynamic structure and a major site of postnatal/adult neurogenesis. Residents in the hippocampus are neural stem cells, self-renewing cells capable of generating neurons, astrocytes, and oligodendrocytes.[35,36] Neurogenesis depends on the presence of a specific neurogenic microenvironment; both endothelial cells and astrocytes can promote/regulate neurogenesis.[20,37] Experimental studies have indicated that brain irradiation results in increased apoptosis,[38] decreased cell proliferation, and a decreased stem/precursor cell differentiation into neurons within the neurogenic region of the hippocampus.[39–41] Rats irradiated with a single dose of 10 Gy produce only 3% of the new hippocampal neurons formed in control animals.[40] Of note, these changes were observed after doses of radiation that failed to produce demyelination and/or white matter necrosis of the rat brain.

Further evidence demonstrating the importance of the microenvironment for successful neurogenesis comes from studies showing that non-irradiated stem cells transplanted into the irradiated hippocampus failed to generate neurons; this may reflect a pronounced microglial inflammatory response, since neuroinflammation is a strong inhibitor of neurogenesis.[42] In contrast to the reduction in neurogenesis, gliogenesis appears to be preserved following irradiation.

A6. Current Thinking on the Pathogenesis of Radiation-Induced CNS Injury

On the basis of the assumption that the CNS has a limited repertoire of responses to injury, the response of the CNS to other forms of insult has been used by Tofilon and Fike[16] to model the pathogenesis of radiation-induced damage. In this model, radiation not only causes acute cell death, but also induces an intrinsic recovery/repair response in the form of specific cytokines and may initiate secondary reactive processes that result in the generation of a persistent oxidative stress and/or chronic inflammation.

A7. Laboratory Studies of Therapeutic Interventions for Radiation-Induced CNS Injury

As noted earlier, radiation-induced CNS injury has been well characterized in terms of histological criteria as well as radiobiological parameters. In contrast, details of the molecular, cellular, and biochemical processes responsible for the expression and progression of radiation-induced CNS injury currently are limited. Thus, the rational application of interventional procedures directed at reducing the severity of late radiation injury is currently problematic. To date, several pragmatic but nonspecific approaches have been used.

Intrathecal administration of the classic radioprotector WR-2721 (Amifostine) before spinal cord irradiation resulted in a dose-modifying factor of 1.3 and a prolongation of median latency to myelopathy by 63% at the ED_{50}.[43] Fike et al. observed that the polyamine synthesis inhibitor α-difluoromethylornithine reduced the volume of radionecrosis and contrast enhancement in the irradiated dog brain;[44] a delayed increase in microglia was also noted.[45] Hornsey et al. hypothesized that treating rats with the iron-chelating agent desferrioxamine would reduce hydroxyl-mediated reperfusion-related injury in the irradiated spinal cord.[46] Rats were fed a low-iron diet from 85 days after local spinal cord irradiation and received desferrioxamine (30 mg in 0.3 mL, sc, 3 times/week) from day 120, the time at which changes in vascular permeability were noted. The onset of ataxia due to white matter necrosis was delayed and the incidence of lesions was reduced after single doses of 25 and 27 Gy. Dexamethasone also delayed the development of radiation-induced ataxia along with a reduction in regional capillary permeability. In contrast, indomethacin did not appear to affect any of these endpoints. In the pig, administration of the polyunsaturated fatty acids γ-linolenic acid (GLA; 18C:3n-6) and eicosapentaenoic acid (EPA; 20C:5n-3), starting the day after spinal cord irradiation, was associated with a reduced incidence of paralysis, from 80% down to 20%.[47] More recently, El-Agamawi et al. reported that GLA significantly reduced the onset of paralysis following spinal cord irradiation in 5-week-old rats.[48] Prophylactic hyperbaric oxygen (HBO) has also been used to try and prevent radiation-induced myelopathy in a rat model. Using a dose of 65 Gy in 10 fractions with or without 30 HBO treatments following the irradiation, Sminia et al. did not demonstrate any preventive value to HBO. In fact, there was a "tendency toward radiosensitization" in the HBO-treated rats.[49] Administration of ramipril, an angiotensin converting enzyme inhibitor, from 2 weeks after stereotactic irradiation with a single dose of 30 Gy, until 6 months postirradiation, was associated with a reduction in the severity of optic neuropathy.[50]

Attempts have been made to rectify the radiation-induced decrease in neurogenesis. Rezvani et al.[51] transplanted neural stem cells 90 days after irradiation of the rat spinal cord with a single dose of 22 Gy. While 100% of the irradiated rats treated with saline exhibited paralysis within 167 days of irradiation, the paralysis-free survival rate of rats treated with neural stem cells was approximately 34% at 183 days. These findings are somewhat controversial; non-irradiated stem cells transplanted into the irradiated rat hippocampus failed to generate neurons, although gliogenesis was spared.[40] Preliminary data suggest that IGF-1 may show efficacy in not only preventing radiation myelopathy in adult rats,[52] but also in ameliorating the radiation-induced cognitive dysfunction observed in the rat following whole brain irradiation.[53]

B. CLINICAL ASPECTS OF CNS RADIATION TOLERANCE

The radiation tolerance of the CNS is dependent on a number of factors, including total dose, dose per fraction, total time, volume, host factors, radiation quality (linear energy transfer), and adjunctive therapies. Table 2 defines the role of these factors in radiation tolerance and injury to the brain, as well as ways they might be modified to increase tolerance (i.e., reduce injury).[54,55]

Table 3 shows partial and whole organ tolerance doses for the brain and spinal cord, and includes doses predicted to result in a 5% and 50% probability of injury 5 years following treatment with radiation (TD 5/5 and TD 50/5, respectively).[56,57] These values are derived from mathematical models of brain and spinal cord tolerance based on the clinical data describing the instances of radiation injury and the total doses and fraction sizes at which they occurred. None of the mathematical models account for the factors listed in Table 2, nor do they adequately predict radiation tolerance or injury.

Table 2. Factors associated with radiation tolerance of the normal central nervous system tissues

Factor*	Factors for increased risk of injury	Tolerance increased by
Total dose	Higher total dose	Decreasing total dose, hyperfractionation‡, radiosensitizers
Dose per fraction	Dose per fraction >180–200 cGy	Decreasing dose/fraction to ≤ 180–200 cGy
Volume	Increased volume, e.g., whole-organ radiation	Decreasing volume, e.g., partial-organ radiation
Host factors	Medical illness, e.g., hypertension, diabetes	Unknown, possibly radioprotectors
Beam quality	High LET radiation beams, e.g., neutrons	Low LET beams, e.g., photons
Adjunctive therapy	Concomitant use of CNS toxic drugs, e.g., methotrexate	Avoid concomitant use of CNS toxic

*Total time is not a major determinant of normal CNS tissue tolerance.
‡Defined as multiple daily fractions, usually two with doses per fraction of ≤180–200 cGy, usually 100–120 cGy, separated by 4–8 hours, to total doses higher than those given with "standard" fractionation.
Data from Leibel and Sheline[54] and Schultheiss et al.[55]

Table 3. Tolerance doses for normal central nervous system tissues*

CNS tissue	TD 5/5 (Gy)	TD 50/5 (Gy)	End point
Rubin, et al.			
Brain			Infarction, necrosis
Whole	60	70	
Partial (25%)	70	80	
Spinal cord			Infarction, necrosis
Partial (10 cm length)	45	55	
Emami, et al.			
Brain			Infarction, necrosis
One-third	60	75	
Two-thirds	50	65	
Whole	40	60	
Brainstem			Infarction, necrosis
One-third	60	–	
Two-thirds	53	–	
Whole	50	65	
Spinal cord			Myelitis, necrosis
5 cm	50	70	
10 cm	50	70	
20 cm	47	–	
Cauda equine	60	75	Clinically apparent nerve damage
Brachial plexus			Clinically apparent nerve damage
One-third	62	77	
Two-thirds	61	76	
Whole	60	75	

*Assumes 2 Gy per fraction, 5 days per week.
Data from Rubin[56] and Emami et al.[57]

The power-law model described by Sheline et al.[58] represents a modification of the Ellis Nominal Standard Dose formula[59]

$$\text{Neuret} = (D)(N^{-0.41})(T^{-0.03}),$$

where D is the total dose, N is the number of fractions, and T is the time.

The linear quadratic model links the response to fractionated irradiation to the fractional reproductive survival of clonogenic target cells. Fractionation data can be analyzed using the formula shown below:[60]

$$E = n(\alpha d + \beta d^2),$$

where the effect (E) is a linear and quadratic function of the dose per fraction (d) and a function of the fraction number (n). This equation allows the determination of the α/β ratio, a measure of the bendiness of the underlying putative target cell survival curve. For the brain and spinal cord, an average α/β ratio of 2 Gy appears appropriate.[61]

On the basis of these various models, the TD 5/5 for the whole brain and for part of the brain is 50 ± 10 Gy and 60 ± 10 Gy, respectively. For a 10-cm segment of the spinal cord, the TD 5/5 is 45–50 Gy (Table 3). Although the TD 50/5 value for the spinal cord is lower than that of the brain, there are not good data to support this difference. Rather, the sequelae of spinal cord radiation injury are perceived as greater than those of

Table 4. Tolerance doses for miscellaneous normal tissues of the cranium

Normal tissue	TD 5/5 (Gy)	TD 50/5 (Gy)	Manifestations of severe injury
Ear (middle/external)	30–55	40–65	Acute or chronic serous otitis
Eye			
Retina	45	65	Blindness
Lens	10	18	Cataract formation
Optic nerve or chiasm	50	65	Blindness

Data from Emami et al.,[57] Sklar and Constine,[65] Gordon et al.,[66] and Cooper et al.[67]

brain injury; therefore, tolerance doses have been arbitrarily lowered. In clinical practice, TD 5/5 and 1/5 values of 60–65 and 50–55 Gy for partial brain irradiation and TD 5/5 and 1/5 values of 55–60 and 45–50 Gy for a limited segment of the spinal cord are commonly used. Clinical data have born out these somewhat empiric dose ranges. In a study of 203 adults with supratentorial low-grade glioma, patients were randomized to partial brain treatment fields with either 50.4 Gy in 28 fractions of 1.8 Gy each or 64.8 Gy in 36 fractions of 1.8 Gy.[62] Radiation necrosis developed in 1% of patients who received 50.4 Gy and 5% of those who had 64.8 Gy. In a retrospective study of 53 head and neck cancer patients undergoing typical posterior cervical treatment fields including the cervical spinal cord to doses of 56–60 Gy in fraction sizes of $\leq$2 Gy, the incidence of radiation myelopathy was 1.9%.[63] In a subsequent study of 1048 lung cancer patients treated with thoracic radiation on three Medical Research Council Lung Cancer Working Party clinical trials, the only patients who developed radiation myelopathy were those treated with 3 Gy fractions or larger. The 2-year risk of radiation myelopathy was 2.2–2.5% among patients receiving thoracic spinal cord doses of 17 Gy in 2 fractions or 39 Gy in 13 fractions. The authors concluded that a total cord dose of 48 Gy given in 2-Gy fractions was safe.[64] These data emphasize the importance of both total dose and dose per fraction in determining CNS tolerance to radiation. These concepts are implied in the neuret model of brain tolerance in which fraction size, which is related to "*N*" (number of fractions), is far more important than "*T*" (time), given that the exponent for *N* is much larger than that for *T*. The TD 5/5s given for brain and spinal cord tolerance assume a fraction size of 180–200 cGy per day. For primary CNS tumor patients being treated with curative intent, fraction size should rarely exceed 200 cGy daily, and in most situations, should be 180–200 cGy (including areas or volumes of "hot spots"). Fraction sizes greater than 200 cGy daily (usually 250–300 cGy) are commonly used for palliation of brain metastases and spinal cord compression, but only because such patients are not expected to live long enough to manifest normal tissue injury.

Table 4 shows the tolerance doses for other normal tissues of the CNS, including the brainstem, eye, ear, optic chiasm, optic nerve, and pituitary gland. The clinical manifestations of severe injury to these structures are listed.[65–67]

C. QUANTITATIVE SCORING OF CNS TOXICITY

Radiation injury is usually described in terms of its time course and severity. Acute injury occurs during the course of brain and spinal cord irradiation, and is extremely

Table 5. RTOG and EORTC central nervous system toxicity tables

1	2	3	4
Acute toxicity grade: brain			
Fully functional status (i.e., able to work) with minor neurological findings; no medication needed	Neurological findings sufficient to require home care; nursing assistance may be required; medications including steroids and anti-	Neurological findings requiring hospitalization for initial management	Serious neurological impairment that includes paralysis, coma, or seizures > 3 per week despite medication and/or hospitalization required
Chronic toxicity grade: brain			
Mild headache; slight lethargy	Moderate headache; great Lethargy	Severe headaches; severe CNS dysfunction (partial loss of power or dyskinesia)	Seizure or paralysis; coma
Chronic toxicity grade: spinal cord			
Mild Lhermitte's syndrome	Severe Lhermitte's syndrome	Objective neurological findings at or below cord level treated	Monoplegia, paraplegia, or quadriplegia

Grade 0 toxicity, none; grade 1, mild; grade 2, moderate; grade 3, severe; grade 4, life threatening; grade 5, fatal.
Data from Cox et al.[68]

uncommon, although acute side effects of radiation do occur, such as fatigue, hair loss, and skin erythema. More common are the early delayed reactions, which occur several weeks to months after radiation has been completed, and the late delayed reactions, which occur beyond several months (and usually between 1 and 2 years) following treatment.

Clinically, radiation-induced toxicities are usually graded as mild, moderate, severe, life-threatening, or fatal, and are defined in an organ-specific manner. Table 5 shows the toxicity tables used for brain tumor clinical research protocols by the Radiation Therapy Oncology Group (RTOG) and its European counterpart, the European Organization for the Research and Treatment of Cancer (EORTC).[68] Alternatively, the National Cancer Institute (NCI) Common Terminology Criteria for Adverse Events version 3.0 can be used (http://ctep.cancer.gov/reporting/ctc.html). To measure quality-of-life in brain tumor patients undergoing combined modality therapy including brain radiation, the Functional Assessment of Cancer Therapy (FACT) scale is used, including the brain subscale.[69]

Early delayed reactions are thought to occur, at least in part, due to the effects of radiation on the oligodendroglial- or myelin-producing cells, resulting in an interruption of myelin synthesis. Myelin forms a concentric sheath that surrounds the axons or nerve fibers. In the brain, this is clinically manifested as somnolence, increased irritability, loss of appetite, and sometimes an exacerbation of underlying tumor-associated symptoms or signs. When this symptom complex occurs in children following whole brain radiation, it is called the "somnolence syndrome". In the spinal cord, symptoms of demyelination include electric shock-like paresthesias radiating into the arms that occur with flexion of the neck, or L'Hermittes syndrome. These early delayed reactions are nearly always transient, lasting several weeks to months, and do not predict for subsequent injury.[70] Late delayed reactions, on the other hand, are usually irreversible. The underlying mechanisms of the late delayed reactions are thought to include (but are not limited to) injury to the capillary endothelium leading to narrowing or obliteration of the arteries supplying blood to the brain or spinal cord, or direct damage of its tissues. For both the early and late delayed reactions, the result is radiation necrosis, which is tissue damage to the substance or white matter of the brain or spinal cord. The clinical symptoms and signs of radiation necrosis are the direct result of the tissue damage, or indirectly result from swelling of the adjacent normal tissues in response to the necrotic material. Brain necrosis may be asymptomatic if it occurs in a non-critical area, but usually is associated with symptoms that are location-specific [e.g., necrosis in the right posterior frontal lobe (motor strip) would result in a left hemiparesis]. Spinal cord necrosis is usually symptomatic, and may include sensory and motor loss in the legs or arms and legs, depending on the level of the injury, as well as sphincter impairment of the bowel and bladder.

D. MANAGEMENT OF RADIATION-INDUCED CNS INJURY

D1. Acute Reactions

The most common acute reactions associated with brain radiation include fatigue, hair loss, and skin erythema. The onset of fatigue is generally several weeks after the first radiation treatment. It is usually mild to moderate in severity. Typically, the fatigue persists for several months after the completion of treatment but may be chronic in a small percentage of patients. One characteristic of the fatigue associated with radiation therapy is a lack of improvement by rest. Methylphenidate (*Ritalin*) can be used to treat the fatigue that usually occurs in patients receiving whole brain radiation.[71] It also improves the cognitive dysfunction and depression in these patients. The usual dose of methylphenidate is 10 mg bid, escalating to 30 mg bid in 1–2-week increments as tolerated. The dose-limiting toxicities are anxiety and insomnia. Hair loss occurs in the same time frame as fatigue, about 2–3 weeks into a course of fractionated whole- or partial-brain radiation. Complete or near-complete hair regrowth is the rule, though it may take 6 months to a year. There are no known treatments to accelerate or maximize hair regrowth. Skin erythema is managed symptomatically with anti-inflammatory and moisturizing creams, typically 1% hydrocortisone or *Aquaphor*, which are applied twice to four times daily or as needed for patient comfort. Moist desquamation behind the ears and in the external auditory canals may develop following whole brain radiation. Treatment usually involves skin creams and *Cortisporin* otic suspension. Rarely, debridement of the external canals by an otolaryngologist may be necessary.

D2. Early Delayed Reactions

There are no known interventions or therapies to prevent or treat the early delayed reactions involving the brain or spinal cord thought to occur because of transient demyelination.

D3. Late Delayed Reactions

Although edema and necrosis of the white matter are classified as late delayed reactions, edema of the brain and spinal cord can occur as an early or late effect of radiation. The treatment of radiation-induced edema is more of an art than a science and typically involves the use of corticosteroid medications. Oral dexamethasone is usually used in initial doses of 4 mg bid for mild symptoms and 4 mg qid for moderate to severe symptoms. Doses in excess of 10 mg qid (40 mg daily) do not increase the likelihood of clinical benefit. The initial dexamethasone dose is usually maintained during the course of radiation, with a slow taper (2–4 mg every 5–7 days) as tolerated thereafter. For life-threatening edema, intravenous dexamethasone is used, 10–25 mg as a bolus followed by 4–10 mg qid. If these patients do not respond to dexamethasone, intravenous mannitol may be required. Patients on dexamethasone should receive gastritis prophylaxis (with ranitidine or an equivalent medication) and appropriate treatments for hyperglycemia (oral hypoglycemic agents or insulin) and oral thrush (fluconazole 200 mg for day 1, then 100 mg daily for 6 days) should they arise. Prophylaxis for pneumocystis pneumonia using one double strength trimethoprim/sulfamethoxizole (*Bactrim*) daily two to three times per week is commonly used in children as well as adults also taking temozolomide (*Temodar*) chemotherapy.[72,73] Patients taking dexamethasone chronically (1 month or longer) usually become Cushingoid, characterized by fatigue, weight gain, facial swelling, central obesity, muscle wasting (particularly in the extremities), striae, and arthralgias. Treatment is symptomatic. The physical manifestations of chronic dexamethasone use can take months to resolve after its discontinuation.

Necrosis of the brain (or spinal cord) can be difficult to clinically and radiographically differentiate from tumor recurrence.[74] Since cerebral radiation necrosis is always accompanied by edema, the initial management of clinically suspected or pathologically proven necrosis is with corticosteroids, as previously described. Several adjunctive medical treatments for cerebral radiation necrosis have been anecdotally described as being helpful to arrest or reverse the process, such as HBO, warfarin (*Coumadin*), and antioxidant vitamins.[75,76] There is no proven value for these interventions in addition to or instead of dexamethasone. In steroid unresponsive patients, surgical resection of the necrotic lesion, provided it can be safely performed, will often allow the dexamethasone dose to be reduced and also provide relief from the symptoms and signs of mass effect associated with the cerebral edema.

The late delayed effect of whole brain radiation, cognitive dysfunction, can occur with total doses as low as 20 Gy in adults and 24 Gy in children given with conventional fractions of 1.8–2 Gy.[77–79] Symptoms range from cognitive slowing, poor concentration, difficulty in multi-tasking, decreased short-term (and eventually long-term) memory, word-finding problems, and decreased IQ (in children), to a progressive Alzheimer's-like dementia, which is also characterized by urinary incontinence and gait disturbance.[29,80–87] There are no proven preventive or therapeutic interventions for radiation-induced cognitive dysfunction. Table 6 lists potential agents derived from the broader literature on brain injury (including radiation-induced injury, stroke, and trauma). The Wake Forest University School of Medicine Comprehensive Cancer

Table 6. Possible preventive and therapeutic interventions for late radiation-induced brain injury

Cytokines (growth factors)
IGF1
CNTF
PDGF
VEGF
bFGF
Antioxidants/free radical scavengers
NAC
Cysteine
Methionine
Glutathione
Sodium thiosulfate
Melatonin
Vitamins C and E
WR2721 (Amifostine)
MnSOD
PUFAs
Other agents
Donepezil
Cox-1 and Cox-2 inhibitors
Vasoactive drugs
Angiotensin inhibitors
DFMO
Ginkgo biloba
Ginseng
Erythropoetin/Darbepoetin
Regenerative approaches
Glial cell transplantation (O-2A progenitor cells, mature oligodendrocytes)
Neural stem cell transplantation
Combined agents/approaches

Center, through its Community Clinical Oncology Program Research Base, has several clinical trials that are addressing therapies for symptomatic late radiation-induced brain injury. In a recently completed Phase II study in 35 patients, donepezil (*Aricept*) 10 mg daily was given for 6 months with serial assessment of quality-of-life and neurocognitive function.[88] A similar study is ongoing using ginkgo biloba 40 mg tid based on the data from randomized trials in dementia.[89]

ACKNOWLEDGEMENTS

Supported by NCI grants CA82722, CA81851, and by an unrestricted educational grant from Elekta Instruments Inc., Norcross, GA.

REFERENCES

1. Levin, VA, SA Leibel, and PH Gutin. 2001. Neoplasms of the central nervous system. In: Devita, VT, Jr, Hellman, S, Rosenberg, SA, eds. Cancer—Principles and Practice of Oncology. Philadelphia, PA: Lippincott Williams and Wilkins.
2. Scally, LT, C. Lin, S Beriwal, and LW Brady. 2004. Brain, Brain Stem, and Cerebellum. In: Perez, CA, Brady, LW, Halperin, EC, Schmidt-Ullrich, RK, eds. Principles and Practice of Radiation Oncology. Philadelphia, PA: Lippincott Williams and Wilkins.

3. Kun, LE. 1994. The brain and spinal cord. In: Cox, JD, ed. Moss' Radiation Oncology—Rationale, Technique, Results. St. Louis, MO: Mosby—Year Book, Inc.
4. Halperin, EC, LS Constine, NJ Tarbell, and LE Kun, eds. 1994. Pediatric Radiation Oncology, 2nd ed. New York: Raven Press.
5. van den Maazen, RWM, BJ Kleiboer, I Berhagen, and AJ van der Kogel. 1993. Repair capacity of adult rat glial progenitor cells determined by an *in vitro* clonogenic assay after *in vitro* or *in vivo* fractionated irradiation. Int J Radiat Biol **63:**661–666.
6. Calvo, W, JW Hopewell, HS Reinhold, and TK Yeung. 1988. Time-and dose-related changes in the white matter of the rat brain after single doses of X rays. Br J Radiol **61:**1043–1052.
7. Schultheiss, TE, and LC Stephens. 1992. Permanent radiation myelopathy. Br J Radiol **65:**737–753.
8. Reinhold, HS, W Calvo, JW Hopewell, and AP van den Berg. 1990. Development of blood vessel-related radiation damage in the fimbria of the central nervous system. Int J Radiat Oncol Biol Phys **18:**37–42.
9. Morris, GM, JA Coderre, A Bywaters, E Whitehouse, and JW Hopewell. 1996. Boron neutron capture irradiation of the rat spinal cord: histopathological evidence of a vascular-mediated pathogenesis. Radiat Res **146:**313–320.
10. Raff, MC, RH Miller, and M Noble. 1983. A glial progenitor cell that develops in vitro into an astrocyte or an oligodendrocyte depending on culture medium. Nature **303:**390–396.
11. van der Maazen, RWM, BJ Kleiboer, I Verhagen, and AJ van der Kogel. 1991. Irradiation *in vitro* discriminates between different O-2A progenitor cell subpopulations in the perinatal central nervous system of rats. Radiat Res **128:**64–72.
12. van der Maazen, RWM, I Verhagen, BJ Kleiboer, and AJ van der Kogel. 1991. Radiosensitivity of glial progenitor cells of the prenatal and adult rat optic nerve studies by an *in vitro* clonogenic assay. Radiother Oncol **20:**258–264.
13. Hornsey, S, R Myers, PG Coultas, MA Rogers, and A White. 1981. Turnover of proliferative cells in the spinal cord after X irradiation and its relation to time-dependent repair of radiation damage. Br J Radiol **54:**1081–1085.
14. Jaenke, RS, MEC Robbins, T Bywaters, E Whitehouse, M Rezvani, and JW Hopewell. 1993. Capillary endothelium: target site of renal radiation injury. Lab Invest **57:**551–565.
15. Moulder, J, MEC Robbins, EP Cohen, JW Hopewell, and WF Ward. 1998. Pharmacologic modification of radiation-induced late normal tissue injury. In: Mittal, BB, Purdy, JA, Ang, KK, eds. Radiation Therapy. Norwell, MA: Kluwer, pp 129–151.
16. Tofilon, PJ, and JR Fike. 2000. The radioresponse of the central nervous system: a dynamic process. Radiat Res **153:**357–370.
17. Hansson, E. 1988. Astroglia from defined brain regions as studied with primary cultures. Prog Neurobiol **30:**369–397.
18. Montgomery, DL. 1994. Astrocytes: form, functions, and roles in disease. Vet Pathol **31:**145–167.
19. Muller, HW, U Junghans, and J Kappler. 1995. Astroglial neurotrophic and neurite-promoting factors. Pharmacol Ther **65:**1–18.
20. Song, H, CF Stevens, and FH Gage. 2002. Astroglia induce neurogenesis from adult neural stem cells. Nature **417:**39–44.
21. Wilson, JX. 1997. Antioxidant defense of the brain: a role for astrocytes. Can J Physiol Pharmacol **75:**1149–1163.
22. Chiang, C-S, WH McBride, and HR Withers. 1993. Radiation-induced astrocytic and microglial cellular hyperplasia. Radiother Oncol **29:**60–68.
23. Vaughan, DW, and A Peters. 1974. Neuroglial cells in the cerebral cortex of rats from young adulthood to old age: an electron microscopic study. J Neurocytol **3:**405–429.
24. Stollg, G, and S Jander. 1999. The role of microglia and macrophages in the pathophysiology of the CNS. Prog Neurobiol **58:**233–247.
25. Mildenberger, M, TG Beach, EG McGeer, and CM Ludgate. 1990. An animal model of prophylactic cranial irradiation: histologic effects at acute, early and delayed stages. Int J Radiat Oncol Biol Phys **18:**1051–1060.
26. Roman, DD, and PW Sperduto. 1995. Neuropsychological effects of cranial radiation: current knowledge and future directions. Int J Radiat Oncol Biol Phys **31:**983–998.
27. Anderson, VA, T Godber, E Smibert, S Weiskop, and H Ekert. 2000. Cognitive and academic outcome following cranial irradiation and chemotherapy in children: a longitudinal study. Br J Cancer **82:**255–262.
28. Moore, BD, III, DR Copeland, H Ried, and B Levy. 1992. Neurophysiological basis of cognitive deficits in long-term survivors of childhood cancer. Arch Neurol **49:**809–817.

29. Crossen, JR, D Garwood, E Glatstein, and EA Neuwelt. 1994. Neurobehavioral sequelae of cranial irradiation in adults: a review of radiation-induced encephalopathy. J Clin Oncol **12:**627–642.
30. Abayomi, OK. 1996. Pathogenesis of irradiation-induced cognitive dysfunction. Acta Oncologica **35:**659–663.
31. Surma-aho, O, M Niemalä, J Vilkki, M Kouri, A Brander, O Salonen, A Paetau, M Kallio, J Pyykkönen, and J Jääskeläinen. 2001. Adverse long-term effects of brain radiotherapy in adult low-grade glioma patients. Neurology **56:**1285–1290.
32. Bassant, MH, and L Court. 1978. Effect of whole-body gamma irradiation on the activity of rabbit hippocampal neurons. Radiat Res **75:**595–606.
33. Pellmar, TC, and DL Lepinski. 1993. Gamma radiation (5–10 Gy) impairs neuronal function in the guinea pig hippocampus. Radiat Res **136:**255–261.
34. Noel, F, GJ Gumin, U Raju, and PJ Tofilon. 1998. Increased expression of prohormone convertase-2 in the irradiated rat brain. FASEB J **12:**1725–1730.
35. Gage, FH, G Kempermann, TD Palmer, DA Peterson and J Ray. 1998. Multipotent progenitor cells in the adult dentate gyrus. J Neurobiol **36:**249–266.
36. Palmer, TD, J Takahashi, and FH Gage. 1997. The adult rat hippocampus contains primordial neural stem cells. Mol Cell Neurosci **8:**389–404.
37. Palmer, TD, AR Willhoite, and FH Gage. 2000. Vascular niche for adult hippocampal neurogenesis. J Comp Neurol **425:**479–494.
38. Bellinzona, M, GT Gobbel, C Shinohara, and JR Fike. 1996. Apoptosis is induced in the subependyma of young adult rats by ionizing irradiation. Neurosci Lett **208:**163–166.
39. Snyder, JS, N Kee, and JM Wojtowicz. 2003. Effects of adult neurogenesis on synaptic plasticity in the rat dentate gyrus. J Neurophysiol **85:**2423–2431.
40. Monje, ML, S Mizumatsu, JR Fike, and T Palmer. 2002. Irradiation induced neural precursor-cell dysfunction. Nat Med **8:**955–961.
41. Mizumatsu, S, ML Monje, DR Morhardt, R Rola, TD Palmer, and JR Fike. 2003. Extreme sensitivity of adult neurogenesis to low doses of X-irradiation. Cancer Res **63:**4021–4027.
42. Monje, ML, H Toda, and TD Palmer. 2003. Inflammatory blockade restores adult hippocampal neurogenesis. Science **302:**1760–1764.
43. Spence, AM, KA Krohn, SW Edmonson, JE Steele, and JS Rasey. 1986. Radioprotection in rat spinal cord with WR-2721 following cerebral lateral intraventricular injection. Int J Radiat Oncol Biol Phys **12:**1479–1482.
44. Fike, JR, GT Goebbel, LJ Martob, and TM Seilhan. 1994. Radiation brain injury is reduced by the polyamine inhibitor alpha-difluoromethylornithine. Radiat Res **138:**99–106.
45. Nakagawa, M, M Bellinzona, TM Seilhan, GT Gobbel, KR Lamborn, and JR Fike. 1996. Microglial responses after focal radiation-induced injury are affected by alpha-difluormethylornithine. Int J Radiat Oncol Biol Phys **36:**113–123.
46. Hornsey, S, R Myers, and T Jenkinson. 1990. The reduction of radiation damage to the spinal cord by postirradiation administration of vasoactive drugs. Int J Radiat Oncol Biol Phys **18:**1437–1442.
47. Hopewell, JW, GJMJ van den Aardweg, GM Morris, M Rezvani, MEC Robbins, GA Ross, EM Whitehouse, and CA Scott. 1993. Unsaturated lipids as modulators of radiation damage in normal tissues. In: Horrobin, DF, ed. New Approaches to Cancer Treatment. London: Churchill Communications Europe, pp 88–106.
48. El-Agamawi, AY, JW Hopewell, PN Plowman, M Rezvani, and D Wilding. 1996. Modulation of normal tissue responses to radiation. Br J Radiol **69:**374–375.
49. Sminia, P, AJ van der Kleij, UM Carl, JJ Feldmeier, and KA Hartmann. 2003. Prophylactic hyperbaric oxygen treatment and rat spinal cord irradiation. Cancer Lett **191:**59–65.
50. Kim, JH, SL Brown, A Kolozsvary, KA Jenrow, S Ryu, ML Rosenblum, et al. 2004. Modification of radiation injury by Ramipril, inhibitor of the angiotensin-converting enzyme, on optic neuropathy in the rat. Radiat Res **161:**137–142.
51. Rezvani, M, DA Birds, H Hodges, JW Hopewell, K Milledew, and JH Wilkinson. 2002. Modification of radiation myelopathy by the transplantation of neural stem cells in the rat. Radiat Res **156:**408–412.
52. Nieder, C, RE Price, B Rivera, and KK Ang. 2000. Both early and delayed treatment with growth factors can modulate the development of radiation myelopathy (RM) in rats. Radiother Oncol **56(Suppl 1):**S15.
53. Lynch, CD, WE Sonntag, and KT Wheeler. 2002. Radiation-induced dementia in aged rats: effects of growth hormone and insulin-like growth factor 1. Neuro-Oncol **4:**354.

54. Leibel, SA, and GE Sheline. 1991. Tolerance of the brain and spinal cord to conventional irradiation. In: Gutin, P, Liebel, SA, Sheline, GE, eds. Radiation Injury to the Nervous System, 1st ed. New York: Raven Press, pp 211–238.
55. Schultheiss, TE, LE Kun, KK Ang, and LC Stephens. 1995. Radiation response of the central nervous system. Int J Radiat Oncol Biol Phys **31:**1093–1112.
56. Rubin, P, and GW Casarett. 1968. Clinical Radiation Pathology, vols 1 and 2. Philadelphia: WB Saunders.
57. Emami, B, J Lyman, A Brown, L Coia, M Goitein, JE Munzenrider, B Shan, LJ Solin, and M Wesson. 1991. Tolerance of normal tissue to therapeutic irradiation. Int J Radiat Oncol Biol Phys **21:**109–122.
58. Sheline, GE, WM Wara, and V Smith. 1980. Therapeutic irradiation and brain injury. Int J Radiat Oncol Biol Phys **6:**1215–1218.
59. Ellis, F. 1969. Dose, time fractionation: a clinical hypothesis. Clin Radiol **20:**1–7.
60. Fowler, JF. 1992. Brief summary of radiobiological principles in fractionated radiotherapy. Semin Radiat Oncol **2:**16–21.
61. van der Kogel, AJ. 1991. The nervous system: radiobiology and experimental pathology. In: Scherer, E, Streffer, C, Trott, KR, eds. Radiopathology of Organs and Tissues. Berlin: Springer-Verlag, pp 191–212.
62. Shaw, E, R Arusell, B Scheithauer, J O'Fallon, B O'Neill, R Dinapoli, D Nelson, J Earle, C Jones, T Cascino, D Nichols, R Ivnik, R Hellman, W Curran, and R Abrams. 2002. A prospective randomized trial of low-versus high-dose radiation therapy in adults with supratentorial low-grade glioma: Initial report of a NCCTG-RTOG-ECOG study. J Clin Oncol **20:**2267–2276.
63. McCunniff, AJ, and AJ Liang. 1989. Radiation tolerance of the cervical spinal cord. Int J Radiat Oncol Biol Phys **16:**675–678.
64. Macbeth, FR, TE Wheldon, DJ Girling, RJ Stephens, D Machin, NM Bleehen, et al. 1996. Radiation myelopathy: estimates of risk in 1048 patients in three randomized trials of palliative radiotherapy for non-small cell lung cancer. The Medical Research Council Lung Cancer Working Party. Clin Oncol (R Coll Radiol) **8:**176–181.
65. Sklar, CA, and LS Constine. 1995. Chronic neuroendocrinological sequelae of radiation therapy. Int J Radiat Oncol Biol Phys **31:**1113–1122.
66. Gordon, KB, DH Char, and RH Sagerman. 1995. Late effects of radiation on the eye and ocular adnexa. Int J Radiat Oncol Biol Phys **31:**1123–1140.
67. Cooper, JS, K Fu, J Marks, and S Silverman. 1995. Late effects of radiation in the head and neck region. Int J Radiat Oncol Biol Phys **31:**1141–1164.
68. Cox, JD, J Stetz, and TF Pajak. 1995. Toxicity criteria of the Radiation Therapy Oncology Group and the European Organization for Research and Treatment of Cancer. Int J Radiat Oncol Biol Phys **31:**1341–1346.
69. Weitzner, MA, CA Meyers, CK Gelke, KS Byrne, DF Cella, and VA Levin. 1995. The Functional Assessment of Cancer Therapy (FACT) scale: Development of a brain subscale and revalidation of the general version (FACT-G) in patients with primary brain tumors. Cancer **75:**1151–1161.
70. Esik, O, T Csere, K Stefantis, Z Lengyel, G Safrany, K Vonoczky, et al. 2003. A review on radiogenic LHermitte's sign. Pathol Oncol Res **9:**115–120.
71. Weitzner, MA, CA Meyers, AD Valentine. 1995. Methylphenidate in the treatment of neurobehavioral slowing associated with cancer and cancer treatment. J Neuropsyc Clin Neurosci **7:**347–350.
72. Wen, PY, and PW Marks. 2002. Medical management of patients with brain tumors. Curr Opin Oncol **14:**299–307.
73. Stupp, R, PY Dietrich, S Ostermann Kraljevic, A Pica, I Maillard, P Maeder, R Meuli, R Janzer, G Pizzolato, R Miralbell, F Porchet, L Regli, N de Tribolet, RO Mirimanoff, and S Leyvraz. 2002. Promising survival for patients with newly diagnosed glioblastoma multiforme treated with concomitant radiation plus temozolomide followed by adjuvant temozolomide. J Clin Oncol **20:** 1375–1382.
74. Forsyth, PA, PA Forsyth, PJ Kelly, TL Casano, BW Scheithauer, EG Shaw, RP Dinapoli, and EJ Atkinson. 1995. Radiation necrosis or glioma recurrence: is computer assisted stereotactic biopsy useful? J Neurosurg **82:**436–444.
75. Liu, CY, BY Yim, and AJ Wozniak. 2001. Anticoagulation therapy for radiation-induced myelopathy. Ann Pharmacother **35:**188–191.
76. Leber, KA, HG Eder, H Kovac, U Anegg, and G Pendl. 1998. Treatment of cerebral radionecrosis by hyperbaric oxygen therapy. Stereotact Funct Neurosurg **70(Suppl 1)**:229–236.
77. Laukkanen, E, H Klonof, B Allan, et al. 1988. The role of prophylactic brain irradiation in limited stage small-cell lung cancer: clinical, neuropsychologic, and CT sequelae. Int J Radiat Oncol Biol Phys **14:**1109–1117.

78. Johnson, BE, B Becker, WB Goff, et al. 1985. Neurologic, neuropsychologic, and computed cranial tomography scan abnormalities in 2- to 10-year survivors of small-cell lung cancer. J Clin Oncol **3:**1659–1667.
79. Roman, D, and P Sperduto. 1995. Neuropsychological effects of cranial radiation: current knowledge and future directions. Int J Radiat Oncol Biol Phys **32:**983–998.
80. Halberg, F, J Kramer, I Moore, W Wara, K Matthay, and A Ablin. 1991. Prophylactic cranial irradiation dose effects on late cognitive function in children treated for acute lymphoblastic leukemia. Int J Radiat Oncol Biol Phys **11:**13–16.
81. DeAngelis, LM, J Delattre, and JB Posner. 1989. Radiation-induced dementia in patients cured of metastases. Neurology **39:**789–796.
82. Frytak, S, JN Shaw, BP O'Neill, RE Lee, RT Eagan, EG Shaw, RL Richardson, DT Coles, and JR Jett. 1989. Leuko-encephalopathy in small cell lung cancer patients receiving prophylactic cranial irradiation. Am J Clin Oncol **12:**27–33.
83. Silber, J, J Radcliffe, V Peckham, G Perilongo, P Kishnani, M Fridman, J Goldwein, and A Meadows. 1992. Whole-brain irradiation and decline in intelligence: the influence of dose and age on IQ score. J Clin Oncol **10:**1390–1396.
84. Ris, M, and R Noll. 1994. Long-term neurobehavioral outcome in pediatric brain-tumor patients: review and methodological critique. J Clin Exp Neuropsychol **16:**21–42.
85. Mulhern, R, J Hancock, D Fairclough, and L Kun. 1992. Neuropsychological status of children treated for brain tumors: a critical review and integrative analysis. Med Pediatr Oncol **20:**181–191.
86. Mulhern, R, D Fairclough, and D Ochs. 1991. A prospective comparison of neuropsychological performance of children surviving leukemia who received 18Gy, 24Gy, or no cranial irradiation. J Clin Oncol **9:**1348–1356.
87. Ochs, J, R Mulhern, D Fairclough, L Parvey, J Whitaker, L Ch'ien, A Mauer, and J Simone. 1991. Comparison of neuropsychologic functioning and clinical indicators of neurotoxicity in long-term survivors of childhood leukemia given cranial radiation or parenteral methotrexate: a prospective study. J Clin Oncol **9:**145–151.
88. Shaw, EG, R Rosdhal, M Culbreth, G Enevold, M Naughton, J Lovato, R D'Agostino, Jr, and S Rapp. 2002. Phase II Study of donepezil (Aricept) in cognitively impaired brain tumor patients (Abstract). Neuro-Oncol **4:**350.
89. Le Bars, PL, MM Katz, N Berman, TM Itil, AM Freedman, and AF Schatzberg. 1997. A placebo-controlled, double-blind, randomized trial of an extract of ginkgo biloba for dementia. JAMA **278:**1327–1332.

2. MANAGEMENT OF RADIATION-INDUCED HEAD AND NECK INJURY

ANGEL I. BLANCO, M.D.
CLIFFORD CHAO, M.D.

The University of Texas M.D. Anderson Cancer Center, Houston, TX

INTRODUCTION

During the treatment of neoplastic diseases, unavoidable toxicities to normal cells may be produced. The mucosal lining of the upper respiratory and gastrointestinal tracts is a prime target for radiotherapy-related toxicity due to its rapid cell turnover rate. The oral cavity is highly sensitive to direct and indirect toxic effects of radiation therapy (RT); this is attributable to multiple factors such as a diverse and complex microflora, trauma to oral tissues during normal oropharyngeal function, and the high mucosal cell turnover rates.

The most common oral complications related to RT are mucositis, infection, salivary gland dysfunction, taste dysfunction, and pain. These complications can lead to secondary complications such as dehydration, dysgeusia, and malnutrition.

Radiation of the head and neck (H&N) can irreversibly injure oral mucosa, vasculature, muscle, and bone. This can result in xerostomia, dental caries, trismus, soft tissue necrosis, and osteoradionecrosis (ORN). Severe oral toxicities can compromise delivery of optimal radiation-therapy protocols. For example, dose reduction or treatment schedule modifications may be necessary to allow for resolution of oral lesions. In cases of severe oral morbidity, the patient may no longer be able to continue cancer therapy; treatment is then usually discontinued. These disruptions in dosing due to oral complications can thus directly affect patient survivorship.

Management of oral complications of cancer therapy includes identification of high-risk populations, patient education, initiation of pretreatment interventions, and timely management of lesions. Assessment of oral status and stabilization of oral disease prior

Table 1. Tolerance doses ($TD_{5/5}$–$TD_{50/5}$) to whole-organ irradiation

Organ	Single dose (Gy)	Fractionated dose (Gy)
Brain	15–25	60–70
Eye (lens)	2–10	6–12
Skin	15–20	30–40
Spinal cord	15–20	50–60
VCTS	10–20	50–60
Mucosa	5–20	65–77
Peripheral nerve	15–20	65–77
Muscle	>30	>70
Bone and cartilage	>30	>70
Thyroid		30–40

VCTS = vasculoconnective tissue systems.
Modified from Rubin P. 1989. The law and order of radiation sensitivity, absolute versus relative. In: Vaeth JM, Meyer JL, eds. Radiation Tolerance of Normal Tissues. Frontiers of Radiation Therapy and Oncology, vol 23. Basel: S. Karger, pp 7–40.

to cancer therapy are critical to overall patient care. This care should be both preventive (i.e., including careful examination of the gingival and assessment of early, treatable periodontal disease) and/or therapeutic (including the extraction of irreversibly damaged teeth) as indicated to minimize risk for oral (i.e., poor wound healing and ORN) and associated systemic complications (such as subacute bacterial endocarditis and associated complications).

Radiation doses traditionally deemed safe should be carefully reevaluated within the context of multidisciplinary management, as these doses can lead to severe late effects in different vital organs. Previously defined radiation tolerance doses[1] ($TD_{5/5}$ and $TD_{50/5}$; Tables 1 and 2) remain as valuable guides by establishing reasonable dose–volume guidelines for two-dimensional radiotherapy. However, these data are being complemented by more modern analyses utilizing three-dimensional dose–volume information. These newer studies and cooperative group protocols place special emphasis on the volume of the organ irradiated, in addition to absolute dose limits, in recognition of the inhomogeneous dose distributions made possible by conformal and intensity-modulated treatment planning. As a prominent example, particular attention has been devoted to the study the dose–volume effects and quality-of-life (QOL) predictors following partial parotid gland irradiation,[2–12] whereas the dosimetric predictors of oral mucositis and esophageal

Table 2. Normal tissue tolerance to therapeutic irradiation

	$TD_{5/5}$ volume			$TD_{50/5}$ volume			
Organ	1/3	2/3	3/3	1/3	2/3	3/3	Selected endpoint
Brain	60	50	45	75	65	60	Necrosis infarction
Brain stem	60	53	50	–	–	65	Necrosis infarction
Spinal cord	5 cm	10 cm	20 cm	5 cm	10 cm	20 cm	Myelitis
	50	50	47	70	70	–	Necrosis

Modified from Emami, B, J Lyman, A Brown, et al. 1991. Tolerance of normal tissue to therapeutic irradiation. Int J Radiat Oncol Biol Phys **21**:109–122.

dysfunction post-RT are in need of further study. In addition, mathematical models such as the nominal standard dose, time–dose factor, and cumulative radiation effect have been supplanted by the linear-quadratic equation[13] using the α/β ratio and its clinical applicability to normal tissue complication probability estimates.

Tables 1 and 2 summarize previously defined whole- and partial-organ tolerances.

A. ETIOLOGY AND PATHOGENESIS

Elimination of preexisting dental/periapical, periodontal, and mucosal infections, institution of comprehensive oral hygiene protocols during therapy, and reduction of other factors that may compromise oral mucosal integrity (e.g., physical trauma to oral tissues) can help reduce the frequency and severity of oral complications in cancer patients. Such complications can be acute (developing during therapy) or chronic (developing months to years after therapy). Radiation is not only associated with acute oral toxicities, but may also induce permanent tissue damage leading to multiple life-long risks of tooth decay, infection, and ORN among others. Multiple prospective studies have demonstrated increased acute toxicities with the addition of chemotherapy to radiation,[14–16] particularly when administered concurrently. However, the contribution of chemotherapy to the late toxicity profile post-RT is in need of further study.

Acute effects of H&N irradiation frequently include ulcerative oral mucositis, clinically similar to that seen with high-dose chemotherapy. In addition, radiation can also induce late tissue damage that results in permanent dysfunction of vasculature, connective tissue, salivary glands, muscle, and bone.[17,18] Loss of bone vitality occurs secondary to injuries to osteocytes, osteoblasts, and osteoclasts as well as from a relative hypoxia due to reduction in vascular supply. These changes can lead to soft tissue necrosis and ORN that result in bone exposure, secondary infection, and severe pain.

Late oral complications of RT are chiefly a result of chronic injury to vasculature, salivary glands, mucosa, connective tissue, and bone. Types and severity of these changes are directly related to radiation dosimetry, including total dose, volume irradiated, fraction size, and duration of treatment. Mucosal changes include epithelial atrophy, reduced vascularization, and submucosal fibrosis. These changes lead to an atrophic, friable barrier. Fibrosis involving muscle, dermis, and/or the temporomandibular joint (TMJ) results in compromised oral function. Salivary tissue changes include loss of acinar cells, alteration in duct epithelium, fibrosis, and fatty degeneration. Compromised vascularization and remodeling capacity of bone leads to risk for ORN.

Unlike that associated with chemotherapy, radiation damage is anatomically site-specific; toxicity is localized to irradiated tissue volumes. The degree of damage is dependent on the treatment regimen-related factors including type of radiation used, total dose administered, and field size/fractionation. Compared with chemotherapy-related effects, an important clinical feature characterizing radiation-induced tissue damage deserves mention. Irradiated tissues tend to manifest permanent damage that places the patient at continual risk for oral sequelae. The oral tissues are thus more easily damaged by subsequent toxic drug or radiation exposure, and normal physiologic repair mechanisms are compromised as a result of permanent cellular damage.

B. PATIENT EDUCATION AND DENTAL EVALUATION PRECEDING IRRADIATION

The severity of oral complications in cancer patients can be reduced significantly when an oral care plan is initiated prior to treatment. Primary preventive measures, such as appropriate nutritional intake, effective oral hygiene practices, and early detection of oral lesions are important pretreatment interventions. The involvement of a dental team experienced with oral oncology may also reduce the risk of oral complications via either direct examination of the patient or in consultation with the community-based dentist. The evaluation should be done as early as possible prior to treatment. The examination allows the dentist to determine the status of the oral cavity prior to cancer therapy, and to initiate necessary interventions that may reduce oral complications during and after that therapy.

C. PRACTICAL ASPECTS OF ACUTE AND LATE EFFECT MANAGEMENT FOLLOWING CANCER THERAPY

C1. Pain Management[19]

Estimated to affect 50–80% of cancer patients and correlating with decreased QOL, pain is frequently multifactorial. Among H&N cancer patients, the etiology of pain may be treatment-related or tumor-related. Recent evidence indicates that cancer pain may be undertreated in many instances.

A number of pain management regimens have been developed. Although the particular drugs and dosing schedules used may vary among institutions, protocols should incorporate the guidelines established by the World Health Organization.[20] According to this system, pain should be evaluated regularly (in the case of RT, weekly or more frequently as needed), classified as mild, moderate, or severe, and treated accordingly.

Mild pain should be treated using acetaminophen-based products, moderate pain should be managed by codeine-based analgesics, and severe pain should be treated with morphine or fentanyl-based regimens.

C2. Oral Hygiene

Routine, systematic oral hygiene is important for reducing the incidence and severity of oral sequelae of cancer therapy. The patient must be informed of the rationale for the oral hygiene program as well as the potential side effects of cancer chemotherapy and RT. Effective oral hygiene is important throughout cancer treatment, with emphasis on oral hygiene beginning prior to initiation of that treatment. Considerable variation exists across institutions relative to specific non-medicated approaches to baseline oral care, given limited published evidence. Most non-medicated oral care protocols utilize topical, frequent (every 4–6 hours) rinsing with 0.9% saline. Additional interventions include dental brushing with toothpaste, dental flossing, ice chips, and sodium bicarbonate rinses. Patients utilizing removable dental prostheses or orthodontic appliances have the risk of mucosal injury or infection.

Dental brushing and flossing represent simple, cost-effective approaches to bacterial dental plaque control.

Periodontal infection causes risk for oral bleeding; healthy tissues should not bleed. Discontinuing dental brushing and flossing can increase risk for gingival bleeding, oral infection, and bacteremia. We recommend the removal of bacterial plaque using gentle debridement via a soft or ultra-soft toothbrush during therapy in order to minimize the risk of infection. Mechanical plaque control not only promotes gingival health, but may also decrease the risk of exacerbation of oral mucositis secondary to microbial colonization of damaged mucosal surfaces.

Oral rinsing with water or saline while brushing will further aid in removal of dental plaque dislodged by brushing. Rinses containing alcohol should be avoided. Since the flavoring agents in toothpaste can irritate oral soft tissues, toothpaste with relatively neutral taste should be considered. Patients skilled in flossing without traumatizing gingival tissues may continue flossing throughout radiotherapy administration. Flossing allows the removal of dental bacterial plaque and thus promotes gingival health.

The oral cavity should be cleaned after meals. If xerostomia is present, plaque and food debris may accumulate secondary to reduce salivary function and more frequent hygiene may be necessary. In addition, it is important to prevent excessive dryness of the lips in order to reduce risk for tissue injury. Mouth breathing and/or xerostomia secondary to anticholinergic medications used for nausea management can induce the condition. Lip care products containing petroleum-based oils and waxes can be useful. Lanolin-based creams and ointments, however, may be more effective in protecting against trauma.

All patients should receive a comprehensive oral evaluation several weeks prior to the initiation of radiation. In accordance with recent studies, we recommend a minimum interval of 2 weeks prior to commencement of RT.[21] This timing provides an appropriate interval for tissue healing in the event invasive oral procedures including dental extractions, dental scaling/polishing, and endodontic therapy are necessary. Such interventions are principally directed at reducing the risks of soft tissue necrosis and ORN.

Candidiasis is the most common clinical infection of the oropharynx in irradiated patients. Patients receiving H&N radiation are frequently colonized with Candida, as demonstrated by an increase in quantitative counts and rates for clinical infection. Candidiasis may exacerbate the symptoms of oropharyngeal mucositis. Treatment of oral candidiasis in the radiation patient has primarily utilized topical antifungals such as nystatin and clotrimazole. Compliance can be compromised secondary to oral mucositis, nausea, and pain and difficulty in dissolving nystatin pastilles and clotrimazole troches. The use of systemic antifungals including ketoconazole and fluconazole to treat oral candidiasis has proved effective and may have advantages over topical agents for patients experiencing mucositis. Bacterial infections may also occur early in the course of head/neck radiation and should be treated with antibiotics appropriately targeted to culture and sensitivity data. It is our recommendation to request cultures in the cases of (a) failed antimicrobial trials when a bacterial, fungal, or combined infectious process is suspected, (b) obvious constitutional symptoms (fever, elevated white count, etc.). In such cases, formal interdisciplinary evaluation (by the Head and Neck Surgery, Medical Oncology, and/or Infectious Disease services) is often sought to rule out competing sources of infection.

The risk of dental cavities increases secondary to a number of factors including shifts to a cariogenic flora, reduced concentrations of salivary antimicrobial proteins, and loss of mineralizing components. Treatment strategies must be directed to each component of the caries process. Optimal oral hygiene must be maintained. Xerostomia should be managed whenever possible via salivary substitutes or replacements. Caries resistance can be enhanced via use of topical fluorides and/or remineralizing agents.

Increased colonization with *Streptococcus mutans* and *Lactobacillus* species increases the risk of cavity formation. Cultural data can be useful in defining the level of risk in relation to colonization patterns. Of interest, topical fluorides or chlorhexidine rinses may lead to reduced levels of *Streptococcus mutans* but not Lactobacilli. Due to adverse drug interactions, fluoride and chlorhexidine dosing should be separated by several hours. Remineralizing agents that are high in calcium phosphate and fluoride have demonstrated salutary in vitro and clinical effects. Delivering the drug via customized vinyl carriers may enhance the intervention. This approach extends the contact time of active drug with tooth structure, which leads to increased uptake into the enamel.

Necrosis and secondary infection of previously irradiated tissue is a serious complication for patients who have undergone radiation for H&N tumors. Acute effects typically involve oral mucosa. Chronic changes involving bone and mucosa are a result of the process of vascular inflammation and scarring that in turn result in hypovascular, hypocellular, and hypoxic changes. Infection secondary to tissue injury and ORN confounds the process.

D. STUDIES ADDRESSING SPECIFIC ISSUES REGARDING TREATMENT-RELATED TOXICITIES IN IRRADIATED H&N CANCER PATIENTS

D1. Xerostomia

Among RT sequelae following the treatment of H&N tumors, reduction in salivary flow due to salivary gland damage is of particular clinical concern. Often permanent and identified by patients as having a negative impact on QOL, xerostomia can result in serious functional impairment and patient discomfort. Clinical experience with conventional irradiation of H&N tumor subsites has demonstrated a steep and rapid reduction in salivary flow rate (FR), ranging from 18% to 50% 1 week after initiation of RT.[22–32] Several strategies have been implemented in an attempt to minimize radiation-induced xerostomia. Randomized trials have documented the benefits of amifostine,[33,34] pilocarpine (PC),[35,36] and, more recently, the pre-RT surgical transfer of submandibular glands to the submental space.[37,38] These treatment options are further described below.

As demonstrated by the prospective studies of Chao et al.[39] and Eisbruch and colleagues,[8,9,40] the reduction in saliva production correlates with the clinical manifestations of xerostomia and its adverse impact on QOL. Frequent signs and symptoms of xerostomia include dryness, burning sensation of the tongue, fissures at lip commissures, atrophy of the dorsal tongue surface, difficulty in wearing dentures, and increased thirst. Saliva is necessary for the normal execution of oral functions such as taste, swallowing, and speech. Unstimulated whole salivary FRs of less than 0.1 mL/minute are considered indicative of xerostomia (normal salivary FR = 0.3–0.5 mL/minute). Xerostomia produces the following changes in the mouth, which collectively cause patient discomfort and increased risk of oral lesions:

- Salivary viscosity increases with resultant impaired lubrication of oral tissues.
- Buffering capacity is compromised with increased risk for dental caries. Oral flora become more pathogenic.

Table 3. Management of the xerostomic patient

Plaque removal	Tooth brushing Flossing Other oral hygiene aids
Remineralization	Topical high concentration fluorides Children: topical and systemic Adults: topical Remineralizing solutions
Antimicrobials	Chlorhexidine solutions (rinses) Povidone iodine oral rinses Tetracycline oral rinses
Sialogogues	Pilocarpine Bethanechol Antholetrithione (Sialor^{TM})

Note: Prescription strength fluorides should be used, non-prescription fluoride preparations are inadequate in the face of moderate to high dental caries risk. If drinking water does not have adequate fluoride content to prevent dental decay, then oral fluoride (i.e., drops, vitamins, etc.) should be provided.
Modified from Schubert, MM, DE Peterson, and ME Lloid. 1999. Oral complications. In: Thomas ED, Blume KG, Forman SJ, eds. Hematopoietic Cell Transplantation, 2nd ed., Malden, Mass: Blackwell Science Inc., pp 751–763.

- Plaque levels accumulate due to the patient's difficulty in maintaining oral hygiene. Acid production after sugar exposure results in further demineralization of the teeth and leads to dental decay.
- Mechanical cleansing ability is affected, thereby contributing to dental caries and progressive periodontal disease. Development of dental caries also is accelerated in the presence of xerostomia due to reduction in delivery to the dentition of antimicrobial proteins normally contained in saliva.

Patients who experience xerostomia must maintain excellent oral hygiene to minimize risk for oral lesions. Periodontal disease can be accelerated and caries can become rampant unless preventive measures are instituted. Multiple preventive strategies should be considered (Table 3).

D2. Dosimetric Predictors of Xerostomia

Important predictors of the degree of dysfunction include radiation dose, technique, and volume of glandular tissue in the radiation field. The clinical implementation of image-based treatment planning, improved patient immobilization, and the introduction of 3-D conformal radiotherapy techniques have allowed significant refinement in portal design. More recently, intensity-modulated RT (IMRT) techniques now permit the concave sculpting of the dose distribution near the parotid gland borders, thereby significantly reducing the mean parotid doses while still permitting the delivery of tumoricidal doses to nearby target regions. As a result, multiple investigators have attempted to characterize the dose–response characteristics of the salivary glands following conformal irradiation.[2,3,5,6,8–10,39,41–49] An updated analysis of a prospective trial evaluating conformal parotid-sparing irradiation conducted at Washington University[50] continues to suggest an exponential reduction in parotid FR as a function of mean dose. The mean dose threshold for stimulated saliva flow expected to result in late grade 4 xerostomia[51] (defined as $<25\%$ of pretreatment level) was 26 Gy. In addition, the study revealed a

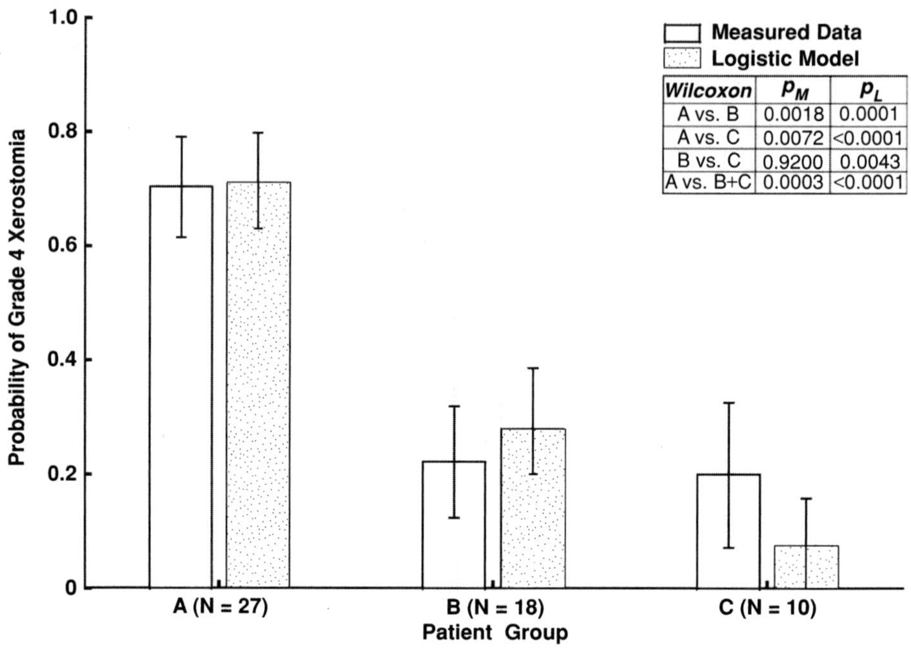

Figure 1. Probability of grade 4 xerostomia as a function of parotid gland mean dose. Patients were divided into three groups according to whether (a) both parotid glands, (b) one parotid gland, or (c) no parotid gland received a mean dose of at least 25.8 Gy. The average measured relative stimulated saliva flow at 6 months was computed for each group and used to calculate the probability of G4 xerostomia. The results were compared with the logistic model prediction for each group. Error bars represent one standard deviation. $P_{M(L)}$ = two-tailed P-values for the intergroup comparisons using saliva measurement (logistic model prediction).

70% incidence of xerostomia for patients in whom both parotid glands received a mean dose of at least 25 Gy; the risk was much smaller for patients in whom one or both parotid glands was spared (Figure 1).

A number of recent clinical publications have validated the potential for decreased late salivary toxicity with the use of conformal parotid-sparing irradiation in a number of H&N treatment subsites. The patterns of failure following parotid-sparing irradiation have also been reported and remain unchanged compared with conventional irradiation,[47,52] suggesting no evidence of tumor protection. In an update of the University of California, San Francisco, experience with treatment of nasopharyngeal cancer, Lee et al.[44] showed excellent loco-regional progression-free and overall survival rates at 4 years of 98% and 88%, respectively, among 67 patients treated with IMRT. They also reported the time-course of post-RT xerostomia (at 12 and 24 months). Remarkably, at 24 months post-RT, less than 10% of patients experienced late RTOG grade >2 xerostomia.[53] Similarly, in a report of 430 patients with oropharyngeal carcinoma comparing conventional radiotherapy versus IMRT, Chao et al.[2] demonstrated equivalent loco-regional control rates at 2 years in comparable cohorts receiving definitive or postoperative radiotherapy. Despite the equivalent tumor control, patients treated with IMRT had significantly lower rates of late grade 2 xerostomia (17–30%) compared with 75% among patients receiving conventional irradiation. More recently, Chao et al.[4] analyzed treatment outcomes following definitive or postoperative IMRT among 74 patients with locally advanced oropharyngeal carcinoma. At 4 years, treatment outcomes were encouraging, with estimated loco-regional control and overall survival rates of 87%. Moreover, rates of late xerostomia were consistent with the prior findings (12% of patients had late grade 2 xerostomia).

D3. Surgical Management of Xerostomia

Jha et al.[37] have conducted a prospective study evaluating the efficacy of surgical transfer of one submandibular salivary gland to the submental space. Among 76 enrolled patients, the salivary gland transfer was done in 60 patients, and 43 had salivary gland transfer and postoperative RT. At a median follow-up of 14 months, 81% experienced none or minimal xerostomia, and 19% developed moderate to severe xerostomia. There were no significant postoperative complications. In response to the encouraging results from this trial, the submental transfer technique is undergoing evaluation in a prospective multicenter study (RTOG 0244).

D4. Mucositis

Oral mucositis results from radiation-induced mitotic death of the basal cells of the oral mucosal epithelium. While it represents[19] an expected side effect of RT to the H&N; its severity varies from mild discomfort to severe pain. Patient-related risk factors for its development include poor nutritional status, poor dental hygiene, dental caries, poorly fitting dentures or oral prosthetics, and habits such as tobacco and alcohol use. Treatment-associated risk factors include RT dose and volume, fractionation regimen,[54] treatment site, use of concurrent chemotherapy, and surgical treatment.

The clinical course of mucositis is well described; characteristic symptoms include erythema, edema, tenderness, pain, difficulty in swallowing, and hoarseness. The typical onset of symptoms is approximately 2 weeks after initiation of RT. Symptoms may persist up to 4 weeks after completion of the therapy, or longer when concurrent chemotherapy is utilized.

Management is directed toward (1) minimizing continued exposure of the affected mucosa by chemical or mechanical irritants (such as tobacco and alcohol, or poorly fitting dentures), (2) maximizing the patients' nutritional status, (3) emphasizing oral hygiene, as discussed previously in this chapter, and (4) maintaining adequate pain management. In addition, specific medical therapy (described below) can be instituted adjunctively when necessary.

E. MEDICAL MANAGEMENT OF XEROSTOMIA AND MUCOSITIS

E1. Amifostine

Unfortunately, some patients treated with conformal parotid-sparing irradiation and the majority of patients receiving bilateral neck RT using conventional methods continue to experience debilitating xerostomia. Therefore, the potential for additional sparing of normal tissues beyond that achievable with IMRT continues to elicit considerable research efforts. One such endeavor involves the joint utilization of IMRT and radioprotectors, chemical compounds that reduce the biological effects of irradiation in normal tissues. As the first cytoprotective drug to attain approval as a radioprotector in the United States and the European Union, WR-2721 (amifostine; Ethyol, MedImmune Pharmaceuticals) is the best studied agent to date. Originally developed by the United States Army in studies conducted at Walter Reed Hospital, amifostine was selected from a group of more than 4400 chemicals screened because of its superior radioprotective properties and safety profile.[55] Of particular relevance to H&N cancer, the drug is known to concentrate in the salivary glands, achieving an estimated dose reduction factor of 2.0 in these organs.

The effectiveness of this radioprotector was recently examined in a multi-institutional, international MedImmune Oncology phase III trial. The study included 315 patients with H&N cancer[33] treated with conventional RT with and without amifostine. Primary end points included the incidence of grade $\geq$2 acute xerostomia, grade $\geq$3 acute mucositis, and grade $\geq$2 late xerostomia and were based on the worst toxicity reported. The amifostine dose was 200 mg/m^2/day intravenously 15–30 minutes before each fraction of RT. Standard fractionated RT (1.8–2.0 Gy/day for 5 days/week for 5–7 weeks, to a total dose of 50–70 Gy) was used in this study. Amifostine significantly reduced grade $\geq$2 acute xerostomia from 78% to 51% ($P < 0.0001$) and grade $\geq$2 chronic xerostomia from 57% to 34% ($P = 0.002$). Median saliva production was greater with amifostine (0.26 g vs. 0.10 g, $P = 0.04$). Amifostine did not reduce mucositis. With and without amifostine, 2-year local-regional control, disease-free survival, and overall survival were 58% versus 63%, 53% versus 57%, and 71% versus 66%, respectively. Side effects associated with amifostine included nausea, vomiting, and hypotension.

Antonadou et al.[34] reported the results of a prospective study designed to determine the efficacy of prophylactic administration of amifostine in protecting against acute and late toxicities from radiochemotherapy in patients with H&N cancer. Fifty patients were randomized to receive CRT (2-Gy fractions, 5 days weekly, to a total of 60–74 Gy, depending on the tumor localization and TNM classification) and carboplatin. Amifostine (300 mg/m^2) was administered in the study group only 15–30 minutes before RT for 6–7.5 weeks. The primary study end point was the grading of acute and late non-hematologic toxicities (mucositis, dysphagia, and xerostomia) induced by chemoradiotherapy. Secondary end points included treatment duration, hematologic toxicity, and clinical outcome. The results showed that treatment duration was significantly shorter in the amifostine-treated group ($P = 0.013$), because treatment interruptions were more frequent in the control group. Acute toxicities (mucositis and dysphagia) were less severe in the amifostine-treated group. By week 3, all in the control group experienced grade 2 mucositis compared with only 9% in the amifostine-treated group ($P < 0.0001$). By week 5, 52.2% of the patients in the control group experienced grade 4 mucositis compared with 4.5% in the amifostine-treated group ($P = 0.0006$). Similar results were obtained for dysphagia. At 3 months of follow-up, only 27% of patients in the study group experienced grade 2 xerostomia compared with 73.9% in the control group ($P = 0.0001$). Eighteen months after therapy completion, the proportion of patients with grade 2 xerostomia was 4.5% versus 30.4% for each respective treatment group ($P = 0.047$). Cytoprotection with amifostine did not affect the treatment outcome. This randomized trial demonstrated the efficacy of amifostine in reducing mucositis and dysphagia resulting from chemoradiotherapy in patients with H&N cancer. Furthermore, amifostine reduced the severity of late xerostomia, a side effect of RT with long-lasting consequences.

In an effort to prevent the need for daily amifostine infusions during irradiation and its associated morbidity, a randomized Phase II trial evaluated the feasibility of subcutaneous (SQ) administration of amifostine during fractionated radiotherapy.[56] Patients were randomized to receive radiotherapy or radiotherapy supported with SQ amifostine. Forty patients with pelvic malignancies, 60 with lung cancer, and 40 with H&N cancer were enrolled into the study. All H&N cancer patients had local or regional disease that justified extended-field irradiation. Overall, amifostine was interrupted in 10 patients (14.2%) for fever, rash, or severe asthenia. A significant reduction of pharyngeal, esophageal, and rectal mucositis was noted in the amifostine arm ($P < 0.04$). Among H&N cancer patients, the experimental group experienced a reduction in grade 3 or 4 mucosal toxicity compared with the control group ($P = 0.02$). Radiation-induced xerostomia was noted in 15 (75%) of 20 patients in the RT-alone arm versus 11 (58%) of 19 patients in the amifostine arm ($P = 0.32$). Response rates could not be assessed among the H&N cancer patients.

E2. Other Cytoprotective Strategies

Saliva substitutes or artificial saliva preparations (oral rinses containing hydroxyethyl-, hydroxypropyl-, or carboxymethylcellulose) are palliative agents that relieve the discomfort of xerostomia by temporarily wetting the oral mucosa.

Pilocarpine

Pilocarpine is the only drug approved by the US Food and Drug Administration for use as a sialogogue (5 mg tablets of PC hydrochloride). The role of PC, a parasympathomimetic agent, in the treatment of radiation-induced xerostomia has been studied extensively during the last two decades. Early, small randomized studies were the first to demonstrate a benefit for the post-RT use of PC. Two subsequent, large, randomized trials by Johnson et al.[36] and LeVeque et al.[35] confirmed the benefits of PC and concluded that approximately 50% of the patients experienced some relief of xerostomia symptoms. The latter study also demonstrated improvement in salivary flow. Interestingly, no correlation was observed between the improvement of salivary flow and the functional improvement demonstrated by the patients. The high response rate to placebo of approximately 25% seen in these studies, however, was not explained. In an attempt to further elucidate the mechanism of action of PC and correlate response with RT parameters, Horiot et al.[57] subsequently conducted a subsequent randomized trial. PC was administered orally at 15 mg/day with a 5 mg optional increase at 5 weeks up to a daily dose of 25 mg beyond 9 weeks. Results indicated 75% compliance; 38 patients (26%) stopped treatment before week 12 for acute intolerance (sweating, nausea, vomiting) or no response. No severe complication occurred. Ninety seven patients (67%) reported significant relief of symptoms of xerostomia at 12 weeks. Within 12 weeks, the size of the subgroup with normal food intake almost doubled, while the size of the subgroup with (nearly) impossible solid food ingestion decreased by 38% (47 vs. 29 patients). The impact on QOL was considered important or very important by 77% of the responders. No difference was found according to dose–volume radiotherapy parameters. The authors concluded that oral PC hydrochloride acts primarily by stimulating minor salivary glands; PC can be of benefit to patients suffering of severe xerostomia regardless of radiotherapy dose–volume parameters; and all responders are identified by 12 weeks post-RT.

The treatment is initiated at 5 mg orally, 3 times daily; the dose is then titrated to achieve optimal clinical response and minimize adverse effects. Some patients may experience increased benefit at higher daily doses; however, incidence of adverse effects increases proportionally with dose. The patient's evening dose may be increased to 10 mg within 1 week after starting PC. Subsequently, morning and afternoon doses may also be increased to a maximum 10 mg/dose (30 mg/day). Patient tolerance is confirmed by allowing 7 days between the increments. The most common adverse effect at clinically useful doses of PC is hyperhidrosis (excessive sweating); its incidence and severity are proportional to dosage. Nausea, chills, rhinorrhea, vasodilation, increased lacrimation, bladder pressure (urinary urgency and frequency), dizziness, asthenia, headache, diarrhea, and dyspepsia are also reported, typically at dosages greater than 5 mg, 3 times daily. Pilocarpine usually increases salivary flow within 30 minutes after ingestion. Maximal response, however, may occur only after continual use. Pilocarpine may exert a radioprotective effect on salivary glands if given during RT to the H&N.

Biafine

Biafine is a hypotonic oil and water emulsion thought to stimulate skin healing mechanisms through the selective recruitment of macrophages and the stimulation of granulation tissue. Biafine products have been used in patients undergoing RT in France for over 25 years. The potential benefit of Biafine may be clinically significant in the H&N patient population because of the proportion of grades 2 and 3 toxicities experienced. RTOG 99-13 is a recently completed study designed to compare Biafine with usual institutional practices and to evaluate its use as a prophylactic agent in reducing skin toxicity. Patients were randomized into one of the three arms: Arm 1, using a pre-declared institutional preference regimen not to include Biafine; Arm 2, with tid application of Biafine at the initiation of therapy; and Arm 3, with tid application of Biafine after the initiation of skin symptoms. Results are pending.

Vitamin E and Pentoxifylline

Vitamin E (VE) is a fat-soluble vitamin existing in a variety of forms in many foods. The most common form of VE in a Western diet is known as alpha-tocopherol. VE is considered to have antioxidant properties and VE supplements have been tested in a number of conditions including: malabsorption disorders, hematologic disorders, cardiovascular disease, and cancer. VE has been proposed as a potential radioprotector. A prospective, double-blind randomized trial in H&N cancer patients treated with RT was designed to test the hypothesis that VE provides oral mucosal protection. An oil solution of either VE (400 mg) or placebo was rinsed twice a day over the oral cavity. Radiation doses ranged from 50 to 70 Gy per 5 to 7 weeks in conventional fractionation. The density of the incidence of severe mucositis was evaluated in both the arms. Results indicated that severe mucositis was more frequent in the placebo group (54 events/161 patients-week = 33.5%) than in the VE group (36 events/167 patients-week = 21.6%, $P = 0.038$). VE reduced the risk of severe mucositis by 36%. The investigators concluded that VE is efficacious in reducing the incidence of severe radiotherapy-induced mucositis in patients with H&N tumors treated with RT.

Pentoxifylline is a xantine derivative that acts by decreasing blood viscosity. Its use is well established in patients with chronic peripheral arterial disease and other cardiovascular conditions. Recent studies have demonstrated a reduction in chronic radiation-induced fibrosis (RIF) among breast and H&N cancer patients[58] receiving pentoxifylline and vitamin E. Pentoxifylline may also have a role in the treatment of chronic trismus.[59] Further studies should be performed to confirm these findings; at present, it is reasonable to consider the use of pentoxifylline and VE in the treatment of RIF.

E3. Skin Toxicity

Analogous to oral mucositis,[19] skin toxicity is an expected, usually temporary side effect of RT to the H&N. Risk factors predictive of its development include poor nutritional status, fair complexion, history of extensive sun exposure, diabetes mellitus, and certain collagen vascular diseases (i.e., scleroderma or lupus). Treatment-associated risk factors include the use of large irradiation fields, treatment with tangential fields, electron beam therapy, altered fractionation regimens, and use of concurrent chemotherapy and surgical treatment.

The clinical course of skin toxicity is also well-characterized; in order of severity, manifestations include erythema, hyperpigmentation, and dry and moist desquamation. The typical onset of symptoms is approximately 2 weeks after initiation of RT; these may persist up to 4 weeks after completion of the therapy.

Management emphasizes (1) careful cleansing of the skin, (2) moisturizing treated skin using a hydrophilic moisturizer (Aquaphor, Eucerin crème, or aloe vera gels), (3) preventing mechanical or chemical irritation of treated skin (such as resulting from tight clothing or perfumes), and (4) maintaining adequate pain management. In the cases of moist desquamation, extra precautions should be taken to minimize the possibility of skin infection and associated treatment delays.

E4. Osteoradionecrosis

The unilateral vascular supply to each half of the mandible results in ORN, most frequently involving mandible versus maxilla. Presenting clinical features include pain, diminished or complete loss of sensation, fistula, and infection. ORN typically occurs within the first 3 years post-diagnosis, although it is thought that patients remain at indefinite risk. The diagnosis of ORN relies on the clinical examination of chronically exposed bone. Radiographic findings include decreased bone density and pathologic fractures. Pathologic fractures can occur, as the compromised bone is unable to appropriately undergo repair at the involved sites. Risk for tissue necrosis is in part related to trauma or oral infection; however, idiopathic cases can also occur.

The incidence of ORN is somewhat difficult to estimate from the retrospective series, as it depends on the primary site and volume irradiated, and degree of comorbidities in the studied patient population. Indeed, review of the literature reveals widely ranging incidence rates from 0.4% to 56%.[60] A recent report by Reuther et al.[61] evaluated the incidence of ORN in a large cohort of 830 patients and showed an overall incidence of 8.2%. The most common location was the body of the mandible. Unfavorable prognostic factors included male gender, advanced stage, segmental mandibular resections, and tooth extractions (found responsible for up to 50% of cases).

Management of Osteoradionecrosis

Patients who develop ORN should be comprehensively managed, including elimination of trauma, avoidance of removable dental prosthesis if the denture bearing area is within the necrosis field, assuring adequate nutritional intake, and discontinuation of tobacco and alcohol use. Topical antibiotics (e.g., tetracycline) or antiseptics (e.g., chlorhexidine) may contribute to wound resolution. Wherever possible, coverage of the exposed bone with mucosa should be achieved. Analgesics for pain control are often effective. Local resection of bone sequestrae may be possible.

Hyperbaric oxygen therapy (HBO)[62–64] is generally recommended for the management of ORN, in that it increases oxygenation of irradiated tissue, promotes angiogenesis, and enhances osteoblast repopulation and fibroblast function. HBO is usually prescribed as 20–30 dives at 100% oxygen and 2–2.5 atm of pressure. If surgery is needed, 10 dives of postsurgical HBO are recommended. Unfortunately, HBO technology is not always accessible to patients who might otherwise benefit.

Partial mandibulectomy may be necessary in severe cases of ORN. The mandible can be reconstructed to provide continuity for aesthetics and function. In a report of 29 cases, Chang et al.[65] reviewed the M.D. Anderson Hospital experience with treatment of advanced mandibular ORN with free flap reconstruction. At a mean follow-up of 33 months, they reported a 21% complication rate and a 14% flap loss rate. A multidisciplinary cancer team including oncologists, oncology nurses, maxillofacial prosthodontists, general dentists, hygienists, and physical therapists is appropriate for management of these patients.

E5. Trismus

Musculoskeletal syndromes may develop secondary to radiation and surgery. Lesions include soft tissue fibrosis, surgically induced mandibular discontinuity, and parafunctional habits associated with emotional stress caused by cancer and its treatment. Patients can be instructed in physical therapy interventions including mandibular stretching exercises as well as use of prosthetic aids designed to reduce severity of fibrosis. It is important that these approaches be instituted prior to the development of trismus. If clinically significant changes develop, several approaches including stabilization of occlusion, trigger point injection and other pain management strategies, muscle relaxants, and/or tricyclic medications can be considered.

E6. Dysphagia and Esophageal Toxicity

Dysphagia can be a prominent symptom in chemotherapy or head/neck radiation patients. Etiology is likely associated with several factors including direct neurotoxicity to taste buds, xerostomia, infection, and psychologic conditioning.

A total fractionated radiation dose of more than 3000 Gy reduces acuity of sweet, sour, bitter, and salt tastes. Damage to the microvilli and outer surface of the taste cells has been proposed as the principal mechanism for the loss of the sense of taste. In many cases, taste acuity returns 2–3 months after completion of RT. However, many other patients develop permanent hypogeusia.

Zinc supplementation (zinc sulfate 220 mg, twice a day) has been considered on a therapeutic basis in view of known antioxidant properties. A recently reported randomized trial[66] showed that the use of zinc supplementation produced a significant reduction in the severity of radiation-induced mucositis and oral discomfort (taste was not evaluated as a primary endpoint). These data are in need of further validation; however, it is reasonable to consider the use of zinc supplementation until such evidence becomes available.

Recent publications have attempted to quantitate the degree of pharyngeal transport dysfunction following chemoradiotherapy.[15] In a series of 15 patients with locally advanced H&N cancer receiving concomitant hydroxyurea and hyperfractionated irradiation, Kotz et al. performed post-RT videofluoroscopic swallow function studies and observed posterior pharyngeal dysfunction characterized by impaired pharyngeal constrictor motility in 12 patients (80%). All patients exhibited pharyngeal abnormalities limiting bolus transport and clearance. In a series of 29 patients with unresectable H&N cancer, Eisbruch et al.[67] performed serial (pretherapy at 1–3 months post-RT and at 6–12 months post-RT) swallowing studies with videofluoroscopy and esophagograms. Posttreatment changes included reduced inversion of the cricopharyngeal muscle and laryngeal closure, promoting aspiration. The rate of aspiration increased significantly in the early and late post-RT studies.

Loss of appetite can also occur in cancer patients concurrent with mucositis, xerostomia, taste loss, dysphagia, nausea, and vomiting. QOL is compromised as eating becomes more problematic. Oral pain upon eating may lead to selection of foods that do not aggravate the oral tissues, often at the expense of adequate nutrition. Modifying the texture and consistency of the diet, adding between-meal snacks to increase protein and caloric intake, and administering vitamin, mineral, and caloric supplements can minimize nutritional deficiencies.

Nutritional counseling may be required during and following the therapy; maintenance of appropriate caloric and nutrient intake should be emphasized. Nasogastric feeding tubes or percutaneous esophageal gastrostomy may be required when swallowing is significantly impaired. Total parenteral nutrition represents a means to provide adequate nutrition but is generally reserved for patients who cannot eat due to mucositis or nausea, as opposed to dysgeusia alone.

When cancer therapy-associated mucositis has resolved, nutritional counseling must consider long-term complications including xerostomia, increased caries risk, altered ability to masticate, and dysphagia. Consideration must thus be given to taste, texture, moisture, calories, and nutrient content.

Cancer patients undergoing high-dose chemotherapy and/or radiation can experience fatigue related to either disease or its treatment. These processes can produce sleep deprivation or metabolic disorders, which collectively contribute to compromised oral status. For example, the fatigued patient will likely have impaired compliance with mouth care protocols designed to otherwise minimize risk of mucosal ulceration, infection, and pain. In addition, biochemical abnormalities are likely involved in many patients. The psychosocial component can also play a major role, with depression contributing to the overall status.

F. SUMMARY

- Toxicity from H&N cancer irradiation is complex and multifactorial. The nature and severity of the side effect profile for a given patient result from the interplay of patient-related, tumor-related, and treatment-factors.
- Among the side effects studied, skin toxicity and mucositis represent the most common acute effects of irradiation. Supportive care is essential to prevent superimposed infection and other complications that might lead to treatment breaks or, in extreme cases, discontinuation of therapy.
- Technological advances with conformal radiotherapy techniques have allowed for increasing salivary gland sparing. Further protection may be achieved with existing and future medical therapies.
- Swallowing dysfunction following chemoradiation for laryngeal cancer is significant and may persist for 1–2 years. Efforts should be made to ensure proper patient education and reassurance in this regard.

REFERENCES

1. Emami, B, J Lyman, A Brown, et al. 1991. Tolerance of normal tissue to therapeutic irradiation. Int J Radiat Oncol Biol Phys **21**:109–122.
2. Chao, KS, N Majhail, CJ Huang, et al. 2001. Intensity-modulated radiation therapy reduces late salivary toxicity without compromising tumor control in patients with oropharyngeal carcinoma: a comparison with conventional techniques. Radiother Oncol **61**:275–280.
3. Chao, KS, M Cengiz, CA Perez, et al. 2001. Superior Functional Outcome with IMRT in Locally Advanced Nasopharyngeal Carcinoma. Chicago, Illinois: ASCO.
4. Chao, KS, G Ozyigit, AI Blanco, et al. 2004. Intensity-modulated radiation therapy for oropharyngeal carcinoma: impact of tumor volume. Int J Radiat Oncol Biol Phys.
5. Cheng, JC, KS Chao, and D Low. 2001. Comparison of intensity modulated radiation therapy (IMRT) treatment techniques for nasopharyngeal carcinoma. Int J Cancer **96**:126–131.
6. Eisbruch, A. 2002. Clinical aspects of IMRT for head-and-neck cancer. Med Dosim **27**:99–104.
7. Eisbruch, A, LA Dawson, HM Kim, et al. 1999. Conformal and intensity modulated irradiation of head and neck cancer: the potential for improved target irradiation, salivary gland function, and quality of life. Acta Otorhinolaryngol Belg **53**:271–275.
8. Eisbruch, A, HM Kim, JE Terrell, et al. 2001. Xerostomia and its predictors following parotid-sparing irradiation of head-and-neck cancer. Int J Radiat Oncol Biol Phys **50**:695–704.
9. Eisbruch, A, JA Ship, LA Dawson, et al. 2003. Salivary gland sparing and improved target irradiation by conformal and intensity modulated irradiation of head and neck cancer. World J Surg.

10. Eisbruch, A, JA Ship, HM Kim, et al. 2001. Partial irradiation of the parotid gland. Semin Radiat Oncol **11:**234–239.
11. Eisbruch, A, JA Ship, MK Martel, et al. 1996. Parotid gland sparing in patients undergoing bilateral head and neck irradiation: techniques and early results. Int J Radiat Oncol Biol Phys **36:**469–480.
12. Roesink, JM, MA Moerland, JJ Battermann, et al. 2001. Quantitative dose–volume response analysis of changes in parotid gland function after radiotherapy in the head-and-neck region. Int J Radiat Oncol Biol Phys **51:**938–946.
13. Fowler, JF. 1989. The linear-quadratic formula and progress in fractionated radiotherapy. Br J Radiol **62:**679–694.
14. Calais, G, M Alfonsi, E Bardet, et al. 1999. Randomized trial of radiation therapy versus concomitant chemotherapy and radiation therapy for advanced-stage oropharynx carcinoma. J Natl Cancer Inst **91:**2081–2086.
15. Forastiere, AA, H Goepfert, M Maor, et al. 2003. Concurrent chemotherapy and radiotherapy for organ preservation in advanced laryngeal cancer. N Engl J Med **349:**2091–2098.
16. Giralt, JL, J Gonzalez, JM del Campo, et al. 2000. Preoperative induction chemotherapy followed by concurrent chemoradiotherapy in advanced carcinoma of the oral cavity and oropharynx. Cancer **89:**939–945.
17. Fajardo, LF. 1989. Morphologic patterns of radiation injury. Front Radiat Ther Oncol **23:**75–84.
18. Fajardo, LF. 1993. Basic mechanisms and general morphology of radiation injury. Semin Roentgenol **28:**297–302.
19. Carper, E, SB Fleishman, and M McGuire. 2004. Symptom management and supportive care for head and neck cancer patients. In: Harrison, LB, Sessions, RB, and Hong, WK, eds. Head and Neck Cancer: A Multidisciplinary Approach. Philadelphia: Lippincott, Williams, and Wilkins.
20. Cancer pain relief. World Health Organization; 1986.
21. Sulaiman, F, JM Huryn, and IM Zlotolow. 2003. Dental extractions in the irradiated head and neck patient: a retrospective analysis of Memorial Sloan-Kettering Cancer Center protocols, criteria, and end results. J Oral Maxillofac Surg **61:**1123–1131.
22. Beumer, J, III, T Curtis, and RE Harrison. 1979. Radiation therapy of the oral cavity: sequelae and management, Part 1. Head Neck Surg **1:**301–312.
23. Beumer, J, III, T Curtis, and RE Harrison. 1979. Radiation therapy of the oral cavity: sequelae and management, Part 2. Head Neck Surg **1:**392–408.
24. Eneroth, CM, CO Henrikson, and PA Jakobsson. 1972. Effect of fractionated radiotherapy on salivary gland function. Cancer **30:**1147–1153.
25. Dreizen, S, LR Brown, S Handler, et al. 1976. Radiation-induced xerostomia in cancer patients. Effect on salivary and serum electrolytes. Cancer **38:**273–278.
26. Dreizen, S, TE Daly, JB Drane, et al. 1977. Oral complications of cancer radiotherapy. Postgrad Med **61:**85–92.
27. Dreizen, S, LR Brown, TE Daly, et al. 1977. Prevention of xerostomia-related dental caries in irradiated cancer patients. J Dent Res **56:**99–104.
28. Shannon, IL, JN Trodahl, and EN Starcke. 1978. Radiosensitivity of the human parotid gland. Proc Soc Exp Biol Med **157:**50–53.
29. Wescott, WB, JG Mira, EN Starcke, et al. 1978. Alterations in whole saliva flow rate induced by fractionated radiotherapy. AJR Am J Roentgenol **130:**145–149.
30. Mossman, KL, AR Shatzman, and JD Chencharick. 1981. Effects of radiotherapy on human parotid saliva. Radiat Res **88:**403–412.
31. Mossman, K, A Shatzman, and J Chencharick. 1982. Long-term effects of radiotherapy on taste and salivary function in man. Int J Radiat Oncol Biol Phys **8:**991–997.
32. Greenspan, D. 1996. Xerostomia: diagnosis and management. Oncology (Huntingt) **10:**7–11.
33. Brizel, DM, TH Wasserman, M Henke, et al. 2000. Phase III randomized trial of amifostine as a radioprotector in head and neck cancer. J Clin Oncol **18:**3339–3345.
34. Antonadou, D, M Pepelassi, M Synodinou, et al. 2002. Prophylactic use of amifostine to prevent radiochemotherapy-induced mucositis and xerostomia in head-and-neck cancer. Int J Radiat Oncol Biol Phys **52:**739–747.
35. LeVeque, FG, M Montgomery, D Potter, et al. 1993. A multicenter, randomized, double-blind, placebo-controlled, dose-titration study of oral pilocarpine for treatment of radiation-induced xerostomia in head and neck cancer patients. J Clin Oncol **11:**1124–1131.
36. Johnson, JT, GA Ferretti, WJ Nethery, et al. 1993. Oral pilocarpine for post-irradiation xerostomia in patients with head and neck cancer. N Engl J Med **329:**390–395.

37. Jha, N, H Seikaly, J Harris, et al. 2003. Prevention of radiation induced xerostomia by surgical transfer of submandibular salivary gland into the submental space. Radiother Oncol **66:**283–289.
38. Jha, N, H Seikaly, T McGaw, et al. 2000. Submandibular salivary gland transfer prevents radiation-induced xerostomia. Int J Radiat Oncol Biol Phys **46:**7–11.
39. Chao, KS, JO Deasy, J Markman, et al. 2001. A prospective study of salivary function sparing in patients with head-and-neck cancers receiving intensity-modulated or three-dimensional radiation therapy: initial results. Int J Radiat Oncol Biol Phys **49:**907–916.
40. Lin, A, HM Kim, JE Terrell, et al. 2003. Quality of life after parotid-sparing IMRT for head-and-neck cancer: a prospective longitudinal study. Int J Radiat Oncol Biol Phys **57:**61–70.
41. Roesnik, JM, MA Moerland, and IJ Battermann. 2001. Xerostomia and its predictors following parotid-sparing irradiation of head-and-neck cancer. Int J Radiat Oncol Biol Phys **50**.
42. Chao, KS, FJ Wippold, G Ozyigit, et al. 2002. Determination and delineation of nodal target volumes for head-and-neck cancer based on patterns of failure in patients receiving definitive and postoperative IMRT. Int J Radiat Oncol Biol Phys **53:**1174–1184.
43. Eisbruch, A, RL Foote, B O'Sullivan, et al. 2002. Intensity-modulated radiation therapy for head and neck cancer: emphasis on the selection and delineation of the targets. Semin Radiat Oncol **12:**238–249.
44. Lee, N, P Xia, JM Quivey, et al. 2002. Intensity-modulated radiotherapy in the treatment of nasopharyngeal carcinoma: an update of the UCSF experience. Int J Radiat Oncol Biol Phys **53:**12–22.
45. Lee, N, C Chuang, JM Quivey, et al. 2002. Skin toxicity due to intensity-modulated radiotherapy for head-and-neck carcinoma. Int J Radiat Oncol Biol Phys **53:**630–637.
46. Ozyigit, G and KS Chao. 2002. Clinical experience of head-and-neck cancer IMRT with serial tomotherapy. Med Dosim **27:**91–98.
47. Chao, KS, G Ozyigit, BN Tran, et al. 2003. Patterns of failure in patients receiving definitive and postoperative IMRT for head-and-neck cancer. Int J Radiat Oncol Biol Phys **55:**312–321.
48. Sultanem, K, HK Shu, P Xia, et al. 2000. Three-dimensional intensity-modulated radiotherapy in the treatment of nasopharyngeal carcinoma: the University of California-San Francisco experience. Int J Radiat Oncol Biol Phys **48:**711–722.
49. ICRU 50. 1993. Prescribing, recording, and reporting photon beam therapy. Bethesda, MD.
50. Blanco, AI, KS Chao, JO Deasy, et al. 2004. Dose–volume modeling of salivary function in patients with head and neck cancer receiving radiation therapy. Int J Radiat Oncol Biol Phys, In press.
51. Pavy, JJ, J Denekamp, J Letschert, et al. EORTC Late Effects Working Group. 1995. Late effects toxicity scoring: the SOMA scale. Radiother Oncol **35:**17–60.
52. Dawson, LA, Y Anzai, L Marsh, et al. 2000. Patterns of local-regional recurrence following parotid-sparing conformal and segmental intensity-modulated radiotherapy for head and neck cancer. Int J Radiat Oncol Biol Phys **46:**1117–1126.
53. Cooper, JS, K Fu, J Marks, et al. 1995. Late effects of radiation therapy in the head and neck region. Int J Radiat Oncol Biol Phys **31:**1141–1164.
54. Wang, CC. 1997. Carcinoma of the oropharynx. In: Wang CC, ed. Radiation Therapy for Head and Neck Neoplasms, 3rd ed. New York: Wiley-Liss, pp xi, 387.
55. Hall, EJ. 2000. Radiobiology for the Radiologist, 5th ed. Philadelphia: Lippincott Williams & Wilkins.
56. Koukourakis, MI, G Kyrias, S Kakolyris, et al. 2000. Subcutaneous administration of amifostine during fractionated radiotherapy: a randomized phase II study. J Clin Oncol **18:**2226–2233.
57. Horiot, JC, F Lipinski, S Schraub, et al. 2000. Post-radiation severe xerostomia relieved by pilocarpine: a prospective French cooperative study. Radiother Oncol **55:**233–239.
58. Delanian, S, S Balla-Mekias, and JL Lefaix. 1999. Striking regression of chronic radiotherapy damage in a clinical trial of combined pentoxifylline and tocopherol. J Clin Oncol **17:**3283–3290.
59. Chua, DT, C Lo, J Yuen, et al. 2001. A pilot study of pentoxifylline in the treatment of radiation-induced trismus. Am J Clin Oncol **24:**366–369.
60. Jereczek-Fossa, BA and R Orecchia. 2002. Radiotherapy-induced mandibular bone complications. Cancer Treat Rev **28:**65–74.
61. Reuther, T, T Schuster, U Mende, et al. 2003. Osteoradionecrosis of the jaws as a side effect of radiotherapy of head and neck tumour patients—a report of a thirty year retrospective review. Int J Oral Maxillofac Surg **32:**289–295.
62. Aitasalo, K. 1986. Bone tissue response to irradiation and treatment model of mandibular irradiation injury. An experimental and clinical study. Acta Otolaryngol Suppl **428:**1–54.
63. Aitasalo, K, J Niinikoski, R Grenman, et al. 1998. A modified protocol for early treatment of osteomyelitis and osteoradionecrosis of the mandible. Head Neck **20:**411–417.

64. Aitasalo, K, R Grenman, E Virolainen, et al. 1995. A modified protocol to treat early osteoradionecrosis of the mandible. Undersea Hyperb Med **22:**161–170.
65. Chang, DW, HK Oh, GL Robb, et al. 2001. Management of advanced mandibular osteoradionecrosis with free flap reconstruction. Head Neck **23:**830–835.
66. Ertekin, MV, M Koc, I Karslioglu, et al. 2004. Zinc sulfate in the prevention of radiation-induced oropharyngeal mucositis: a prospective, placebo-controlled, randomized study. Int J Radiat Oncol Biol Phys **58:**167–174.
67. Eisbruch, A, T Lyden, CR Bradford, et al. 2002. Objective assessment of swallowing dysfunction and aspiration after radiation concurrent with chemotherapy for head-and-neck cancer. Int J Radiat Oncol Biol Phys **53:**23–28.

3. RADIATION PNEUMONITIS AND ESOPHAGITIS IN THORACIC IRRADIATION

JEFFREY BRADLEY, M.D.

Alvin J. Siteman Cancer Center, Washington University School of Medicine, St. Louis, MO

BENJAMIN MOVSAS, M.D.

Henry Ford Hospital, Detroit, MI

INTRODUCTION

Without regard to normal tissue complications, most tumors could likely be eradicated by irradiation through escalating the dose. However, normal tissue complications limit our ability to administer the dose necessary for tumor control. Tumor control probability (TCP) for a given tumor is represented by a sigmoid curve in which an increase in dose results in greater tumor cell kill. Likewise, the normal tissue complication probability (NTCP) is represented by a second sigmoid curve sitting to the right of the TCP curve (Figure 1). The relationship between these two sigmoid curves is called the therapeutic ratio (see Figure 1). Ideally, the TCP and NTCP curves are separated so that a tumoricidal dose can be delivered without concern for toxicity. A clinical example is irradiating the para-aortic lymphatics in patients with resected stage I seminomas, in which tumoricidal dose (25 Gy) is less than the $TD_{5/5}$ for adjacent normal tissues. On the other hand, epithelial malignancies, such as carcinomas, require doses between 45 and 50 Gy for subclinical disease, and 65 and 80 Gy or higher doses for gross disease, which are beyond tolerance for most organs. Potential means of modifying the therapeutic ratio include radiation sensitizers that can shift the TCP curve to the left, and protectors that can shift the NTCP curve to the right. Examples of sensitizers include chemotherapy, oxygen, and hypoxic cell sensitizers. Examples of radiation-sparing approaches include amifostine and conformal or intensity modulated radiation therapy (IMRT) (see Figure 1). This review describes treatment-related pneumonitis and esophagitis; parameters for predicting these complications, their prevention, and management.

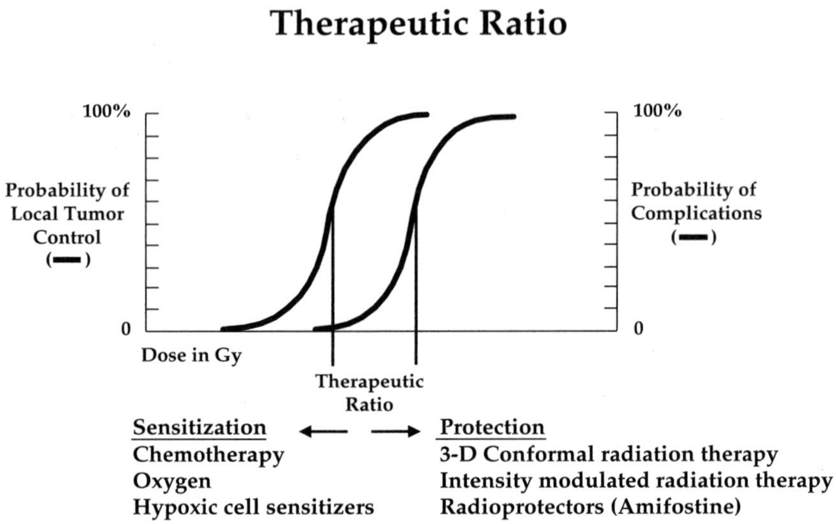

Figure 1. The relationship between the sigmoid curves representing tumor control probability (TCP) and normal tissue complication probability (NTCP) is termed the therapeutic ratio.

A. COMPLICATIONS OF IRRADIATION TO THE THORAX

Emami et al.[1] published partial-volume irradiation parameters for various organs in a report from an NCI designated task force. The parameters were derived from a review of the literature and from clinical opinions of experienced radiation oncologists. The parameters for lung and esophagus are given in Table 1. These dose limits have defined partial organ tolerances. Toxicity end points are a 5% complication rate at 5 years ($TD_{5/5}$) and a 50% complication rate at 5 years ($TD_{50/5}$) for different volumes irradiated. These toxicity parameters are incomplete. At the time of publication, the task force acknowledged that the current information leading to these parameters was "less than adequate". For normal tissues within the thorax, radiation tolerance data were compiled in an era before the use of biological modifiers and conformal radiation therapy.

Table 1. Normal tissue tolerance of therapeutic irradiation: traditional estimates

Organ	1/3	2/3	3/3	Selected end point
$TD_{5/5}$ volume				
Lung	4500	3000	1750	Pneumonitis
Esophagus	6000	5800	5500	Clinical stricture/perforation
$TD_{50/5}$ volume				
Lung	6500	4000	2450	Pneumonitis
Esophagus	7200	7000	6800	Clinical stricture/perforation

*$TD_{5/5}$ and $TD_{50/5}$ represent the estimated dose for each organ volume or partial organ volume resulting in a 1–5% risk and a 50% risk, respectively, at 5 years. From Emami et al.[1], with permission.

The pathophysiology of radiation injury is generally categorized as acute or late toxicity. Acute toxicity occurs during or immediately after a course of radiation therapy. It typically resolves within 4–6 weeks after completion of therapy. Late toxicity occurs months to years after a course of irradiation. Both types may lead to significant morbidity and/or mortality.

Chemotherapy alters the therapeutic ratio by shifting the TCP and NTCP curves to the left, enhancing the cytotoxic effect on both tumor cell and normal cell populations. Three-dimensional conformal radiation therapy (3D CRT) shifts the NTCP curve to the right, enabling tumor dose escalation while keeping the NTCP relatively constant. 3D CRT enables the radiation oncologist to precisely determine the dose–volume relationship delivered and therefore to analyze toxicity more accurately than was previously possible.

B. LUNG TOXICITY

The lungs are particularly sensitive to irradiation. Lung injury by irradiation is related to both dose and volume effects. The $TD_{5/5}$ for one-third, two-thirds, and three-thirds lung is 45, 30, and 17.5 Gy, respectively.[1] The acute complication of lung injury by irradiation is radiation pneumonitis. The late effect of lung injury is lung fibrosis. Both can be severely debilitating or even fatal.

This section reviews our present understanding of the biology of lung injury by irradiation, updates the dose–volume lung tolerances given in Table 1, and discusses areas of potential modification of the therapeutic ratio in favor of enhancing TCP.

B1. Radiation-Induced Lung Damage

Before we describe the pathophysiology of lung damage, it is important to clarify the distinction between damage and morbidity. Although these terms are often used interchangeably, they refer to different concepts. Damage refers to structural changes within the organ that occur as a result of irradiation. Morbidity is a clinical term describing signs or symptoms that develop in a patient as a result of the damage. Irradiation damage may be detected on biopsy or subsequent x-rays, or may remain subclinical.

The need to clarify this important difference relates to anatomic considerations. The lung is a system of branching ducts and accompanying blood vessels that ultimately terminate in alveoli, the sacs at which gas exchange takes place. The functional subunit of the lung is the acinus, which includes the terminal bronchiole and the respiratory bronchioles, which terminate in the alveolar sac, each bearing many alveoli. Lung damage in response to irradiation becomes clinical (i.e., morbidity develops) after a critical number of acini are destroyed.

Lung damage by irradiation was first documented as early as the 1920s.[2] The two main phases of radiation injury, radiation pneumonitis and fibrosis, were described by Evans and Leucutia in 1925.[3] Radiation pneumonitis is the acute injury phase and lung fibrosis is the resultant chronic injury.[1] These two phases of damage are clearly separated in time. Radiation pneumonitis occurs within the first 6 months after the organ is treated, and fibrosis occurs after 1 year. The study of lung injury by radiation in animals has identified two additional subclinical phases of injury, the latent and intermediate phases.

The weeks to months that precede the appearance of radiation pneumonitis are referred to as the latent period. No overt histopathologic, radiographic, or clinical signs or symptoms of radiation damage are observed during this period. However, electron microscopic examination of tissues from animals irradiated previously shows degranulation and loss of type II pneumocytes with loss of surfactant and loss of basal laminar proteoglycans, resulting in swelling of the basement membrane and transudation of proteins into the alveolar spaces, indicating increased capillary permeability and suggesting a loss of endothelial cells within the first month after whole-lung irradiation.[4–6] The endothelial cells become vacuolated and pleomorphic and may slough, leading to denudation of the basement membrane and increased capillary permeability.[7] With the advent of new molecular techniques, knowledge of the latent phase changes has increased. Depending on the radiation dose, latent phase changes may resolve or may progress to the next phase of radiation pneumonitis.

Classic radiation pneumonitis occurs within the first 6 months after lung irradiation (Figure 2). Tables 2 and 3 show the grading definitions for acute and late lung toxicity, respectively. The characteristic histologic findings are acute inflammatory changes, including a prominent inflammatory cell infiltrate in the alveoli and in the pulmonary interstitium. The inflammatory infiltrate consists of macrophages, lymphocytes, and mononuclear cells, and is not predominantly neutrophils. Characteristically, pneumonitis occurs 2–3 months after radiation and persists for up to 7 months. Generally speaking, as the radiation dose increases the latent period becomes shorter and the onset of classic pneumonitis occurs earlier. Because it takes months for the characteristic symptoms and corresponding microscopic changes of classic radiation pneumonitis to develop, it has been hypothesized that the target cells in which radiation injury is initiated represent a slowly dividing cell population. The leading candidates are the

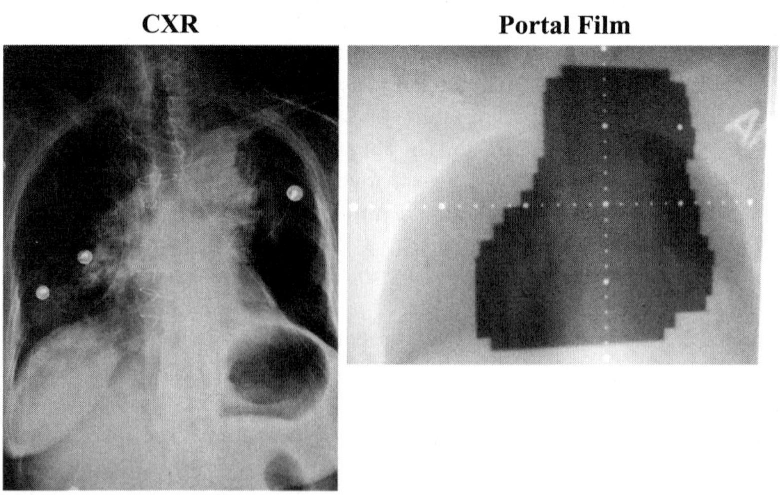

Figure 2. Chest x-ray and portal film correlating classic radiation pneumonitis.

Table 2. NCI/CTC (version 3) acute pneumonitis/pulmonary infiltrates

Grade	Description
0	No change over baseline
1	Asymptomatic, radiographic findings only
2	Symptomatic, not interfering with activities of daily living
3	Symptomatic, interfering with activities of daily living; O_2 indicated
4	Life-threatening; ventilatory support indicated
5	Death

Table 3. RTOG/EORTC late lung morbidity grading criteria

Grade	Description
0	No change over baseline
1	Asymptomatic or mild symptoms (dry cough), slight radiographic appearances
2	Moderate symptomatic fibrosis or pneumonitis (severe cough), slight radiographic appearances
3	Severe symptomatic fibrosis or pneumonitis, dense radiographic changes
4	Severe respiratory insufficiency/continuous oxygen/assisted ventilation

type II pneumocyte[8] and the vascular endothelial cell.[9–11] The type II pneumocyte is suspected because of measured dose-dependent changes in the phospholipid component of lavage fluid as early as 24 hours after irradiation.[12] The vascular endothelial cell is suspected on the basis of observations that it is the cell most likely to divide soon after irradiation and that edema is a consistent finding in the interstitium and air spaces after irradiation.

Patients who survive the acute pneumonitis phase of damage enter the intermediate phase, which is characterized by the resolution of acute exudative pneumonitis. Light microscopy reveals the presence of foamy macrophages in the air spaces, along with hyperplasia of type II pneumocytes.

Radiation fibrosis develops insidiously months to years after irradiation. The pathogenesis of this process remains largely unknown. Two forms of fibrosis have been described in mice and humans. Interstitial fibrosis is characterized by collagen deposition in the alveolar wall, bounded by the basement membrane of the lung epithelium on one side and the basement membrane of the endothelium on the other. The second form of fibrosis is an intra-alveolar process characterized by masses of collagen in the alveolar spaces.

Classic radiation pneumonitis characteristically occurs within the irradiated portal. However, approximately 10–15% of patients may experience signs or symptoms of radiation pneumonitis that do not fit the classical definition. A sporadic form of radiation pneumonitis has been described.[13] Several factors suggest that this syndrome may be different from the classical form of radiation-induced lung damage: (a) it affects 10–15% of patients; (b) the symptoms frequently resolve without sequelae; (c) it frequently develops within 2–6 weeks after completion of radiation; and (d) unirradiated lung may show infiltrates on x-ray. Sporadic radiation pneumonitis is believed to represent an immune-mediated hypersensitivity pneumonitis. At present there is no animal model in which this entity could be studied.

B2. Predicting Radiation Pneumonitis

Normal lung tissue is highly sensitive to low doses of irradiation (Table 1). Therefore, whereas TCP may be predicted by the high dose distribution around the tumor target, NTCP is predicted by the dose–volume relationship of the low-dose region. Several authors have contributed to our fund of knowledge about this complex problem. As a result, several parameters have been reported to be predictive of pneumonitis. Mean lung dose (MLD) is the simplest parameter and is clinically useful. The volume of total lung receiving above a certain dose is reported as V_{20} ($\geq$20 Gy)[14] or V_{30} ($\geq$30 Gy).[15] The MLD, V_{20} and V_{30}, parameters have the advantage of being easily calculated. Other more complicated calculations involve DVH reduction techniques which reduce the DVH of an organ to a single effective uniform dose (EUD): effective lung dose (V_{eff}),[16] the NTCP calculation model,[17,18] and the functional subunit model of Niemierko.[19] These parameters are technically more difficult to calculate and, thus, are not as widely applied.

Kwa et al.[20] performed mathematical modeling to compare two DVH reduction techniques, the NTCP (Kutcher model) and functional subunit models, predicting pneumonitis. The two techniques provided predictions that were very similar to those predicted by MLD for total doses up to 80 Gy.

A pooled analysis of 540 patients who received thoracic irradiation at five institutions reported that 73 patients developed grade 2 or greater pneumonitis.[20] After α/β calculation adjustments for fraction size, the physical dose distribution was converted to the biologically equivalent dose distribution given in fractions of 2 Gy, dose–volume histograms were calculated, and an MLD was derived, which was the only factor analyzed in the study. In all five centers, a higher MLD was correlated with an increased risk for pneumonitis (Figure 3). On the basis of this large pooled analysis, MLD appears to be a good indicator of pneumonitis risk.

Investigators from the Netherlands Cancer Institute and the University of Michigan pooled dosimetric and toxicity data for 382 patients treated to the thorax for lymphoma, lung, and breast cancers.[21] Thirty-seven and 7 patients developed $\geq$grade 2 and $\geq$grade 3 pneumonitis, respectively. Different NTCP models were compared for the ability to predict pneumonitis, including the general parallel model, the Lyman–Kutcher–Burman (LKB) model, the MLD model, and the volume above threshold (V_{Dth}) model. The general parallel and LKB models are mathematical reductions of a sigmoid-shaped dose–volume histogram to an equivalent uniform dose. The V_{Dth} model is a special case of the parallel model. Examples include V_{20} and V_{30}. The MLD is a special case of the LKB model. The investigators concluded that MLD was the most accurate parameter of these models.

Prospective data from Washington University reported on 99 patients treated with definitive conformal irradiation to doses ranging from 50 to 70 Gy (1.8–2 Gy per day).[14] This population consisted mainly of patients with locally advanced disease: 22% had stage I cancers, 5% stage II, and 72% stage III. Most patients received elective nodal

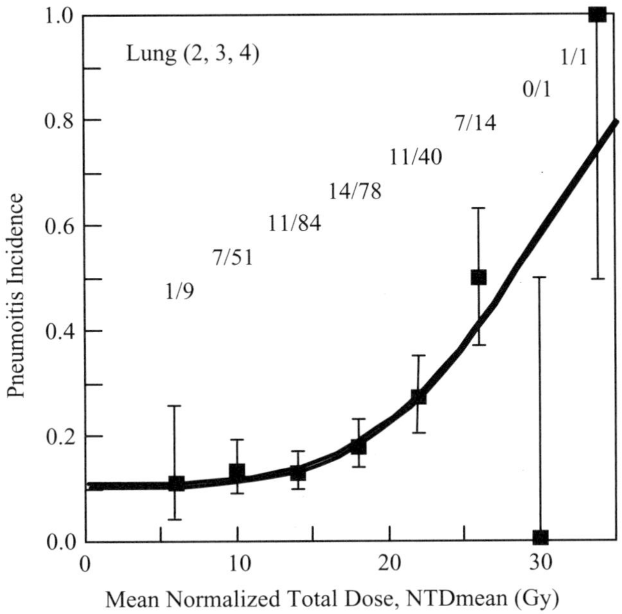

Figure 3. Curve representing the incidence of radiation pneumonitis by mean lung dose. From Kwa et al.[64] with permission from Elsevier Science Publishing.

irradiation to 50 Gy to treat microscopic tumor, followed by a boost to the planning target volume encompassing gross disease. The development of grade 2 or greater pneumonitis was 14% at 6 months, 17% at 12 months, and 24% at 24 months. The most important prognostic factors for radiation pneumonitis, in order of statistical significance, were percent volume of total lung receiving a dose greater than 20 Gy (V_{20}), total MLD, effective lung dose (V_{eff}), and location of the primary tumor (lower lobe worse). On multivariate analysis, V_{20} was the single best predictor of this complication. There was a strong correlation between V_{20} and severity of pneumonitis. When V_{20} was less than 22% there was no clinical grade 2 or greater pneumonitis. When V_{20} was 22–31% the incidence was 8%, and when V_{20} was greater than 32% grade 3 pneumonitis was encountered. In patients with a V_{20} of ≥40%, there was a 36% incidence of grades 2–5 pneumonitis. Three patients in this group died of unequivocal radiation-induced pneumonitis (Table 4). On the basis of these data, the RTOG conducted a phase I/II dose escalation study in patients with non-small cell lung cancer (NSCLC) for whom the total dose prescribed to the PTV depended on V_{20} (RTOG 93-11).[22] The incidence of ≥grade 3 late pneumonitis or fibrosis was approximately 7% and 15% for patients with a V_{20} <25% receiving 70.9 Gy and >70.9 Gy, respectively. Likewise, the incidence of ≥grade 3 late pneumonitis or fibrosis was 15% for patients with a V_{20} between 25% and 36% receiving doses of 70.9 Gy or greater. Investigators from Duke University[23] reported lung toxicity data in 201 patients treated with conformal

Table 4. Predicting radiation pneumonitis

Variable	Cut-offs ≥ grade 2	Incidence of pneumonitis (%)
% Total lung Volume >20 Gy (V_{20})	<22	0
	22–32	7
	32–40	13
	>40	36
Total lung mean dose	<20 Gy	8
	>20 Gy	24

radiation therapy for thoracic tumors. Chemotherapy was delivered in 120 patients. Concurrent chemotherapy and radiation therapy were given in 37 patients. Radiation therapy doses ranged from 26 to 86.4 Gy with 85% of patients receiving >60 Gy. A minimum follow-up of 6 months was required. Of 201 patients, 39 developed radiation pneumonitis, including 1 grade 4, 27 grade 2, and 8 grade 3. Comparison of multiple dosimetric factors in their database showed that V_{30}, MLD, or NTCP (LKB model) alone was the best predictors of radiation pneumonitis. Comparisons of the incidence of radiation pneumonitis for each of these parameters are illustrated in Figure 4. Each of the above studies reported dosimetric parameters that are based on the total lung volume. Investigators from Memorial Sloan-Kettering Cancer Center chose to evaluate both the total and subtotal lung volumes (ipsilateral and contralateral lung, upper and lower lung zones).[24] Dosimetric parameters included EUD (V_{eff}), the functional subunit model (F_{dam}), MLD, V_{20}, and NTCP. Of the 49 patients studied, 9 developed grade 3 or greater radiation pneumonitis. Significant predictors for RP were MLD, D_{eff}, and F_{dam} when total lung volumes were considered. For ipsilateral lung volumes, RP risk

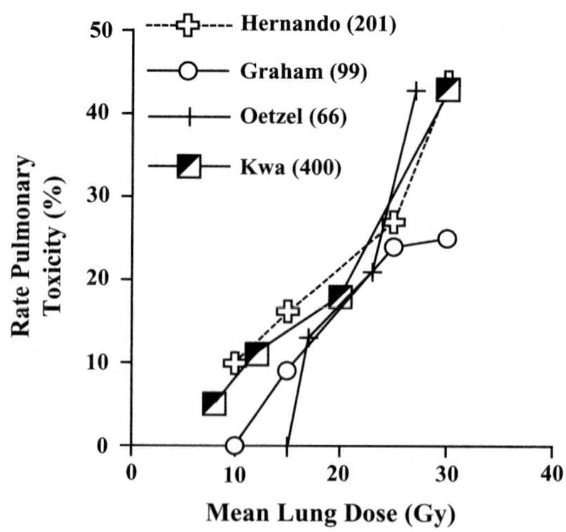

Figure 4. Curves correlating pulmonary toxicity rates with mean lung dose, NTCP, and V_{20} or V_{30}. From Hernando et al.[23] with permission from Elsevier Science Publishing.

correlated with MLD, D_{eff}, F_{dam}, and V_{20}. When the lower half of the lungs were considered, MLD, D_{eff}, and NTCP were predictors of RP. Values calculated for the upper lung zones and for the contralateral lung did not correlate with RP risk.

The administration of concurrent chemotherapy with radiation therapy appears to increase the risk of radiation pneumonitis compared to sequential chemoradiation or radiation therapy alone. Patients with NSCLC treated on the RTOG 9311 dose escalation study did not experience increased acute or late complications whether or not 2 cycles of chemotherapy were delivered prior to definitive radiation therapy.[22] Tsujino et al.[25] reported a retrospective review that included 65 patients who received concurrent chemotherapy using various doublets. Grade 2 or greater radiation pneumonitis rates for V_{20} values of $\leq$20%, 21–25%, 26–30%, and $\geq$31% were 8.7%, 18.3%, 51%, and 85%, respectively. These rates are slightly higher than what has been reported without concurrent chemotherapy. Onishi et al.[26] reported 3 deaths from radiation pneumonitis in 32 patients treated with radiation therapy and weekly docetaxel for stage III NSCLC. Although these two studies identify this problem, further investigation will be necessary to quantify acceptable dosimetric parameters in the setting of concurrent chemoradiation.

Our clinical practice is to limit normal lung doses as much as possible for each patient, while delivering a tumoricidal dose of 60–70 Gy, depending on the clinical scenario. The rates of severe pneumonitis are very high for patients with V_{20} values exceeding 36% or MLDs exceeding 25 Gy. Therefore, such patients are not treated with these plans, but are often referred for chemotherapy to volume-reduce and/or treated with the smallest possible radiation field (e.g., gross tumor volume only).

In summary, several dosimetric factors appear to be effective in predicting radiation pneumonitis, including MLD, V_{20}, V_{30}, V_{eff}, and NTCP calculations. Which parameter to use remains a matter of debate. For ease of calculation and predictability, MLD and the volume of lung receiving 20 Gy are reliable. Each of the above parameters needs to be re-tested in databases of lung cancer patients treated with concurrent chemotherapy and radiation therapy in order to confirm or modify predictions of pneumonitis risk.

B3. Management of Radiation Pneumonitis

There is a surprising lack of literature to guide the management of this complication. Therefore, the following represents the management strategy of our own institutions. The typical patient returns to the medical and/or radiation oncology clinic for follow-up evaluation complaining of a cough, low-grade fever, shortness of breath, or any combination of these symptoms. The differential diagnosis includes infectious pneumonitis, pulmonary embolism, tumor recurrence, and radiation pneumonitis. A thorough history is obtained, paying particular attention to the timing, severity, and duration of symptoms. Radiation pneumonitis generally occurs 1–6 months following completion of the radiation therapy. Patients should be asked about any recent medical interventions, including surgical procedures, chemotherapy, or antimicrobial therapy. Patients continuing to receive chemotherapy may be at risk for development of infectious pneumonia. Patients having surgery may be at greater risk for pulmonary embolism. The presence of hemoptysis is concerning for central tumor recurrence or pulmonary embolism. The physical examination should concentrate on the vital signs (temperature, pulse, respiratory rate, and blood pressure), and the examination of the chest. The laboratory work-up should initially consist of a complete blood count (with differential) and a chest x-ray. A thin-cut CT using the pulmonary embolism protocol can be helpful. Patients receiving chemotherapy and experiencing a neutropenic fever are admitted to the hospital and placed under neutropenic precautions. Patients with a productive cough, a high white blood cell count, and infiltrates on chest x-ray are given antibiotics and should be monitored closely for persistent symptoms.

If the cough is non-productive, the white blood cell count is normal, and the x-ray shows infiltrates in the distribution of the radiotherapy portals, the patient is usually initiated on prednisone with a presumed diagnosis of radiation pneumonitis. The typical prescription is 50–60 mg per day for 1 week, decreasing slowly by 10 mg/week. The dose is tapered slowly because some patients experience a rebound pneumonitis with a faster tapering schedule. In some cases, patients may need to maintain a low-dose prednisone schedule for more extended periods of time. Referral to pulmonary medicine should be considered, as clinically indicated.

It has been our experience that some patients experience a rapid decline in pulmonary function as a result of overwhelming respiratory failure. Radiation pneumonitis is almost always on the list of differential diagnoses including adult respiratory distress syndrome, infectious pneumonia, pulmonary embolism, and broncholitis obliterans with organizing pneumonia (BOOP). Patients experiencing respiratory failure may require intensive care and mechanical ventilation. As such, patients presenting with symptoms of cough, fever, and shortness of breath should be managed cautiously.

C. FUTURE DIRECTIONS RELATED TO LUNG TOXICITY

Much more needs to be learned in order to avoid or minimize lung toxicity from radiation therapy. The possible mechanisms can be broken down into improved radiation delivery, medical interventions designed to impede the inflammatory response of normal lung to irradiation, and the ability to predict inflammatory response based on genetic predisposition.

IMRT has the potential to concentrate the prescribed radiation dose within the target volume and reduce the dose to surrounding normal structures. Clinical experience with IMRT techniques is growing but is mainly limited to head and neck, brain, and pelvic malignancies. Thoracic and abdominal malignancies are problematic with respect to tumor excursion secondary to ventilatory and/or heart motion. IMRT can be applied but the beam apertures must be large enough to account for this motion. Larger beam apertures irradiate more normal tissue and negate any potential advantage of IMRT. Investigations are under way to control respiratory motion,[27–30] to gate the linear accelerator to "beam on" during selected phases of the ventilatory cycle,[31,32] or to track tumor excursion by dynamic movement of multileaf collimators during therapy.[31,33] Investigations in four-dimensional imaging of the lung (*x*, *y*, and *z* coordinates with time) will undoubtedly enhance the ability to gate the linear accelerator or track individual tumors for radiation therapy delivery.[34,35]

Captopril is an angiotensin-converting enzyme (ACE) inhibitor that may protect target endothelial cells against radiation-induced cell killing. Preclinical studies show that captopril reduces endothelial dysfunction after irradiation and reduces radiation-induced lung fibrosis in rats.[36,37] On the basis of these exciting data, a randomized phase II clinical trial is open through the Radiation Therapy Oncology Group (RTOG 0123) in which patients are randomized to maintenance captopril or not following completion of radiation therapy. The role of amifostine, the radioprotector, in lung cancer will be reviewed in the next section.

There is a wide clinical variation in the degree of acute pneumonitis and lung fibrosis among patients who have been treated similarly. These differences suggest a variation in lung radiosensitivity from person to person. Investigators at Duke University[38] have shown that the cytokine transforming growth factor-β1 (TGF-β1) can be used to predict the risk of radiation-induced lung injury. They recently reported the results of a clinical trial in which patients achieving normal TGF-β1 plasma levels following 73.6 Gy of accelerated hyperfractionated radiation therapy received a boost to total doses of 80 and 86.4 Gy, respectively. Grade 3 or greater complications occurred in 4 of 24 patients treated to 73.6 Gy, 1 of 8 patients treated to 80 Gy, and 2 of 6 patients treated to 86.4 Gy, respectively. There were 3 grades 4–5 complications, each of which occurred in patients treated to the lower dose (i.e., persistently elevated TGF-β1 levels), suggesting that persistently elevated plasma TGF-β1 identifies patients who are at a greater risk of severe complications. Subsequent trials confirming this relationship are being planned.

D. ESOPHAGEAL TOXICITY

The radiotherapeutic management of thoracic malignancies often exposes the esophagus to high levels of ionizing radiation. After 2–3 weeks of conventionally fractionated radiotherapy, patients often complain of dysphagia and/or odynophagia. This acute reaction to radiation can cause significant morbidity from dehydration and weight loss that can lead to treatment interruptions. In rare instances, patients may experience perforation or obstruction. The late reactions of the esophagus to radiation usually involve fibrosis of the organ, which can lead to strictures. Patients may experience various degrees of dysphagia and may require endoscopic dilatation. As with the acute reaction, rare cases may involve perforation or fistula formation. Tables 5 and 6 define the grading of acute and late esophageal toxicity, respectively.

Table 5. NCI/CTC (version 3) acute esophagitis grading criteria

Grade	Description
0	No change over baseline
1	Asymptomatic pathologic, radiographic, or endoscopic findings only
2	Symptomatic, altered eating/swallowing (e.g., altered dietary habits, oral supplements); IV fluids indicated <24 hours
3	Symptomatic and severely altered eating/swallowing (e.g., inadequate oral caloric or fluid intake); IV fluids, tube feedings, or TPN indicated >24 hours
4	Life-threatening consequences
5	Death

Table 6. RTOG/EORTC late esophagitis morbidity grading criteria

Grade	Description
0	No change over baseline
1	Mild fibrosis; slight difficulty in swallowing solids; no pain on swallowing
2	Unable to take solid food normally; swallowing semisolid food; dilatation may be indicated
3	Severe fibrosis; able to swallow only liquids; may have pain on swallowing; dilatation required
4	Necrosis/perforation, fistula

Emami et al.[1] have reported $TD_{5/5}$ and $TD_{50/5}$ values for stricture and perforation of the esophagus. The issue of acute and late esophagitis was not addressed. Even with the limited end points of stricture/perforation, the authors acknowledged: "The data . . . are quite soft . . . especially since few authors have attempted to define a dose volume relationship."

Data regarding the clinical and dosimetric predictors of acute and late esophagitis have become particularly important in this era of radiation therapy dose escalation and combined chemo-RT regimens. Further intensification of these therapy regimens will require further characterization of dose-limiting toxicities such as esophagitis. This further characterization must include the dose limits for radiation only and also elucidation of the effect of sequential and concurrent chemotherapy on these dose limits.

D1. Clinical Studies

The occurrence of esophagitis first became evident once skin toxicity was no longer limiting, after the advent of megavoltage radiation therapy. In 1957, Seaman and Ackerman[39] at the Mallinckrodt Institute of Radiology reported on 20 patients with various degrees of esophagitis after treatment for lung cancer delivered via a betatron with 24 MEV photons. Four cases were severe. Some of the patients underwent autopsy. They appeared fairly unremarkable, but thickening was noted in the muscularis and submucosa.[39]

Seaman and Ackerman also noted that radiologic findings were rare and that, when apparent, narrowing of the esophageal lumen was most common. They suggested that the tolerance of the esophagus is 6000 rad given at 1000 rad/week. These figures are similar to those suggested by Emami et al.[1]

Goldstein et al.[40] reported on 30 patients who developed esophagitis after thoracic irradiation. Most had no abnormality on barium swallow; however, among those with any findings altered motility was most common. Lepke and Lipshitz[41] reported on 250 patients treated with thoracic irradiation. Forty patients had abnormal esophagrams. Only 1.6% (1/63) of those treated with radiation therapy only had esophageal abnormality. This compared to 7.7% (10/132) or nearly a fivefold increased incidence among those treated with combined chemotherapy and RT.

Several large trials have shown that the esophagus is able to tolerate relatively high doses of radiation therapy alone with conventional fractionation. Furthermore, platinum-based induction chemotherapy does not appear to significantly lower esophageal tolerance. Dillman et al.[42] reported the results of a randomized trial comparing induction vinblastine and cisplatin followed by 60 Gy versus 60 Gy alone. There was a similar incidence of esophageal toxicity (<1%) in both arms. These incidences were similar in the comparable arms of the RTOG 88-08 study.[43]

The addition of concurrent chemotherapy to radiation therapy lowers the tolerance of the esophagus to radiation therapy. This has resulted in markedly higher incidences of esophagitis with concurrent chemotherapy and radiation therapy with conventional fractionation versus radiation therapy alone with conventional fractionation. Most investigators have reported their results according to the RTOG/EORTC grading scale. Hirota et al. validated this scale via endoscopy performed at the end of a course of radiation therapy, with or without chemotherapy, in patients treated with thoracic malignancies (Spearman rank correlation coefficient = 0.428; $P < 0.0001$). Endoscopic grade 3 esophagitis was observed in none of the patients receiving radiation alone and in 27% of patients treated with concurrent chemoradation therapy ($P = 0.004$).

Choy et al.[44] have reported a 46% incidence of acute grades 3–4 esophagitis during treatment with concurrent chemo-RT consisting of weekly paclitaxel and carboplatin and 66 Gy of RT in 2-Gy daily fractions. Byhardt et al.[45] described the toxicity results from five RTOG trials for patients with lung cancer using radiation- and cisplatin-based chemotherapy. The investigators divided patients into three groups according to treatment: (a) neoadjuvant chemotherapy and definitive radiation; (b) neoadjuvant chemotherapy followed by concurrent chemoradiation; and (c) concurrent chemotherapy and hyperfractionated radiation. The incidence of grade 3 or greater acute esophagitis was significantly higher for group c versus groups a and b (Figure 5). Similarly, late esophagitis showed a trend toward significance in the hyperfractionated group (8% vs. 2% and 4%; $P = 0.077$).

Data from Washington University on patients treated with definitive radiotherapy or chemoradiation indicate that concurrent chemotherapy was the predominant factor leading to treatment-related esophagitis.[46] Overall, 16 patients (8%) developed acute or late grades 3–5 esophagitis. Fourteen of the 16 patients who developed esophagitis received concurrent chemoradiation. The other two patients developing grade 3 esophagitis received maximum esophageal doses of >69 Gy. The use of concurrent chemotherapy and a maximum point dose to the esophagus of >58 Gy was predictive of grade 3 or greater esophagitis on multivariate analysis.

D2. Dosimetric Studies

Recent publications have attempted to define the clinical and dosimetric predictors of esophagitis. Much of this work continues to evolve. Maguire et al.[47] have reported on 91 patients, of whom 10 had acute grade 3 or higher esophagitis. Twelve patients had late grade 3 or higher esophagitis. Forty-eight percent of patients were treated with concurrent chemotherapy. Fifty-seven percent of patients were treated with hyperfractionated RT. No factors were found to significantly associate with acute esophagitis on univariate analysis. Factors significantly associated with late esophagitis on multivariate analysis included percent organ volume treated greater than 50 Gy and maximum percent treated greater than 80 Gy. In addition, length of 100% circumference treated greater than 50 Gy was significant on univariate analysis only.

Werner-Wasik et al.[48] also analyzed clinical and dosimetric predictors of esophagitis in 105 patients treated for lung cancer, 58 of whom received concurrent chemotherapy

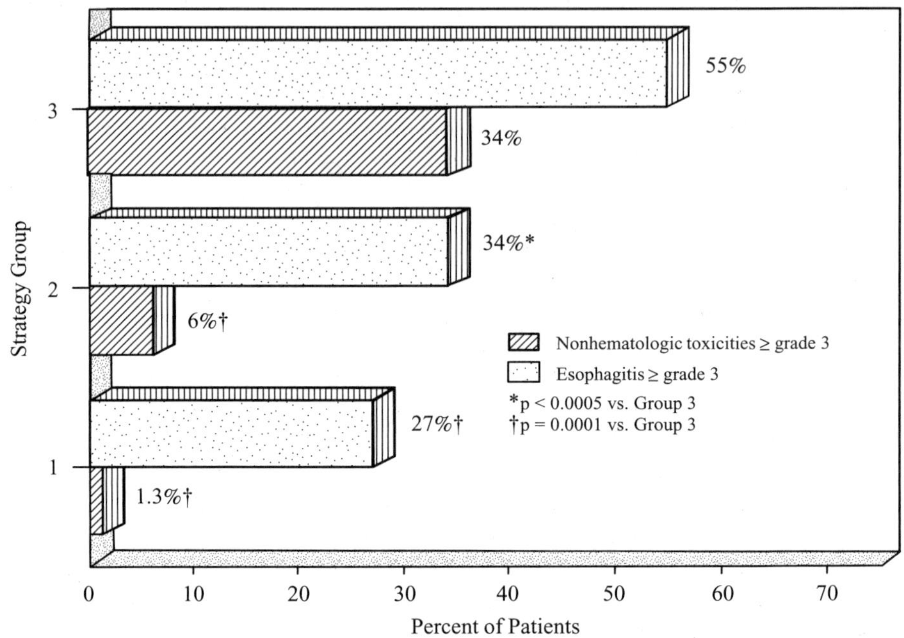

Figure 5. Incidence of ≥grade 3 esophagitis according to chemoradiation strategy grouping. From Byhardt et al.[45] with permission from Elsevier Science Publishing.

and seven of whom were treated with twice-daily fractionation. The median time to first occurrence of esophagitis was 15 days for all patients; 16 days for patients receiving conventional RT alone; 17 days for patients receiving induction chemotherapy followed by conventional RT; 19 days for patients receiving concurrent chemotherapy with conventional RT; and 13 days for patients receiving concurrent chemotherapy with hyperfractionated RT. The median duration of acute esophagitis was 14 days for patients treated with RT alone; 19 days for patients receiving induction chemotherapy followed by RT; 29 days for patients treated with concurrent chemotherapy with conventional RT ($P = 0.004$ compared to RT alone); and 87 days for patients treated with concurrent chemotherapy with hyperfractionated RT ($P = 0.002$ compared to RT alone). Figure 6 shows the esophagitis index (EI) (area under the curve) for each risk group. Specific rates of ≥ grade 3 esophagitis by treatment groups were 6%, 0%, 18%, and 43% for RT alone, induction chemotherapy followed by radiation, concurrent chemotherapy with daily RT, and concurrent chemotherapy with twice-daily RT, respectively.

The problem with predicting acute esophagitis risk using irradiated length or full circumference methods is that the boost fields often treat a portion of the esophageal circumference. Thus, the partial circumferential dose is neglected with these methods. Bradley et al.[49] published a dosimetric analysis or esophagitis risk in 166 patients treated with radiation alone, induction chemotherapy followed by radiation therapy, or concurrent chemoradiation therapy. Clinical esophagitis was scored by RTOG/EORTC

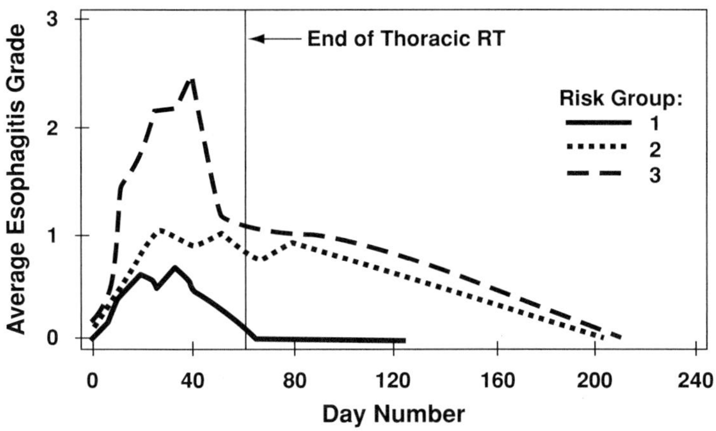

Figure 6. Esophagitis Index in different treatment groups (group 1 = daily fractionated radiation therapy with or without induction chemotherapy; group 2 = daily fractionated radiation therapy with concurrent chemotherapy; group 3 = twice-daily radiation therapy with concurrent chemotherapy.[48]

criteria during weekly visits during the course of therapy. Dosimetric data were reconstructed to produce both dose–surface area and dose–volume histograms for each patient. On multivariate analysis, the most predictive parameters for ≥ grade 2 acute esophagitis were the surface area receiving ≥55 Gy ($P \leq 0.0005$), the volume receiving ≥ 60 Gy ($P \leq 0.001$), and the use of concurrent chemotherapy ($P = 0.001$). Specific predictions of ≥grade 2 acute esophagitis by irradiated surface area or volume with or without concurrent chemotherapy are shown in Figures 7 and 8.

D3. Management of Acute Esophagitis

Literature regarding the management of acute esophagitis is scarce. As such, the following reflects the practice of our institutions. Patients generally begin to complain of burning or pain on swallowing during the third to fourth week of a course of radiation therapy and during the second and third week of a course of chemoradiation. The pain described may be similar to heartburn from gastroesophageal reflux disease. Findings at the time of physical examination may be normal. Patients may have signs of dehydration including weight loss, increased heart rate, orthostatic hypotension, dry mucosa, and skin tenting. A thorough examination should be performed to look for signs of oropharyngeal candidiasis.

The management of chemoradiation-induced esophagitis will vary based on the patient's symptoms and physical signs. Early symptoms are managed medically. Patients are typically given a prescription for "magic mouthwash", a cocktail consisting of cherry maalox (4 oz), benadryl elixer (4 oz), viscous lidocaine (100 ml), and mycostatin oral suspension (1 oz). Instructions are to swallow 5–10 ml every 2–3 hours as needed. For patients who cannot tolerate this mixture, narcotics are prescribed (i.e., MSIR liquid or fentanyl patches). Oropharyngeal candidiasis should be treated with oral antifungal therapy (nystatin or fluconazole). It may be helpful to initiate a proton pump inhibitor

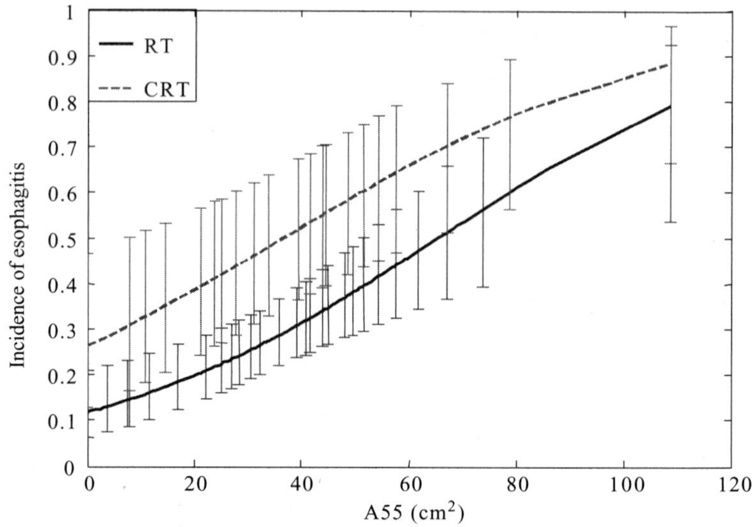

Figure 7. Curves representing the incidence of ≥grade 2 acute esophagitis by the surface area of the esophagus receiving ≥55 Gy ($p \leq 0.0005$). RT = radiation therapy with or without induction chemotherapy. CRT = radiation therapy with concurrent chemotherapy. From Bradely et al.[49] with permission from Elsevier Science Publishing.

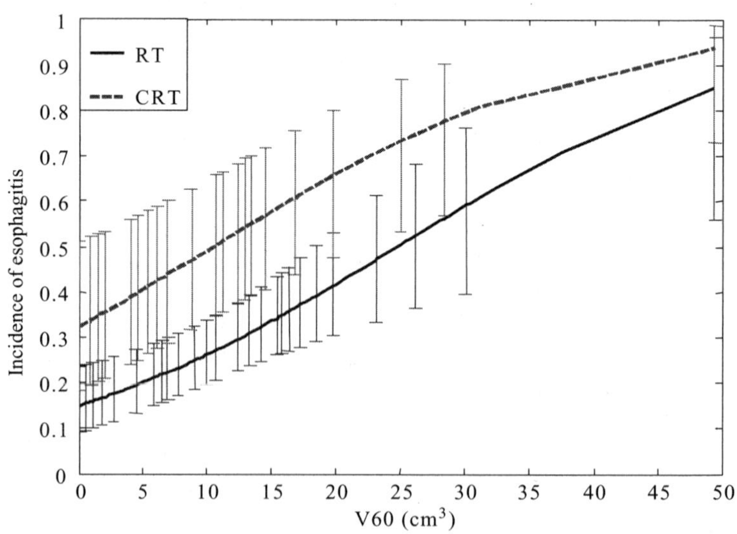

Figure 8. Curves representing the incidence of ≥grade 2 acute esophagitis by the volume of the esophagus receiving ≥60 Gy ($p = 0.001$). RT = radiation therapy with or without induction chemotherapy. CRT = radiation therapy with concurrent chemotherapy. From Bradely et al.[49] with permission from Elsevier Science Publishing.

to decrease acid reflux irritation. Indeed, some investigators begin such therapy at the outset, prior to the development of any symptoms. Examples of proton pump inhibitors include omeprezole, esomeprazole, lansoprazole, and pantoprazole. If dehydration occurs, rehydration is usually best managed by encouraging the patient to increase oral fluid intake. For patients who cannot sustain oral hydration, intravenous fluids are indicated. On occasion, some patients will be unable to maintain adequate hydration despite the management outlined above. Alternative considerations include a gastrostomy tube or a break from radiation therapy.

McGinnis et al.[50] studied the utility of sucralfate suspension in preventing acute esophagitis in a prospective, double-blind randomized trial involving patients who received thoracic radiotherapy. Surprisingly, 58% of patients in the experimental arm dropped out of the study, mainly because of nausea and vomiting ascribed to sucralfate. The incidence of esophagitis was similar in the two arms. It was noted that the sucralfate suspension used in the study was not identical to the commercially available formulation.

D4. Preventive Strategies

Although accurate volumetric parameters have yet to be defined, minimizing the amount of esophagus irradiated is an obvious means of limiting radiation esophagitis. Unfortunately, this is often impossible in the treatment of thoracic malignancies due to the anatomic distribution of the GTV and clinical target volume (CTV).

Recently, several randomized trials have studied the role of amifostine, a radioprotector, in the setting of lung cancer. Amifostine (*Ethyol; WR-2721*) is an organic thiophosphate selected from over 4400 compounds screened by the US Army as the best radioprotective compound. Amifostine is dephosphorylated at the tissue site to its active metabolite (*WR-1065*) by alkaline phosphatase.[51] Once inside the cell, WR-1065, the free thiol, acts as a potent scavenger of oxygen free radicals induced by ionizing radiation.[52]

Randomized phase II or III studies of amifostine in lung cancer have demonstrated mixed results regarding the ability of this agent to reduce esophagitis and/or pneumonitis. Antonadou et al.[53] randomized 146 lung cancer patients receiving standard thoracic radiation to ±amifostine (340 mg/m^2 prior to daily RT). They found significant reductions in grade ≥2 esophagitis and pneumonitis ($P < 0.001$). In a subsequent randomized phase II trial by the same group,[54] 73 stage III NSCLC patients receiving concurrent chemotherapy (either paclitaxel 60 mg/m^2 or carboplatin AUC 2) once weekly during standard RT were randomized to ±amifostine (300 mg/m^2 IV daily prior to treatment). They reported a significant reduction in grade ≥3 esophagitis and pneumonitis.[54] Komaki et al.[55] reported the results of a randomized trial of amifostine in 60 patients performed in the context of concurrent chemotherapy (cisplatin and oral etoposide) and hyperfractionated radiation therapy (1.2 Gy BID to 69.6 Gy). In this study, amifostine was administered 500 mg IV daily (prior to the AM RT fraction) for 2 days each week during the chemoRT. Komaki et al.[55] reported that morphine intake to reduce severe esophagitis was significantly lower in the amifostine arm (7.4% vs. 31%, $P = 0.03$), as was the rate of acute pneumonitis (13.7% vs. 23%, $P = 0.04$). As a follow-up to this trial, Gopal et al.[38] reported that the administration of amifostine had a protective effect on residual pulmonary function following treatment. They found a sharp decline in DLCO (diffusion capacity of carbon monoxide) values at radiation doses above 13 Gy given without amifostine, and above 36 Gy when amifostine was administered. In a randomized phase II study testing subcutaneous amifostine (500 mg daily before RT), Koukourakis et al.[56] reported a reduction in esophageal toxicity among 60 patients receiving thoracic RT (WHO grade 0/1 vs. 3/4, $P = 0.08$; grade 0/1 vs. 2–4, $P = 0.02$).

Other randomized phase III trials of amifostine in stage III NSCLC, however, have not demonstrated a significant benefit to amifostine. Leong et al.[57] studied 60 patients who were treated with 2 cycles of paclitaxel (175 mg/m^2) and carboplatin (AUC 6) followed by radiation (64 Gy) with concurrent weekly paclitaxel (60 mg/m^2). In this double-blinded study, patients were randomized to receive 740 mg/m^2 of amifostine versus placebo before each dose of paclitaxel and carboplatin. Although Leong et al. noted a trend toward reducing the severity of esophagitis in the amifostine arm, this finding did not reach statistical significance.[57] Moreover, the preliminary results of another randomized phase III trial in stage III NSCLC ($N = 100$) of concurrent RT (64.8 Gy) with weekly paclitaxel (50 mg/m^2) and carboplatin (AUC) followed by 2 cycles of consolidation gemcitabine and cisplatin ±amifostine (200 mg/m^2 IV daily prior to RT and 500 mg IV weekly before chemotherapy) have so far demonstrated no cytoprotective benefit of amifostine.[58]

Of all of the studies testing the role of amifostine in lung cancer, RTOG 98-01 is the largest trial ($N = 243$) and the only one that was performed in the setting of a multi-institutional cooperative group. Eligibility criteria stipulated medically inoperable stage II or unresectable stage IIIA/B NSCLC patients with a KPS >70, age >18, and weight loss <5%. Two hundred and forty-three patients received induction paclitaxel (P) 225 mg/m^2 IV: day 1, 22; carboplatin (C) AUC 6: day 1, 22 followed by concurrent weekly paclitaxel (50 mg/m^2 IV); carboplatin (AUC 2) and hyperfractionated RT (69.6 Gy @ 1.2 Gy BID) starting day 43. Patients were randomized at registration to ±amifostine (A) 500 mg IV four times per week (mostly before the afternoon RT fraction). Toxicity was assessed via NCI-CTC & EORTC/RTOG criteria, physician dysphagia logs (PDL), daily patient swallowing diaries and QOL (EORTC QLQ C30/LC-13). Swallowing area under the curve (AUC) analyses were calculated from patient diaries and PDL. Two hundred and forty-three patients were enrolled from 9/98–3/02. One hundred and twenty patients were randomized to amifostine, 123 to no amifostine (1 patient was ineligible). Baseline demographics were comparable for each arm. Seventy-three percent received amifostine per protocol or with a minor deviation. Grade ≥3 esophagitis rate was 30% with amifostine versus 34% without amifostine ($P = 0.9$). Similarly, there was no reduction in the rates of pneumonitis. However, based on patient diaries, the swallowing AUC dysfunction during chemoradiation was lower with amifostine (Z-test $P = 0.03$), especially among females ($P = 0.006$) and patients >65 years ($P = 0.003$). RTOG 98-01 is unique in that it is the only study of amifostine in lung cancer that included a prospective, validated quality-of-life instrument (EORTC-QLQ-C30 and QLQ-LC-13 questionnaires).[59,60] While overall QOL was not significantly different between the two arms, it is noteworthy that the symptom of pain showed significantly more clinically meaningful improvement and less deterioration at 6 weeks of follow-up (vs. pre-treatment) on the amifostine arm ($P = 0.003$). This is despite the fact that the amifostine arm was associated with significant increases in nausea and vomiting (mostly grades 1 and 2), cardiovascular toxicity (mostly transient hypotension), and fever/febrile neutropenia. The median survivals on both arms were comparable (A: 15.5 months vs. no-A: 15.6 months, $P = 0.65$).

Overall, RTOG 98-01 does not support the hypothesis that amifostine reduces esophagitis (or pneumonitis) in the context of chemotherapy and twice-daily radiation for patients with locally advanced/inoperable NSCLC. At the same time, some of the secondary endpoints (e.g., patient-derived self-assessments) suggest a possible advantage to amifostine that should be further explored with alternative dosing/administration schedules. Preliminary results in this context appear promising with subcutaneous amifostine[56] which is certainly more "user-friendly" to use in the radiation clinic. At this time, the role of amifostine in lung cancer remains unclear.

Other strategies to minimize esophagitis should also be investigated. Emerging data utilizing 3-D conformal radiation with chemotherapy suggests that promising results can be obtained with significantly less esophagitis.[61] Ultimately, further improvements may be obtained with more sophisticated technology, such as IMRT, making sure to account for tissue inhomogeneity and respiratory/target motion.[62] An entirely different "biologic" strategy under development involves the use of manganese superoxide dismutase.[63] Ultimately, the goal of treatment must be to improve not only the quantity, but also the quality of survival of patients with lung cancer.

E. CONCLUSION

Three-dimensional conformal radiation therapy has greatly enhanced our understanding of partial organ tolerances of lung and esophagus to radiotherapy. Concurrent chemotherapy appears to shift the TCP and NTCP dose–response curves to the left for both lung and esophagus. Much additional work remains to be performed before biological modifiers, either radiosensitizers or radioprotectors, become a more integral part of therapy. Summaries of clinical data indicate that both patient-related and treatment-related factors contribute to normal tissue toxicity in these organs.

REFERENCES

1. Emami, B, J Lyman, A Brown, L Coia, M Goitein, JE Munzenrider, B Shank, LJ Solin, and M Wesson. 1991. Tolerance of normal tissue to therapeutic irradiation. Int J Radiat Oncol Biol Phys **21:**109–122.
2. Groover, TA, AC Christie, and EA Merritt. 1922. Observations on the use of a copper filter in the roentgen treatment of deep-seated malignancies. South Med J **15:**440.
3. Evans, WA and T Leucutia. 1925. Intrathoracic changes induced by heavy radiation. Am J Radiol **13:**203.
4. Gross, NJ. 1977. Pulmonary effects of radiation therapy. Ann Intern Med **86:**81.
5. MacDonald, S, P Rubin, and Maasilita P. 1989. Response of normal lung to irradiation. Front Radiat Ther Oncol **23:**255–276.
6. Rosiello, RA and Merrill WW. 1990. Radiation-induced lung injury. Clin Chest Med **11:**65–71.
7. Penney, D, D Siemann, P Rubin, D Shapiro, J Finkelstein, and R Cooper. 1982. Morphologic changes reflecting early and late effects of irradiation on the distal lung of the mouse review. Scan Electron Microsc **1:**413–425.
8. Rubin, P, D Shapiro, J Finklestein, and D Penney. 1980. The early release of surfactant following lung irradiation of alveolar type II cells. Int J Radiat Oncol Biol Phys **6:**75–77.

9. Law, MP and RG Ahier. 1989. Vascular and epithelial damage in the lung of the mouse after x-rays or neutrons. Radiat Res **117:**128–144.
10. Law, MP. 1981. Radiation induced vascular injury and its relation to late effects on normal tissues. Adv Radiat Biol **9:**37.
11. Gross, N. 1980. Experimental radiation pneumonitis IV. Leakage of circulatory proteins onto the alveolar surface. J Lab Clin Med **45:**19–31.
12. Shapiro, DL, JN Finkelstein, DP Penny, DW Seimann, and P Rubin. 1982. Sequential effects of irradiation on the pulmonary surfactant system. Int J Radiat Oncol Biol Phys **8:**879–882.
13. Holt, JAG. 1964. The acute radiation pneumonitis syndrome. J Coll Radiol Aust **8:**40.
14. Graham, MV, JA Purdy, B Emami, W Harms, W Bosch, MA Lockett, and CA Perez. 1999. Clinical dose–volume histogram analysis for pneumonitis after 3D treatment for non-small cell lung cancer (NSCLC). Int J Radiat Oncol Biol Phys **45:**323–329.
15. Munley, MT, LB Marks, C Scarfone, GS Sibley, EF Patz, TG Turkington, RJ Jaszczak, DR Gilland, MS Anscher, and RE Coleman. 1999. Multimodality nuclear medicine imaging in three-dimensional radiation treatment planning for lung cancer: challenges and prospects. Lung Cancer **23:**105–114.
16. Kutcher, GJ and C Burman. 1991. Calculation of complication probability factors for non-uniform normal tissue irradiation: the effective volume method. Int J Radiat Oncol Biol Phys **2:**137–146.
17. Kutcher, GJ, C Burman, L Brewster, M Goitein, and R Mohan. 1991. Histogram reduction method for calculating complication probabilities for three-dimensional treatment planning evaluations. Int J Radiat Oncol Biol Phys **21:**137–146.
18. Lyman, JT and B Wolbarst. 1989. Optimization of radiation therapy; IV: a dose–volume histogram reduction algorithm. Int J Radiat Oncol Biol Phys **17:**433–436.
19. Niemierko, A. 1993. Reporting and analyzing dose distributions: a concept equivalent to uniform dose. Med Phys **24:**103–110.
20. Kwa, SL, JC Theuws, and A Wagennar. 1998. Evaluation of two dose–volume histogram reduction models for prediction of radiation pneumonitis. Radiother Oncol **48:**61–69.
21. Seppenwoold, Y, J Lebesque, K Jaeger, J Belderbos, L Boersma, C Schilstra, G Henning, J Hayman, K Martel, and RT Haken. 2003. Comparing different NTCP models that predict the incidence of radiation pneumonitis. Int J Radiat Oncol Biol Phys **55:**724–735.
22. Bradley, JD, WL Thorstad, S Mutic, TR Miller, F Dehdashti, BA Siegel, W Bosch, and R Bertrand, Impact of FDG-PET on Radiation Therapy Volume in Non-Small Cell Lung Cancer. International Journal of Radiation Oncology Biology Physics 2004; **59(1)**:78–86
23. Hernando, M, L Marks, G Bentel, S Zhou, D Hollis, S Das, M Fan, M Munley, T Shafman, M Anscher, and P Lind. 2001. Radiation-induced pulmonary toxicity: a dose–volume histogram analysis in 201 patients with lung cancer. Int J Radiat Oncol Biol Phys **51:**650–659.
24. Yorke, E, A Jackson, K Rosenzweig, S Merrick, D Gabrys, E Venkatraman, C Burman, S Leibel, and C Ling. 2002. Dose–volume factors contribution to the incidence of radiation pneumonitis in non-small-cell lung cancer patients treated with three-dimensional conformal radiation therapy. Int J Radiat Oncol Biol Phys **54:**329–339.
25. Tsujino, K, S Hirota, M Endo, K Obayashi, Y Kotani, M Satouchi, T Kado, and Y Takada. 2003. Predictive value of dose–volume histogram parameters for predicting radiation pneumonitis after concurrent chemoradiation for lung cancer. Int J Radiat Oncol Biol Phys **55:**110–115.
26. Onishi, H, K Kuriyama, M Yamaguchi, T Komiyama, S Tanaka, T Araki, K Nishikawa, and I Ishihara. 2003. Concurrent two-dimensional radiotherapy and weekly docetaxel in the treatment of stage III non-small cell lung cancer: a good local response but no good survival due to radiation pneumonitis. Lung Cancer **40:**79–84.
27. Stromberg, JS, MB Sharpe, LH Kim, VR Kini, DA Jaffray, AA Martinez, and JW Wong. 1999. The use of active breathing control (ABC) to reduce margin for breathing motion. Int J Radiat Oncol Biol Phys **44:**911–919.
28. Stromberg, JS, MB Sharpe, LH Kim, VR Kini, DA Jaffray, AA Martinez, and JW Wong. 2000. Active breathing control (ABC) for Hodgkin's disease: reduction in normal tissue irradiation with deep inspiration and implications for treatment. Int J Radiat Oncol Biol Phys **48:**–806.
29. Hanley, J, MM Debois, D Mah, GS Mageras, A Raben, K Rsenzweig, B Mychalczak, LH Schwartz, PJ Gloeggler, W Lutz, CC Ling, SA Leibel, Z Fuks, and GJ Kutcher. 1999. Deep inspiration breath-hold technique for lung tumors: the potential value of target immobilization and reduced lung density in dose escalation. Int J Radiat Oncol Biol Phys **45:**603–611.
30. Rosenzweig, KE, J Hanley, D Mah, G Mageras, M Hunt, S Toner, C Burman, CC Ling, B Mychalczak, Z Fuks, and SA Leibel. 2000. The deep inspiration breath-hold technique in the treatment of inoperable non-small-cell lung cancer. Int J Radiat Oncol Biol Phys **48:**81–87.

31. Shirato, H, S Shimizu, T Kunieda, K Kitamura, M van Herk, K Kagei, T Nishioka, S Hashimoto, K Fujita, H Aoyama, K Tsuchiya, K Kudo, and K Miyasaka. 2000. Physical aspects of a real-time tumor-tracking system for gated radiotherapy. Int J Radiat Oncol Biol Phys **48:**1187–1195.
32. Kubo, H, P Len, S Minohara, and H Mostafavi. 2000. Breathing-synchronized radiotherapy program at the University of California Davis Cancer Center. Med Phys **27:**346–353.
33. Neicu, T, H Shirato, Y Seppenwoolde, and S Jiang. 2003. Synchronized moving aperture radiation therapy (SMART): average tumor trajectory for lung patients. Phys Med Biol **48:**587–598.
34. Low, D, J Bradley, J Dempsey, D Politte, K Islam, M Mutic, J Deasy, C Zakarian, and G Christensen. 2002. A method for the four-dimensional measurement of normal and cancerous lung during free breathing (Abstract). Int J Radiat Oncol Biol Phys **54:**199.
35. Low, D, M Nystrom, E Kalinin, P Parikh, J Dempsey, J Bradley, S Mutic, S Wahab, T Islam, G Christiansen, D Politte, and B Whiting. 2003. A method for the reconstruction of four-dimensional synchronized CT scans acquired during free breathing. Med Phys **30:**1254–1263.
36. Ward, W, Y Kim, A Molteni, and N Soliday. 1988. Radiation-induced pulmonary endothelial dysfunction in rats: modification by an inhibitor of angiotensin converting enzyme. Int J Radiat Oncol Biol Phys **15:**135–140.
37. Ward, WF, A Molteni, CH Ts'ao, and JM Hinz. 1990. Captopril reduces collagen and mast cell accumulation in irradiatated rat lung. Int J Radiat Oncol Biol Phys **19:**1405–1409.
38. Gopal, R, S Tucker, R Komaki, Z Liao, K Forster, C Stevens, J Kelly, and G Starkschall. 2003. The relationship between local dose and loss of function for irradiated lung. Int J Radiat Oncol Biol Phys **56:**106–113.
39. Seaman, WB and LV Ackerman. 1957. The effect of radiation on the esophagus: a clinical and histologic study on the effects produced by the betatron. Radiology **68:**534–541.
40. Goldstein, HM, LF Rogers, and GH Fletcher. 1975. Radiological manifestations of radiation-induced injury to the normal upper gastrointestinal tract. Radiology **117:**135–140.
41. Lepke, RA and HI Lipshitz. 1983. Radiation-induced injury of the esophagus. Radiology **148:**375–378.
42. Dillman, RO, SL Seagren, KJ Propert, J Guerra, WL Eaton, MD Perry, RW Carey, DF Frei, and MR Green. 1990. A randomized trial of induction chemotherapy plus high-dose radiation versus radiation alone in Stage III non-small cell lung cancer. N Engl J Med **323:**940–945.
43. Sause, W, P Kolesar, S Taylor, D Johnson, R Livingston, R Komaki, B Emami, W Curran, R Byhardt, AR Dar, and A Turrisi. 2000. Final results of phase III trial in regionally advanced unresectable non-small cell lung cancer: Radiation Therapy Oncology Group, Eastern Cooperative Oncology Group, and Soutwest Oncology Group. Chest **117:**358–364.
44. Choy, H, W Akerley, and S Graziano. 1998. Multiinstitutional phase II trial of paclitaxel, carboplatin, and concurrent radiation therapy for locally advanced non-small-cell lung cancer. J Clin Oncol **16:**3316–3322.
45. Byhardt, RW, C Scott, WT Sause, B Emami, R Komaki, B Fisher, JS Lee, and C Lawton. 1998. Response, toxicity, failure patterns, and survival in five radiation therapy oncology group (RTOG) trials os sequential and/or concurrent chemotherapy and radiotherapy for locally advanced non-small-cell carcinoma of the lung. Int J Radiat Oncol Biol Phys **42:**469–478.
46. Singh, AK, MA Lockett, and JD Bradley. 2003. Predictors of radiation-induced esophageal toxicity in patients with non-small cell lung cancer treated with three-dimensional conformal radiation therapy. Int J Radiat Oncol Biol Phys **55:**337–341.
47. Maguire, P, G Sibley, S Zhou, T Jamieson, K Light, P Antione, JI Herndon, M Anscher, and L Marks. 1999. Clinical and dosimetric predictors of radiation-induced esophageal toxicity. Int J Radiat Oncol Biol Phys **45:**97–103.
48. Werner-Wasik, M, E Pequignot, and D Leeper. 2000. Predictors of severe esophagitis include use of concurrent chemotherapy, but not the length of the irradiated esophagus: a multivariate analysis of patients with lung cancer treated with nonoperative therapy. Int J Radiat Oncol Biol Phys **48:**689–696.
49. Bradley, J, J Deasy, S Bentzen, and IE Naqa. 2002. Dosimetric correlates for acute esophagitis in patients treated with radiation therapy for lung carcinoma. Int J Radiat Oncol Biol Phys **54:**105.
50. McGinnis, WL, CL Loprinzi, SJ Buskirk, JA Sloan, RG Drummond, AR Frank, TG Shanahan, SP Kahanic, RL Moore, SE Schild, and SL Humphrey. 1997. Placebo-controlled trial of sucralfate for inhibiting radiation-induced esophagitis. J Clin Oncol **15:**1239–1243.
51. Calabro-Jones, P, R Fahey, G Smoluk, and J Ward. 1985. Alkaine phosphatase promotes radioprotection and accumulation of WR-1065 in V79-171 cells incubated in medium containing WR-27821. Int J Radiat Oncol Biol Phys **47:**23–27.
52. Tannehill, S and M Mehta. 1996. Amifostine and radiation therapy: past, present, and future. Semin Oncol **23:**69–77.

53. Antonadou, D, N Coliarakis, M Synodinou, H Anthanassiou, A Kouveli, C Verigos, G Georgakopoulos, K Panoussaki, P Karageorgis, and N Throuvalas. 2001. Randomized phase III trial of radiation treatment +/− amifostine in patients with advanced-stage lung cancer. Int J Radiat Oncol Biol Phys **51:**915–922.
54. Antonadou, D, N Thruvalas, A Petridis, N Bolanos, A Sagriotis, and M Synodinou. 2003. Effect of amifostine on toxicities associated with radiochemotherapy in patients with locally advanced non-small-cell lung caner. Int J Radiat Oncol Biol Phys **57:**402–408.
55. Komaki, R, J Lee, B Kaplan, P Allen, J Kelly, Z Liao, and C Stevens. 2002. Randomized phase III study of chemoradiation with or without amifostine for patients with favorable performance status inoperable stage II–III non-small ell lung cancer: preliminary results. Semin Radiat Oncol **12:**46–49.
56. Koukourakis, MI, G Kryrias, S Kakolyris, C Kouroussis, C Frangiadaki, A Giatromanolaki, G Retalis, and V Georgoulias. 2000. Subcutaneous administration of amifostine during fractionated radiotherapy: a randomized phase II study. J Clin Oncol **18:**2226–2233.
57. Leong, SS, EH Tan, KW Fong, E Wilder-Smith, YK Ong, BC Tai, L Chew, SH Lim, J Wee, KM Lee, KF Foo, and PT Ang. 2003. Randomized double-blind trial of combined modality treatment with or without amifostine in unresectable stage III non-small-cell lung cancer. J Clin Oncol **21:**1767–1774.
58. Senzer, N. 2002. Rationale for a phase III study of erythropoietin as a neurocognitive protectant in patients with lung caner receiving prophylactic cranial irradiation. Semin Oncol **29:**47–52.
59. Aaronson, NK, S Ahmedzai, B Bergman, M Bullinger, A Cull, N Duez, A Filiberti, H Flechtner, SB Fleishman, and JC de Haes. 1993. The European Organization for Research and Treatment of Cancer QLQ-C30: a quality-of-life instrument for use in international clinical trials in oncology. J Natl Cancer Inst **85:**365–376.
60. Bergman, B, NK Aaronson, S Ahmedzai, S Kaasa, and M Sullivan. 1994. The EORTC QLQ-LC13: a modular supplement to the EORTC Core quality of life questionnaire (QLQ-C30) for use in lung cancer clinical trials. EORTC Study Group on Quality of Life. Eur J Cancer and Clinical Oncology **30A:**635–642.
61. Rosenman, JG, JS Halle, MA Socinski, K Deschesne, DT Moore, H Johnson, R Fraser, and DE Morris. 2002. High-dose conformal radiotherapy for treatment of stage IIIA/B non-small cell lung cancer: technical issues and results of a phase I/II trial. Int J Radiat Oncol Biol Phys **54:**348–356.
62. Grills, I, D Yan, A Martinez, F Vicini, J Wong, and L Kestin. 2003. Potential for reduced toxicity and dose escalation in the treatment of inoperable non-small cell lung cancer: a comparison of intensity-modulated radiation therapy (IMRT), 3D conformal radiation, and elective nodal irradiation. Int J Radiat Oncol Biol Phys **57:**875–890.
63. Greenberger, JS, MW Epperly, J Gretton, M Jefferson, S Nie, M Bernarding, V Kagan, and HL Guo. 2003. Radioprtective gene therapy. Curr Gene Ther **3:**183–195.
64. Kwa, SLS, JV Lebesque, JCM Theuws, LB Marks, MT Munley, G Bentel, D Oetzel, U Spahn, MV Graham, RE Drzymala, JA Purdy, AS Lichter, MK Martel, and RK Ten Haken. 1998. Radiation pneumonitis as a function of mean dose: an analysis of pooled data of 540 patients. Int J Radiat Oncol Biol Phys **42:**1–9.

4. TOXICITY FROM RADIATION IN BREAST CANCER

JULIA WHITE, MD

Medical College of Wisconsin, Milwaukee, WI

MICHAEL C. JOINER, Ph.D.

Karmanos Cancer Institute and Wayne State University, Detroit, MI

Breast cancer is probably among the most common diagnoses found on daily patient treatment lists in the majority of Radiation Oncology departments. This makes understanding what type of toxicity to expect from radiation for breast cancer and its management of prime importance, since it affects significant numbers of patients daily. Radiation for breast cancer is predominantly to the intact breast for early stage disease with post-mastectomy radiation comprising a smaller proportion of radiation delivered for this diagnosis. The acute toxicity that develops as well as the type of late sequelae that can occur in each of these treatment scenarios is similar. During intact breast or chest-wall radiation, the organs commonly at risk for radiation injuries that manifest as acute and late toxicity include skin, chest wall, lung, and heart. When regional nodal irradiation is added, the shoulder, brachial plexus, and axillary lymphatics are also at risk for potential injury.

In general, radiation for breast cancer post-lumpectomy and post-mastectomy is very well tolerated by most patients and does not significantly impair their daily activities. Acute side effects of treatment are generally common in occurrence, self-limiting, and resolve within 4–6 weeks after the treatment is completed. Skin reactions and the constitutional symptom of fatigue dominate the early toxicity profile. Late toxicity or permanent sequelae can be divided into two groups: the more common effects on the appearance of the breast such as persistent breast edema, hyperpigmentation, and fibrosis and those that are very uncommon but can have significant health consequences as a result of permanent injury to other organs such as brachial plexopathy, radiation pneumonitis, cardiac morbidity, or secondary malignancy.

A. ACUTE REACTIONS

A1. Skin

Skin reaction is the most common side effect during breast cancer radiation. Over 90% of women who receive radiation for breast cancer will as a result develop some skin changes during their course of treatment.[1]

Skin is divided into two main sections: the outermost layers or epidermis and the deeper layers or dermis. Acute radiation changes in the skin primarily reflect injury to the epidermis.[2,3] The epidermis is composed of several layers. The stratum corneum is the outer most layer, which is made up of flattened dead cells and comprises approximately 25% of the total epidermal thickness. Beneath the stratum corneum is a thin layer called the stratum granulosum, which is a transitional layer between the non-viable stratum corneum above and the viable layers below. The viable layers include the stratum spinosum, which contains mostly post-mitotic cells. The deepest layer, where the majority of the cell division occurs, is the basal cell layer. The basal cell layer is the primary target for radiation injury that results in the clinically visible acute radiation skin reactions.

Approximately half the cells produced in the basal layer undergo the process of terminal transition.[2] From the basal layer, post-mitotic cells enter the more superficial viable layer stratum spinosum, then into the transitional region or the stratum granulosum. In this layer, the cells become flattened, lose the nucleus and other organelles, and ultimately become mature, keratinized, or cornified cells of the stratum corneum. From the stratum corneum, cells detach and desquamate, but are continually replaced by cells produced in the basal layer that undergo terminal transition. The entire epidermis turns over on average in about 30 days.

The thickness of the dermis varies from 1 to 3 mm and contains blood vessels, nerves, hair follicles, and various glands. The dermis is subdivided into two layers: the superficial papillary layer and the deeper reticular dermis. The papillary layer is highly vascularized. The reticular dermis has the characteristic bundles of collagen fibers that give the skin its biomechanical properties.[2,3]

Radiation-induced changes in the skin are characterized by several phases. A transient early erythema can be seen within a few hours after radiation and subsides after 24–48 hours.[2] This is believed to be an inflammatory response, i.e., histamine-like substances are released that cause dermal edema and skin erythema from the permeability and dilatation of capillaries. The main erythematous reaction occurs 3–6 weeks after the radiation begins and reflects a varying severity of loss of epidermal basal cells. It has been shown that the fields treated with 2 Gy daily fractionation do not show changes in the basal cell density until total doses of 20–25 Gy are delivered.[3] The reddening of the skin is thought to represent a secondary inflammatory reaction or hyperemia.[2,3] With higher radiation doses, there is a marked reduction in the number of mitotic cells and an increase in degenerate cells. If cells are not being reproduced at the same rate in the basal cell layer and the normal migration of cells to the stratum corneum continues, the epidermis becomes denuded in the time equivalent to its natural turnover, or approximately 30 days. When sufficient numbers of clonogenic cells in the basal layer persist to sustain repopulation, atypical thickening of the stratum corneum may be seen and the patient will experience dry flaking skin in the treated area, or dry desquamation. This is typically seen at doses ≥45 Gy. If new cell proliferation is inadequate, moist desquamation with exposed dermis and oozing of serum occurs. The repopulation of the basal layer of the epidermis after irradiation is predominantly from the surviving clonogenic cells within the irradiated area. This is typical of moist desquamation that occurs between the does of 45 and 50 Gy with 2 Gy fractionation. Total skin doses of ≥60 Gy are associated with moist desquamation that does not heal as well.[2,3] When an area of irradiated skin is completely denuded of clonogenic epithelial cells, the healing of moist desquamation must occur totally as a result of the division and migration of viable cells from the skin around the irradiated area. When large areas of skin are irradiated to high doses such that the reproductive cells in the basal layer are depleted, cell migration from the edges of the field can be ineffective. In such situations, secondary ulceration involving the loss of dermal tissue can occur as a result of infection or trauma.

If radiation continues at a time when moist desquamation is evident, then further injury may lead to dermal and subcutaneous necrosis. Necrosis has been characterized by the damage of blood vessels in the dermis and is evidenced by the loss of endothelial cells and reduction in dermal blood flow prior to the onset of necrosis.

The radiation doses utilized for breast cancer treatment are typically 45–50.4 Gy with 1.8–2.0 Gy fractionations to larger fields for the intact breast, chest wall, or nodal sites. Cumulative doses of 60–66 Gy may be given to smaller boost volumes of the lumpectomy site or chest wall. With this standard dosing, breast radiation will result in 80–90% of patients developing some skin erythema and dry desquamation; in 30–50% of patients, the erythema is more severe and is associated with skin tenderness; in 5–10% of patients, patchy moist desquamation confined mostly to skin folds can be seen; and in <5% of patients, confluent moist desquamation occurs.[1]

An understanding of what to expect for a typical acute skin reaction from standard breast cancer radiation is important so that a foundation exists for evaluating products and techniques that hope to prevent or treat these symptoms. A useful prospective study was done that carefully documented the skin reactions each week of 126 breast cancer patients receiving breast radiation after lumpectomy and axillary node dissection.[1] In this study, the whole breast received 45 Gy in daily fractions of 1.8 Gy with a 20 Gy electron boost delivered by 1 field daily with 2 Gy fractions. Patients were treated 5 days/week. A modified Radiation Therapy Oncology Group (RTOG) scoring system for acute skin reactions was used, which made patchy moist desquamation limited to skin fold scored as 2.5 instead of 2 (Table 1). The irradiated breast was divided into eight sections for observation: sternum, axilla, UOQ, UIQ, LOQ, LIQ, nipple, and inframammary fold. In addition to the skin observations, a VAS pain score and written description of topical agents used was recorded as well. The range of skin reactions recorded in the nine regions of the breast is shown in Table 2. This demonstrated that during weeks 1–2, skin reactions are uncommon. During week 3, almost 50% of the patients had developed mild erythema and for up to 12% more severe erythema was seen. By week 4, about 80% of the patients demonstrated skin changes with 20% of these being more severe. The emergence of patchy moist desquamation in skin folds was also

Table 1. RTOG acute toxicity scoring for skin[4]

Toxicity score	0	1	2	3	4
Description	No change over baseline	Follicular, faint or dull erythema, dry desquamation, epilation, decreased sweating	Tender or bright erythema, patchy moist desquamation,* moderate edema	Confluent moist desquamation, other than skin folds, pitting edema	Ulceration, hemorrhage, necrosis

*Confined to skin folds.

Table 2. Acute skin toxicity (range) in 126 breast cancer patients during a course of breast radiation after lumpectomy.[1] Patients (%) demonstrating modified RTOG toxicity score

	Score					
Week	0	1	2	2.5	3	4
1	98–100*	0–1	0–1	0	0	0
2	94–98	0–5	0–1	0	0	0
3	33–46	40–48	4–18	0	0	0
4	16–22	49–65	4–18	0	0	0
5	4–8	52–67	24–40	1–8	0–2	0
6	6–16	38–63	6–33	2–10	0–2	0
7	8–28	41–57	6–38	0–10	0–2	0

*All percentages estimated from bar graph.

Table 3. Worse observed skin toxicity with best supportive care during a course of breast radiation following lumpectomy. Patients (%) with RTOG SCORE

Study	*N*	0	1	2	3	4
Porock[1,*]	126	8	63	31	2	0
Fischer[17]	89	7	58	32	3	0

*Weeks 5 and 6.

seen in week 4. The frequency of reactions was at its worse during weeks 5–6. Patchy moist desquamation occurred in four sites: sternum, axilla, UOQ, and inframammary fold during the radiation course, and confluent moist desquamation occurred only in the axilla. This description of the acute skin reaction for breast radiation is confirmed when one looks at the best supportive care arm of the RTOG 97-13 study (Table 3) and finds very similar percentages of acute toxicity scores.

The pain scores associated with the acute skin reactions in the Podrock study are listed in Table 4. From this it is seen that, overall, the vast majority of patients did not develop significant pain associated with their course of breast radiation. The highest frequency of pain scores >0 occurred during week 6. At that time, 17% of patients developed pain: 9.6% scored their pain as 1–3 or mild, 6.3% scored it at 4–6 or moderate, and 0.9% had

Table 4. Distribution of 126 breast cancer patients according to VAS pain scores during a course of breast radiation following lumpectomy[1]

	Pain VAS (%)								
Week	0	1	2	3	4	5	6	8	9
1	99.2	0.8							
2	98.4	0.8	0.8						
3	96.8		2.4	0.8					
4	92.8	0.8	0.8	1.6	3.2			0.8	
5	87.3	1.6	2.4	3.2	1.6	2.4	0.8	0.8	
6*	83.2	2.7	6.0	0.9	1.8	1.8	2.7		0.9
7†	88.6		4.4	0.9	1.8	1.8	2.7		

*$N = 115$.
†$N = 114$.
Reprinted with permission.

severe pain scored at 9. By week 7, this fell to 12% scoring >0 on the pain scale and 6 was the highest pain level scored.

Multiple factors in this population were found to be associated with more severe acute skin reactions. These included mean patient weight, breast size ≥D-cup, lymphocele aspiration, and being a current smoker.[1]

The use of topical agents was also recorded in this study. The percent of patients using a topical agent by week was 0%, week 1; 11%, week 2; 37%, week 3; 53%, week 4; 56%, week 5; 57%, week 6; and 39%, week 6. The choice of cream in this study was based on the nurse's assessment. These experiences lead them to recommend light moisturizers in the early phase of treatment, with a switch to thicker oil-based products for the peak of the reaction if necessary.

There have been numerous studies evaluating the benefit of applying a topical agent to the skin during the course of breast radiation (Table 5). Although studies examining various topical agents appeared shortly after x-ray therapy emerged a century ago,[5] this discussion will focus on studies primarily in breast cancer patients published since 1990. The intention of most of these studies has been prevention of, instead of treatment for, acute radiation skin toxicity.

A Canadian study evaluated the impact of not washing versus washing the skin on the acute skin reactions for 100 breast cancer patients.[6] The washing patients had significantly lower worst RTOG acute toxicity scores ($P < 0.04$), and less frequently developed moist desquamation (14% vs. 33%, $P < 0.03$). No significant difference between arms for the occurrence of dry desquamation was seen—74% no washing and 56% washing arm. On univariate analysis, washing, chemotherapy, concomitant chemotherapy schedule, weight >165 lb, and dosimetric hotspot were all predictors ofworse acute skin toxicity. On multivariate analysis, concomitant chemotherapy schedule, weight >165 lb, and dosimetric hotspot remained the strongest predictors of increased skin toxicity. Non-washing was weakly associated ($P = 0.06$).

Another study from Norway evaluated no cream versus the use of Bepanthen® cream during radiotherapy in 86 patients with each patient serving as their own control.[7]

Table 5. Prospective trials in breast cancer patients evaluating topical agents for reduction of acute radiation skin reaction

Topical agents	*N*	Author	Study design	Toxicity scoring	Results	*P*
Washing versus no washing	100	Roy[6]	Randomized	RTOG	Washing: less skin reaction less moist desquamation	0.03
Bepanthen versus placebo	86	Lokkevik[7]	Randomized double blind	Institution*	Less desquamation	
Hyalurenic acid versus placebo†	130	Ligouri[10]	Randomized	Institution	Reduced skin toxicity wks 3–7	<0.001
Chamomile cream versus almond oil	50	Maiche[8]	Pt own control	Institution	No significant difference in maximal toxicity score	NS
Sucralfate cream versus placebo	50	Maiche[9]	Pt own control, physician blinded	Institution	Reduced grade II toxicity with faster recovery time	0.05
Aloe vera versus placebo	194	Williams[11]	Randomized double blind	Modified RTOG	No difference maximal radiation reaction or weekly scores	NS
Aloe vera versus observation	106	Williams[11]	Randomized double blind	Modified RTOG	No difference maximal radiation reaction or weekly scores	NS
					No difference erythema, moist desquamation	<0.001
Aloe vera versus aqueous cream	208	Heggie[12]	Randomized double blind	Institution	Aloe vera: more dry desquamation, more pain	0.003
Aloe vera versus soap	77	Olsen[13]	Randomized	RTOG	Aloe vera may delay onset skin reactions	NS
MMF‡ (steroid) versus emollient cream	49	Bostrom[14]	Randomized double blind	Institution	MMF: < maximal erythema	0.011
					< burning	0.069
					< itching	0.087
0.1% Methyl prednisone versus 0.5% dexpanthenol versus control	36	Schmuth[15]	Randomized double blind	Institution	Reduced mean toxicity severity with steroids	<0.005
0.2% Hydrocortisone versus placebo†	21	Potera[16]	Pt own control	Institution	No significant difference	NS
Biafine versus best supportive care	172	Fisher[17]	Randomized	RTOG	No difference in maximal skin toxicity	NS
Biafine versus Lipiderm versus control	74	Fenig[19]	Randomized	RTOG	No difference in maximal skin toxicity	NS
Biafine	60	Szumacher[18]	Prospective single arm	RTOG	Less severe toxicity than expected when giving chemotherapy concomitantly	
Biafine versus Calendula	245	Pommier[20]	Randomized	RTOG	Calendula: < grade 2–3 toxicity	0.001
					< pain	0.003

*Institution developed and used its own toxicity scoring scale.
†Small percentage of breast cancer patients.
‡Mometasone furoate cream (Elocon®).

Bepanthen®, or dexpanthenol cream, had been used extensively at the reporting institution for acute skin reactions. Eighty percent of the patients were breast cancer patients and the rest were laryngeal cancer patients. Each patient applied the Bepanthen® cream twice-daily beginning with the first day of treatment to half the field and none to the other half. The evaluators were kept blinded. Three patients discontinued the Bepanthen® cream because of "untoward or allergic" reactions. There was a statistically significant reduction in desquamation with the use of the cream. With further analysis, this effect on desquamation was mainly for "low-grade lesions." The authors concluded that there was no overall significant effect of the ointment. Chamomile cream and almond ointment have also been studied in breast cancer patients in a similar fashion using the patient as her own control. Neither agent had a significant overall effect, but the almond ointment did reduce grade II toxicity.[8]

An interesting study reported a significant reduction in high-grade skin toxicity with the use of hyaluronic acid 0.2% cream (Ialugen®) compared to placebo in a population of predominantly head and neck cancer patients.[10] A double-blind randomized trial was performed in 134 patients (68% had head and neck cancer, 22% breast cancer, and 10% pelvic cancer) with the agents applied twice daily (1–2 hours after treatment and evening) for 10 weeks. No concomitant medications were allowed. The hyaluronic acid group had significantly delayed onset of skin reactions, overall less severity in toxicity, and faster resolution of reactions than the placebo group.

Aloe vera has been used by various institutions for radiation-induced skin toxicity.[11–13] Aloe vera is an extract derived from the tropical cactus genus, Aloe. It is available over the counter in a variety of preparations and used generally for other types of dermatitis such as sunburn. The North Central Cancer Treatment Group (NCCTG) and the Mayo Clinic collaboratively conducted a randomized, prospective trial evaluating aloe vera gel as a prophylactic agent for acute skin toxicity in breast cancer patients receiving either intact breast or chest-wall irradiation.[11] Two separate studies were conducted: the first was randomized in a double-blinded manner to aloe vera gel or a placebo gel, and then 108 women were randomly assigned aloe vera gel or observation. Gel application was BID and began within the first 3 days of RT and continued for 2 weeks afterward. The study allowed treatment with other topical agents once a skin reaction was demonstrated. Patients with marked erythema and pruritus were to use 1% hydrocortisone cream. An acute toxicity scoring system, somewhat similar to the one established by RTOG (Table 1) was used; however, only dry desquamation was scored as grade 2 and any moist desquamation was scored as grade 3. No significant differences were found between the two arms in either of the study leading the authors to conclude that aloe vera was unable to decrease radiation-induced dermatitis. No mention was made of the agents used for the "treatment" of dermatitis during the study and no analysis was performed to evaluate if this may have confounded the study's results. The scores of health care providers and patients were examined and revealed that they were highly correlated. It is notable that 36% of the time, patients judged their dermatitis to be more severe than did their health care provider, and for only 7% did patients judge their dermatitis as less severe than the physician ($P < 0.0001$).

Another randomized trial found some benefit from aloe vera gel in reducing erythema associated with radiation but inferior to an aqueous cream for relief of dry desquamation and pain.[12] In this study, 225 patients after lumpectomy for early stage cancer were randomized in a double-blinded fashion to use aqueous cream or 98% aloe vera gel on their skin during breast radiation. The aloe vera or aqueous cream was applied three times daily beginning with RT and continued for 2 weeks post-treatment. This study found that the cumulative probability for pain (26% vs. 16%, $P = 0.03$) and dry desquamation (70% vs. 41%, $P \leq 0.001$) was greater in the aloe vera arm compared to aqueous cream. The cumulative probability for pruritus was also higher in the aloe vera arm but did not reach statistical significance. However, statistical significance was obtained for increased >grade 2 erythema in the aqueous cream arm ($P = 0.06$). Subjects in either arm with a bra cup ≥ size D were significantly more likely to experience severe erythema when compared to smaller breast sizes.

Finally, a third study compared aloe vera gel plus mild soap to mild soap alone in a randomized blinded manner in a heterogeneous group of cancer patients receiving RT.[13] This study reported that for patients who had not shown skin reactions by 27 Gy, those patients using aloe vera had a significant delay in the onset of skin reactions ($P = 0.013$). This led the authors to speculate that aloe vera is protective for radiation dermatitis in some people.

Topical steroids have also been commonly used for the management of acute radiation skin reactions for breast cancer patients.[14–16] A small double-blind randomized study from Sweden compared mometasone furoate MMF (Elocon®) with an emollient cream in 50 breast cancer patients.[14] The agents were applied once daily, 3 times a week until 24 Gy, and then once daily until 3 weeks post-treatment. Patients using the steroid cream had statistically lower maximal erythema scores, $P = 0.011$. Less itching and burning symptoms were reported with the MMF, but it did not reach statistical significance and there was no difference in VAS pain scores between the two agents.

Another smaller double-blind randomized trial compared 0.1% methylprednisolone (Advantan®) to 0.5% dexpanthenol (Bepanthen®) in 31 breast cancer patients receiving breast radiation after lumpectomy.[15] Using a 15-point scoring system, there were fewer patients with scores ≥4 in the steroid group ($P < 0.05$), and slightly lower mean scores with methylprednisolone treatment. A skin-specific quality-of-life (QOL) tool (Skindex) demonstrated significant reduction in the dimension of embarrassment ($P < 0.05$) and approached significance for the dimensions of fear ($P = 0.06$) and physical discomfort ($P = 0.057$). The authors concluded that the use of corticosteroid reduced the clinical severity of radiation dermatitis and lessened its negative impact on the patients skin-related QOL.

Biafine is a water-based emulsion for dermal wound healing that has been used widely in France for the management of acute radiation skin reactions. Four recent studies have evaluated its efficacy in this role.[17–20] The RTOG conducted a randomized phase III trial comparing Biafine to the best supportive care for preventing or reducing acute skin toxicity in 172 women receiving breast radiation after lumpectomy.[17] There was no statistical difference in maximum toxicity, time to development of ≥grade 2 toxicity, or resolution of toxicity between the two arms. Large-breasted women (D-cup or larger) had a higher frequency of ≥grade 2 toxicity, overall. Biafine use was associated with statistically less toxicity at 6 weeks post-RT in large-breasted women ($P = 0.002$). Patients with ≥grade 2 toxicity had significantly worse QOL ($P = 0.048$).

A phase II study evaluated Biafine for 60 breast cancer patients receiving concomitant breast radiation with CMF chemotherapy.[18] Eighty-three percent had grade 2 toxicity and 2% grade 3. The authors concluded that this was less than what would probably occur with no topical therapy in this clinical scenario.

A small prospective study from Israel evaluated acute skin toxicity in 74 women receiving breast radiation after lumpectomy randomly assigned to Biafine, Lipiderm, or observation.[19] Lipiderm is a moisturizing cream popular in Israel. Patients could have additional topical therapies for radiation skin reaction if clinically warranted. There was no significant difference between the three arms for the %grades 3–4 reactions or the mean maximal score.

Finally, Biafine was compared to Calendula in 254 breast cancer patients undergoing radiation following lumpectomy or mastectomy in a Phase III randomized study from Lyon, France.[20] Calendula is fabricated from a plant of the marigold family and commercially available in France. It is used for the topical treatment of irritant dermatitis, skin lesions, and superficial burns.[20] The radiation to the intact breast was 52 Gy in 2 Gy fractions with 5 MV accelerator and a 10 Gy boost to the tumor bed with electrons. After mastectomy, the chest wall received 46 Gy with electrons. The ointment was applied at the beginning of RT, twice daily until completion. No other prophylactic agent was allowed, but treatment of > grade 2 toxicity with other topical agents was permitted. Acute skin toxicity was evaluated according to the RTOG scale in four regions: breast or chest wall, inframammary fold when present, axilla, and within the supraclavicular field. There was a lower incidence of grades 2–3 acute skin toxicity with the use of Calendula compared to Biafine, 41% versus 63%, respectively ($P < 0.001$). Grade 3 toxicity was observed in 7% who used Calendula, and in 20% who used Biafine ($P = 0.034$). When these results were examined by treated region, it was found that significant reductions in acute toxicity were primarily in the inframammary fold, axilla, and the supraclavicular field. There were no significant reductions in acute skin toxicity over the breast, chest wall, or internal mammary regions. The mean maximal pain score on the VAS was 1.54 for the Calendula and 2.1 with Biafine ($P = 0.03$). A multivariate analysis of factors associated with radiation-induced skin reactions during breast cancer treatment found that a body mass index ≥ 25 ($P < 0.001$) and type of ointment used ($P < 0.001$) were most predictive. For patients undergoing lumpectomy, chemotherapy prior to RT ($P < 0.001$), BMI ≥ 25 ($P<0.001$), and ointment used ($P= 0.001$) were risk factors for skin toxicity. The authors conclude that Calendula should be proposed as preventative treatment for patients undergoing radiation for breast cancer.

In summary, the multiple studies above that examined primarily prophylaxis of acute skin toxicity by a topical agent demonstrated some reduction in toxicity with hyaluronic acid and Calendula application. Washing the irradiated skin was also associated with less severe skin reactions. In general, topical steroids reduced symptoms, particularly erythema and pruritus. Aqueous cream application reduced the occurrence of dry desquamation in comparison to aloe vera.

At the Medical College of Wisconsin, all the breast cancer patients are put on a light moisturizer (Clean and Moist®) during their first week of treatment to be used twice daily and continued until 4 weeks post-radiation. If patients cannot tolerate this product, they are instead given Biafine or some other comparable moisturizer. A switch is made to a thicker oil-based product (typically Aquaphor®) as necessary later in the treatment course depending on the severity of reactions that develop. Patients are asked to apply the moisturizer at least 2 hours before each radiation treatment to minimize a potential bolus effect. A steroid cream (e.g. Synalaar, Lidex) is prescribed for those patients who develop significant pruritus and/or a raised bumpy follicular rash associated with their skin erythema. Patients are encouraged to take acetaminophen, ibuprofen, or other over-the-counter non-steroidal pain relievers as directed for breast discomfort. For that small percentage of patients who develop pain >3/10 on the VAS scale that does not respond to the measures above, a narcotic analgesic is prescribed. We have commonly used Ultracet or Tylenol with codeine for this as tolerated. We find the most common need for narcotic type pain medication is to help patients sleep more comfortably at night. It is our observation that patients experience two different types of breast discomfort during radiation. The first type is associated with the skin reaction and is localized to the most severe skin changes. This is the discomfort for which analgesics are most often prescribed. The second type is sharp shooting pains in the breast that patients tend to report in the latter half of treatment that are unrelated to the severity of the skin reaction. Patients refer to these as "zingers," or "electric shock" type pains. These become less frequent following the completion of treatment and resolve over the next several weeks.

On average, >80% of acute skin toxicity during breast radiation is grades 1–2 with moist desquamation confined to the skin fold areas such as the axilla or the inframammary fold. The incidence of grade 3 acute skin toxicity in the studies detailed above (and in Table 5) averaged about 11% (range 0–40%). When moist desquamation does occur, it is recommended that the RT is held or, if possible, the affected area of the skin is blocked out of the field, particularly when radiating for breast conservation. Moist desquamation is associated with an increased risk of late telangiectasia development that can contribute to cosmetic failure.

Very little information exists examining the optimal method for managing radiation-induced moist desquamation. Instead, moist desquamation has been approached with the general principles of wound healing that applies to injuries from other mechanisms. The prevailing philosophy has been that wound healing is more rapid in a moist environment. As a result, hydrocolloid (HC) dressings have been used increasingly for radiation-induced moist desquamation. HC dressings are pliable sheets made of material such as pectin or gelatin with a polyurethane backing. Studies have demonstrated their benefit in a wide range of injuries including pressure sores, leg ulcers, donor sites, and minor burns.[21,22] The HC dressing absorbs wound exudate and forms a gel that keeps the wound surface moist. It has also been shown to be an effective barrier for bacteria. They are best for low to moderate exudate wounds. There are limited data examining their efficacy in radiation-induced moist desquamation. One study compared a Tegaderm type dressing to a conventional dressing (hydrous lanolin gauze) in 16 patients and found shorter overall healing time in patients where the Tegaderm type dressing was used.[23] Other studies have demonstrated that occlusive HC dressings reduced healing time for management of moist desquamation.[24] An interesting study from Hong Kong randomly assigned 42 patients with mostly head and neck cancers who had developed moist desquamation to a HC dressing or application of gentian violet for management.[25] There was no significant difference in the overall healing time between the two therapies. However, although patients assigned to HC dressings experienced increased discomfort associated with dressing changes, patients were more satisfied with the HC dressings and rated them with a higher mean comfort score ($P = 0.0002$) and a better aesthetic acceptance ($P = 0.007$).

When moist desquamation occurs from breast radiation, our clinic uses HC dressings. The challenge is to get these dressings to conform and stick to areas such as the axillary, inframammary, or supraclavicular folds. Frequently, a secondary dressing such as dry gauze or an ABD is placed over the HC dressing and then gauze mesh tubes (Stockinette) or gauze bandage (kerlex) is fitted around the thorax to keep everything in place. The dressing is removed for treatment. After treatment, the nursing staff gently cleans and débrides as much as possible any necrotic material within the desquamating area with normal saline and reapplies the dressing. Patients change the dressings again at home as necessary depending on the amount of exudate. It has been our experience, as well as others,[1] that patients with tender, dry desquamation are more comfortable with the application of a HC dressing.

Avoidance of moist desquamation is a major goal of the skin care strategy during radiation therapy for breast cancer. In review of the studies above, larger BMI, patient size, and/or breast size, and skin folds were consistent predictors of more severe skin reactions. It is crucial that this be taken into consideration at the time of simulation when the patient's treatment position is set and immobilization established. When establishing the patient's treatment position, techniques should be used to minimize significant inframammary or axillary redundant skin folds where the incidence of moist desquamation is high. This can be a challenge to accomplish for larger and/or ptotic breasts that tend to hang laterally on the chest wall or inferiorly on the abdominal wall. A breast ring and cup have been advocated for this purpose.[26] These are fitted around or over the breast and fastened to keep the breast upright on the chest wall to avoid skin redundancies. These have been shown to have some bolus effect and can worsen acute skin toxicity.[26] Our institution and others have used a prone breast radiation technique in this group of women with larger and/or ptotic breasts.[27,28] Using a 3-dimensional radiation therapy technique, a homogenous dose distribution can be achieved comparable to the supine position in patients with smaller breasts.

Concurrent chemotherapy with breast radiation has also been associated with worse acute skin toxicity in many series.[29–34] Select series are shown in Table 6 demonstrating a higher rate of grade 3 skin toxicity with combined modality therapy. Anthracycline-based chemotherapy in particular has been associated with severe acute skin toxicity when given concomitantly with breast radiation.[31,34] Conflicting results are observed with concomitant CMF and paclitaxel chemotherapy. Caution is advised in delivering chemotherapy together with breast radiation given the potential for worse acute toxicity and no consistent evidence that it offers a benefit in terms of survival and/or local regional recurrence rates over sequential therapy.

Table 6. Acute skin toxicity from concurrent radiation and chemotherapy for breast cancer

Regimen evaluated	Author	Patient population	% Grade 3 toxicity	% Other toxicity	Conclusion
Paclitaxel every 3 weeks	Ellerbroeck[29]	24 BCT s/p AC × 4	0%*	8 pts with treatment break >3.5 days	Well tolerated
Paclitaxel every 3 weeks	Hanna[30]	20 stage II–III 6 6 BCT/14 MRM s/p AC × 4	33%*	20% clinical RT pneumonitis	Approach cautiously
Paclitaxel twice weekly	Formenti[31]	44 stage IIB–III neoadjuvant	7%*	14% post-MRM complications	Well tolerated
Paclitaxel every 3 weeks	Bellon[32]	29 stage III or recurrent	10%*	Bolus associated w/↑ toxicity	Concurrent therapy feasible
Docataxel every 3 weeks		15 Stage III or recurrent	40%*	One case of acute pericarditis	
CMF every 3 weeks	Isaac[33]	220 stage I–III BCT 75% MRM 25%	1.5%*		Acceptable adjuvant regimen
CMF (classic) every 21 days	Fiets[34]	51 (73% BCT)	41%†	4% Clinical pneumonitis	Too toxic
AC every 21 days		61 (56% BCT)	70%†	17% Hospitalization	

*RTOG acute toxicity.
†Common toxicity criteria version 2.
BCT, breast conserving therapy; MRM, modified radical mastectomy; AC, Adriamycin and Cytoxan; CMF, Cytoxan, methotrexate, 5-FU.

A2. Fatigue

During radiation for breast cancer, patients will commonly report that they feel fatigued. Fatigue in breast cancer patients receiving radiation seems to be mild to moderate in intensity and develops in a characteristic pattern. This is illustrated in a small study that reported on 15 women who demonstrated mild fatigue (2–4 on a 10-point scale) during a course of radiation for early stage breast cancer. The intensity of fatigue peaked at the 4th week, plateaued through the 7th week, and then dropped beginning with the 11th week.[35] Similarly, a different study in 30 breast cancer patients receiving radiation reported that fatigue peaked at weeks 4–6 and returned to baseline level 1 month after treatment.[35] Another study examining fatigue with a FACT fatigue subscale demonstrated that 43% of 52 women receiving breast radiation developed significant fatigue (score >37) and in 54% minimal or no fatigue was found. They reported that fatigue increased during the first few weeks of breast radiation, peaked at week 4 and then remained stable until 2 weeks after RT and was beginning to return to the baseline levels by 6 weeks post-treatment.[37]

Although radiation-related fatigue may be mild to moderate and dissipate within several weeks after the treatment is completed, when present, it can have a significant effect on patients' daily functions and overall QOL. This is demonstrated in a study evaluating fatigue with the Fatigue Severity Scale in 35 patients with prostate cancer and 34 with breast cancer, comparing scores prior to treatment and 1 week afterward.[38] Using this tool, 69% of the patients report of subjective fatigue that was relatively modest, and 28% demonstrated an increase in severe fatigue (score of >42) from a baseline of 19%. Measures by the EORTC QOL scale demonstrated significant decreases in role, cognitive, and social functioning as well as global QOL during radiation. In this and the previous study, an important predictor of fatigue level after radiation was the baseline fatigue prior to starting the treatment. A different study evaluated fatigue in 76 breast cancer patients at 6 time points: pre-RT, 2 weeks into treatment course, end of RT, and 3 and 6 months post-RT using Pearson Byars Fatigue Feeling Checklist.[39] This study, in contrast to previous ones, demonstrated fatigue onset in the first week of treatment, stabilizing thereafter, and resolving by the end of RT. Fatigue scores were back to pre-treatment level by the 3 and 6 month follow-up. Subjects in this study had significant alterations in functional activities from the start of radiation until its completion. Alteration in functional activities returned to baseline by 3 months after treatment. This study also evaluated Fatigue Relief Strategies to determine how patients managed their fatigue. Seventeen self-initiated strategies were assessed. The strategy of sit and sleep were consistently the most frequently used strategy and scored as the most effective.

During a course of breast radiation, patients should be guided about self-management of fatigue, that is, prioritizing essential activities and deferring, postponing, or delegating activities that are non-essential. Patients who work full-time are advised that they may need to reduce their work hours during the last 2 weeks of breast radiation and for 2 weeks afterward. A discussion about what type of documentation a patient needs to reduce work hours if necessary may be in order. Treatment of specific causes related to fatigue should be done, e.g., anemia, depression, anxiety, and insomnia.[40] In addition, convincing clinical evidence has emerged that exercise can be an effective strategy for management of fatigue related to breast cancer treatment.

One such study examined the effect of exercise on fatigue levels by randomizing 46 women aged 35–64 receiving breast radiation after lumpectomy[41] to an exercise program versus usual care during treatment. In the exercise group, 86% reported exercising for at least 30 minutes ≥3 times per week and the usual care tended to decrease their activity level as the treatment progressed. One hundred percent of patients in the study reported fatigue during treatment, but the fatigue scores were lower for the exercise group. Anxiety, depression, and difficulty sleeping were common for both groups; however, greater symptom intensity was found in the usual care group.

On the basis of this, we guide our patients to rest when they feel tired and to be active when they feel good. All the patients are counseled about the benefits of exercise for minimizing fatigue symptoms during treatment. Patients are encouraged to maintain their exercise routines when they feel well and given support if they express interest in beginning the exercise programs during treatment.

B. LATE TOXICITY

B2. Breast Appearance

The main goals of breast conservation therapy in early stage breast cancer are to provide primary tumor control comparable to mastectomy and to preserve an acceptable cosmetic appearance of the breast. An unsatisfactory cosmetic outcome should be considered as a potential late toxicity. The rate of poor or fair cosmetic outcome in most series is 15–20% or less.[42–46,48–50] It has been demonstrated in many studies that surgical factors including the extent or volume of surgical resection[45,46] and scar orientation,[45] have the largest impact on breast appearance and the cosmetic outcome.[42–47] The use of chemotherapy and patient factors such as breast size, older age, and race have also been associated with more frequent cosmetic failures.[42–47] However, several radiation treatment factors are associated with poorer cosmetic outcomes as well. It is important to consider these factors when planning radiation treatment to minimize the late toxicity rate. Table 7 lists the cosmetic outcomes from single institution retrospective studies that have analyzed the impact of radiation techniques on subsequent cosmetic outcome.

Wazer et al. from New England Medical center at Tufts demonstrated an increase in fair/poor cosmetic outcomes with larger chest-wall separations (24 cm mean) and

Table 7. Physician assessed cosmetic results from breast conservation therapy

Institution	*N*	F/U (years)	Excellent (%)	Good (%)	Fair (%)	Poor (%)	Radiation factors associated with poorer cosmesis
Tufts U[46]	234	4.2	41	47	9	3	Heterogeneous RT dose; Boost; use of >2 fields
Harvard/JCRT[44,49]							Breast dose >50 Gy; use of >2 fields; boost dose >18 Gy; implant boost
<1981	504	8.9	58	28	10	4	
1982–1985	655	5.6	73	23	3.5	0.5	
Washington U[45]	458	4.4	38	44	15	4	Use of >2 fields; breast dose >50 Gy; no compensator filters

greater maximal dose inhomogeneity (13% mean) at the central axis.[46] The use of a boost and a supraclavicular and/or axillary field were the other factors associated with a higher proportion of fair/poor cosmetic outcomes. In this study, an electron boost, but not an interstitial implant boost, was associated with the decline in cosmetic outcome. Patients in this study were treated with 6 MV photons, 81 patients with an implant boost, and it is not stated what proportion were treated to >2 fields.

The effect of radiation technique on the cosmetic result was demonstrated by the Joint Center for Radiation Therapy and Harvard Department of Radiation Therapy when it compared cosmetic results in two different cohorts of patients treated between 1970–1981 and 1981–1985.[44] In the earlier cohort, 85% received a 3-field technique, 95% an implant for boost, 33% ≥ 50 Gy breast dose, and 85% >18 Gy boost dose. The institution had previously found that the use of >2 fields, an implant boost, boost dose >18 Gy and a breast dose >50 Gy were associated with poorer cosmetic outcomes.[48,49] Treatment techniques had changed during the latter time interval, such that 55% received a 3-field technique, 47% an implant for boost, 5% ≥50 Gy breast dose, and 42% >18 Gy boost dose. The cosmetic results were significantly better with the techniques used in the latter period (Table 7). When examined, there was no influence of the boost, number of fields treated, and/or the daily dose on cosmetic outcome in the latter cohort.[44]

Washington University[45] similarly found that the percentage of excellent/good cosmetic outcomes decreased with the use of more than 2 fields ($P = 0.034$), and increasing radiation dose to the entire breast ($P = 0.024$). With increasing separations at the central axis, a relative deterioration occurred in excellent/good ratings, especially with the use of lower energy, 4 MV photons. This is inferred to be from the dose inhomogeneity that occurs with the larger chest-wall separation. The effect of dose homogeneity on cosmetic outcome is again demonstrated in this study by a significantly higher frequency of excellent/good cosmetic scores (82%) that occurred with the use of compensating filters compared with no use of compensating filters (59%) ($P = 0.002$). Daily fraction size (1.8 vs. 2.0 Gy), boost versus no boost, and the type of boost did not influence cosmetic outcome in this series.[45] Other studies have confirmed the influence of radiation therapy factors on cosmetic outcomes. For instance, Ryoo et al.[43] reported that the use of a wedge in the breast tangents was a significant factor for obtaining a good cosmetic result.

The cosmetic failure rates reported in all of these studies reflect treating physician observation. Studies that include patient-rated cosmetic evaluations demonstrate fairly good concordance with physician-rated cosmesis and satisfaction with a range of cosmetic outcomes.[45,50]

In an attempt to objectively measure cosmetic outcome, Pezner et al. developed a Breast Retraction Assessment (BRA) that quantified the amount of retraction of the treated breast in comparison to the untreated one by measuring the lateral and vertical displacement of the nipple.[42] On multivariate analysis in order of descending importance, patient age >60, extensive breast resection, patient weight >150 pounds, and upper quadrant primary site were the most significant factors related to breast retraction after BCT. None of the RT parameters studied were associated with breast retraction. Subset analysis related that the volume of the boost had some relation to retraction, but did not reach statistical significance.

Table 8. Cosmetic outcome from EORTC 22881/10882 Boost versus no boost trial[51]

	No boost		Boost	
Score (%)	Post-OP	3-YEAR	Post-OP	3-YEAR
Excellent	37.4	41.7	34.8	32.7
Good	47.3	43.9	45.0	38.2
Fair	13.7	13.1	18.8	25.8
Poor	1.6	1.4, $P = 0.23$	1.4	3.3, $P < 0.001$

The effect of the boost on the cosmetic result was evaluated in a randomized trial, EORTC 22881/10882.[51] In this trial, 5569 stage I and II breast cancer patients who had received lumpectomy, axillary dissection, and breast radiation up to 50 Gy over 25 fractions were randomized between a boost of 16 Gy or no boost if the lumpectomy resection margins were negative. Cosmetic outcome in each arm was assessed by two methods postoperatively and at 3 years: by a 5-physician panel evaluating photographs in a sample of 713 patients (Table 8) and by the percentage BRA relative to a reference length in a sample of 1141 patients.

Postoperatively, there was no significant difference in cosmetic assessment between the two arms, but by 3 years, the patients in the boost arm had a significantly lower rate of excellent/good cosmetic outcome and nearly double the rate of fair outcomes (13% no boost vs. 25.8% boost) ($P = 0.0001$). Very few patients in either arm had a poor result at either time period. By the panel assessment, the boost group had significantly worse median scores for all the items evaluated—appearance of the surgical scar, breast size, breast shape, nipple position, and areola shape. Interestingly, despite the observations of the panel, the difference in the percentage BRA was small, less than 1% between the two arms. Even in the larger sample size, this difference reached only borderline statistical significance ($P = 0.04$).

In contrast, radiation did not have a deleterious effect on cosmetic outcome in a subset of 101 women accrued to the Milan III trial that randomized women with breast cancers $\leq$2 cm in size to quadrantectomy (QUAD) or quadrantectomy plus breast irradiation (QUART).[52,53] Radiation consisted of 50 Gy whole breast dose followed by a "scar" boost of 10 Gy, all delivered with 2 Gy fractionation. This study also evaluated cosmesis with two separate measures: an objective measurement of nipple and breast displacement to assess symmetry; and second, with a subjective rating by physicians and patients. There was not a statistical difference in cosmetic outcome between the QUAD versus QUART by either measure.[53] The absence of a negative effect from radiation in this trial may be as a result of the lower total dose to the boost area of 60 Gy versus 66 Gy in the ETORTC trial.

In summary, there is a whole host of patient and treatment factors that can contribute to cosmetic failure as a late toxicity from breast conservation therapy. However, the radiation factors that influence the cosmetic outcome in most series are the use of a boost, greater than 2 fields (i.e., the addition of a supraclavicular, axillary, or internal mammary field), the total dose, and dose heterogeneity in the breast fields. Newer radiation therapy planning methods such as 3-dimensional conformal therapy or intensity-modulated radiation therapy can produce more homogeneous dose distributions through the breast. However, CT-based treatment planning for breast cancer is still emerging. In 1999, the Patterns of Care Study demonstrated that a CT was used for radiation treatment planning in only 17% of intact breast cases and 15% of those irradiated post-mastectomy.[54,55]

The efficacy of the boost for improving local control, particularly in certain subsets of patients, has been demonstrated.[56,57] Care should be taken that the boost is delivered using the appropriate techniques to minimize morbidity. Careful image-guided localization of the cavity will help reduce excess breast tissue being taken to higher doses unnecessarily.

B2. Augmented or Reconstructed Breast Appearance

Breast cancer patients who receive radiation to an augmented breast following lumpectomy or a reconstructed breast following mastectomy have a higher risk of cosmetic failure.

Augmentation

Breast augmentation preceding the diagnosis and treatment of a breast cancer can create a clinical conundrum. The appearance of the breasts is, typically, particularly important in this patient group; yet, their risk for cosmetic failure following breast conservation therapy is higher in some studies. Table 9 lists the rate of excellent or good cosmetic results in multiple studies demonstrating a wide range of outcomes.[58–63] Three studies demonstrate acceptable rates of 85–100% excellent/good cosmesis, but in the other 3, only 27–45% of patients achieved this result. Fairly uniform radiation techniques were used among these studies with the augmented breast receiving on average a range of 45–50 Gy with cobalt, 4 or 6 MV photons and subsequent boosts of 10–20 Gy delivered in most cases. The primary cause of cosmetic failure in irradiated augmented breasts is capsular contracture, which has been demonstrated to occur in 57–65% of cases.[59–62] The average time interval for onset of capsular contracture was reported at 22 weeks.[62] Mark et al. reported that the capsular contracture seemed related to the type of the implant (silicone 64% and saline 40%) and was more likely with sub-muscular (64%)

Table 9. Cosmetic outcome following lumpectomy and breast irradiation in women with previous breast augmentation

Institution (author)	N	Mean follow-up (mo.s)	% Excellent/good or % Bakers 1–2* cosmetic outcome
Beaumont (Victor)[56]	8	32	100
Van Nuys (Handel)[59]	26	NA	27*
Memorial SK (Ryu)[66]	3	24	33[†]
Cornell U. (Chu)[64]	7	43	85
USC, UCLA (Mark)[62]	21	22	43
John Wayne Cancer Institute (Guenther)[63]	20	45	85

[†]66% ultimate after one patient had surgical revision for capsular contracture.
NA means not available.

versus sub-glandular (50%) placement.[62] Baker's classification provides an assessment of capsular contracture. Baker I is a soft breast or implant with no deformity, II—the implant has a slightly thickened consistency with slight deformation, III—the implant is firm to hard and moderate deformity of the breast is noted, and IV—the implant is hard and there is severe breast deformity. There is an inherent risk of capsular contracture from breast implants in general unrelated to radiation. The overall incidence of capsular contracture after cosmetic breast augmentation with implants is 12% and is significantly greater for breast reconstruction following mastectomy for cancer treatment (34%) or cancer prophylaxis (30%).[64]

Surgical revision can improve the cosmetic outcome from capsular contracture in an augmented breast in some cases. At Memorial Sloan Kettering, Ryu reported that 2 patients underwent surgical revision with a subsequent excellent result.[60] Eight patients in the Van Nuys experience underwent revision surgeries after capsular contracture. Five patients had a capsulectomy and a new implant placed and 4 (80%) subsequently had an excellent cosmetic outcome.[59]

Reconstruction

An increasing percentage of breast cancer patients who are ineligible for breast conserving therapy or who have more locally advanced breast cancer are seeking reconstruction of the breast following mastectomy.[65] The options for breast reconstruction are tissue expansion with subsequent prosthetic implant placement or autologous tissue reconstruction. Immediate breast reconstruction during the same surgical period as the mastectomy provides the psychological benefit of waking-up post-procedure with a breast mound in place. However, a dilemma has emerged in that there is clinical evidence that breast reconstructions that undergo radiation have a higher risk of cosmetic failure,[58–62,66–71] while even a larger percentage of mastectomy patients may now be considered candidates for treatment since publication of a survival advantage in a subset of women who receive post-mastectomy RT.[72,73]

Table 10 lists the cosmetic outcome from immediate expander/implant breast reconstruction that underwent a course of post-mastectomy irradiation. In three of these studies, there was a low rate of acceptable cosmetic outcome.[58,60,66] The radiation treatment was similar in these studies with the chest wall/reconstructed breast receiving

Table 10. Cosmetic outcome following mastectomy with implant reconstruction and subsequent irradiation for primary or recurrent breast cancer

Institution (author)	*N*	Cancer	Mean follow-up (months)	% Excellent/good cosmetic outcome
Beaumont (Victor)[58]	13	Primary	32	54
Cornell (Chu)[61]	27	Recurrent	30	93
Washington U. (Kuske)[66]	65	68% Primary	48	45
Memorial SK (Ryu)[60]	11	Recurrent	24	56
Memorial SK (Cordeiro)[67]				
RT	68	Primary	34	80
No RT	81	Primary	34	88 (P = ns)

on average of 50 Gy with cobalt, 4 or 6 MV photons, standard fractionation, and an electron boost to the chest wall was used for many. A similar radiation technique was used at MD Anderson Cancer Center for 12 patients, 6 post-mastectomy with implant reconstruction, and 6 cancers arising in a previously augmented breast.[68] Comparable results were noted with no excellent, 33% good, and 42% poor cosmetic outcomes. In two studies,[58,66] the use of bolus application during radiation was associated with a significantly worse cosmetic outcome. At Beaumont Hospital,[58] 87% of patients who were treated without bolus application had a good to excellent result compared to 37% who were treated with bolus application ($P = 0.016$). Similarly, Kuske et al.[66] from Washington University reported that the use of a bolus layer was the only radiotherapy factor found to influence cosmetic results: 81% of patients with no bolus had an excellent/good cosmetic result versus 37% of patients for whom bolus was used during radiation ($P = 0.003$). In this study, the use of bolus also resulted in a higher complication rate (51% vs. 23%, $P = 0.048$). The use of compensators or wedges was associated with a lower complication rate but did not have a significant effect on cosmesis. Eight of 70 reconstructed breasts in this study were treated without a compensator or wedge and all of these patients experienced complications ($P = 0.036$).

Two studies in Table 10 reported a high rate of acceptable cosmetic outcome from irradiation of expander/implant reconstructions.[61,67] Chu et al. from New York Hospital, Cornell University Medical Center, reported a 93% excellent/good and 7% fair/poor cosmetic result in 27 patients with recurrent breast cancer 1 month to 10 years following mastectomy and silicone implant reconstruction.[61] Nine patients in this study received "wide-local field technique" and were not treated to the entire reconstructed breast.

The other study with acceptable cosmetic results was recently reported from Memorial Sloan Kettering and looked at 687 breast cancer patients who underwent immediate tissue expander/implant reconstruction following mastectomy.[67] At this institution, patients underwent mastectomy with placement of the tissue expander. Tissue expansion was continued during chemotherapy; and then 4 weeks following the completion of chemotherapy, the tissue expander was exchanged for the permanent implant. Post-mastectomy radiation began 4 weeks after this exchange. Eleven percent of 81 irradiated implants were subsequently removed versus 6% of 542 non-irradiated cases. The ultimate success rate for implant reconstruction was 90% versus 99% for irradiated and non-irradiated cases, respectively ($P = 0.001$). The 81 irradiated cases were matched to 75 non-irradiated control cases. There was an 80% excellent/good cosmetic result after post-mastectomy radiation that was not statistically different from the 88% noted in the non-irradiated cases.[67] Non-irradiated cases did have a higher rate of very-good/excellent cosmetic result. Overall, 68% of the irradiated patients developed a capsular contracture compared with 40% of those non-irradiated ($P = 0.006$). Irradiated patients were more likely to develop a Baker's grade III contracture (33.3% vs. 9.3%), but there was no significant increase in grade IV or severe contracture. Sixty-seven percent of irradiated patients were satisfied with their reconstructions and 72% stated that they would choose the same form of reconstruction again. The authors concluded that although irradiation increased the incidence of implant complication and contracture, the rates of reconstructive success and patient satisfaction remained high.

The long-term cosmetic consequences of irradiation following an autologous breast reconstruction have been contradictory. Kuske et al. reported that cosmetic results in 8 patients who underwent PMR after immediate transverse rectus abdominis myocutaneous (TRAM) flap reconstruction were good/excellent in 87% despite a 63% complication rate.[66] Similarly, a study by Zimmerman et al. from UCLA, reported 90% patient-rated good/excellent cosmesis in 21 patients who underwent radiation following immediate free TRAM flap breast reconstruction and had a mean follow-up interval of 19 months.[69] Other series have demonstrated worse complication rates from radiation after TRAM flap reconstruction.[71] This inconsistency is illustrated by two reports with similar outcomes but different conclusions. Nineteen patients who received radiation after pedicled TRAM flap reconstruction were compared to 108 patients who underwent radiation prior to a similar reconstruction at Emory University.[70] Thirteen or 68% of the 19 cases irradiated post-TRAM reconstruction had local recurrence of cancer requiring radiation. There was no significant difference in the rate of complication for an irradiated TRAM (31%) versus radiation pre-TRAM (25%) flap reconstruction. There was a 17% complication rate for 572 non-irradiated TRAM flap reconstructions at the institution overall. The authors concluded that the complication rate does not change whether a patient receives radiation before or after her TRAM flap reconstruction, only the nature of the complication changes (fat necrosis instead of fibrosis). A similar retrospective study from MD Anderson Cancer Hospital also compared the complication rate for post-mastectomy radiation after ($n = 32$) and before ($n = 70$) free TRAM flap breast reconstruction.[71] The delayed reconstruction was performed an average of 43 months post-completion of radiation. There was no difference in the rates of early complications (vessel thrombosis, partial flap loss, total flap loss, and mastectomy flap necrosis) between the two groups. There were significantly more late complications (fat necrosis 43.8%, flaps with volume loss 87.5%, and flaps with contracture 75%) in the immediate reconstruction group compared to the group that underwent reconstruction after completion of radiation (fat necrosis 8.6%, flaps with volume loss 0%, and flaps with contracture 0%). Twenty-eight percent of the 32 flaps that were irradiated required additional flap or an external prosthesis to correct the volume loss. On the basis of this experience, the authors concluded that patients who are candidates for free TRAM flap breast reconstruction and need post-mastectomy radiation, reconstruction should be delayed until radiation therapy is complete. Unfortunately, neither of these studies provided physician- or patient-rated cosmetic data or patient satisfaction scores.

An interesting study from the Michigan Breast Reconstruction Outcome Study evaluated factors that influenced complication rates in a prospective cohort of 326 women who underwent breast reconstruction after mastectomy from 1994 to 1998. Twenty-three plastic surgeons from 12 centers in Michigan, Pennsylvania, Louisiana, and Ontario contributed patients to the survey.[74] Sixty-four percent were immediate reconstructions and 24% were expander/implant, 55% were pedicle tram flap, and 21% were free TRAM flap reconstructions. No significant differences were observed across procedure types with regard to patient demographics or comorbidities. Complication data were collected 2 years after reconstruction. Overall, there were no complications in 54.6%, 1 complication in 29.1%, and 2 complications in 16.3%. Twenty-three percent had one major complication, and 8% had 2–3. Multivariate analysis to assess the effect of reconstruction type and timing while controlling for patient age, body mass index, smoking, chemotherapy, and radiation demonstrated that only immediate reconstruction and body mass index were significantly associated with higher total complication rates. For TRAM flap reconstructions, the major complication rates were 36% in the immediate group and 18% in the delayed group ($P = 0.002$). Trends for higher complication rates were noted with radiation therapy and chemotherapy in separate analyses. Radiation before or after surgery for an expander/implant reconstruction was associated with higher overall complication ($P = 0.08$) and major complication ($P = 0.07$) rates. Chemotherapy was associated with significantly higher major complications in TRAM flap procedures ($P = 0.03$).

B3. Chronic Pain

Breast cancer patients can report pain in the irradiated breast, chest wall, or nodal regions for years after treatment. A survey of 127 breast cancer survivors who were on average 3 years post-treatment was done and revealed that 27% reported chronic pain.[75] The pain was rated mild in severity for 90% of patients. The sites of pain affected were breast 86%, ipsilateral arm 69%, and ipsilateral axilla 81%. Pain in all three sites was reported in 58%. The prevalence of pain was 27% after lumpectomy with RT, and 23% after mastectomy alone. The impact of irradiation on breast pain has been reported from two randomized studies. A companion study to assess breast pain was done at Princess Margaret Hospital during a prospective trial that randomized breast cancer patients older than 50 years to tamoxifen alone or tamoxifen and breast RT after lumpectomy.[76] This study found that radiation did not adversely affect breast pain up to 12 months post-treatment. Another QOL study that accompanied a randomized trial of observation versus breast RT after lumpectomy demonstrated that patients did have increased breast pain during irradiation and up to 2 years post-treatment. At 2 years no difference between the treatment groups could be detected in the rates of skin irritation, breast pain, and being upset by the appearance of the breast.[77]

B4. Fibrosis

Skin thickening or fibrosis of the breast or chest wall can occur after radiation for breast cancer. An analysis was done for complications after BCT in 294 patients treated at MD Anderson Cancer Center from 1990 to 1992.[78] Breast radiation was delivered with standard fractionation to a total prescribed dose of 50 Gy. Fibrosis was noted to develop in 29%, but only 3.7% experienced grade 2 (moderate) and 0.3% grade 3 (impaired ROM) fibrosis.[78] Similar to the findings associated with cosmetic failure, breast fibrosis developed more commonly in patients treated with additional radiation fields (38% vs. 21%, $P = 0.001$) and in patients who received a boost (33% vs. 22%, $P = 0.04$).

The influence of total dose and fraction size on the development of subsequent breast fibrosis is demonstrated by a study from the University of Hamburg that evaluated long-term radiation sequelae using LENT-SOMA criteria[80] in three groups of women who had undergone BCT with a minimum of 6 years follow-up: group 1 received 60 Gy total breast dose with 2.5 Gy fractions (1983–1987, $n = 45$); group 2—55 Gy total dose with 2.5 Gy fractions (1988–1993, $n = 345$); and group 3—55 Gy total dose in 2 Gy fractions (1993–1995, $n = 200$). Grades 2–3 breast fibrosis developed in 58%, 51%, and 20% of patients in groups 1– 3, respectively.[79]

The effect of hypofractionation and the latency for developing subcutaneous fibrosis was studied by Bentzen et al. from Aarhus, Denmark. Fractionation studies compared two groups of breast cancer patients treated with post-mastectomy irradiation between 1978 and 1982: 163 women treated with a minimum target dose of 36.6 Gy to mid-axilla in 12 fractions of 3.05 Gy delivered twice weekly versus a sample of 66 women treated with a total dose of 40.92 Gy to mid-axilla over 22 fractions of 2.04 Gy delivered 5 fractions per week.[81] This study found that the incidence of fibrosis increased with time during the first 4 years of follow-up. By 3.2 years, 90% of the fibrosis had been expressed. A longer latency was demonstrated for the most severe fibrosis at 4.4 years, in comparison to grade 1 fibrosis which had developed by <2 year. The incidence of moderate to severe fibrosis was nearly double in the hypofractionated, 2 fraction per week schedule, 96% versus 45% in the 5 fraction per week schedule.[81]

Certain patient populations may be at risk for developing exaggerated fibrotic reactions following radiation. Patients with certain collagen vascular diseases (CVDs) may represent such a subset and are discussed later. Breast cancer patients who are heterozygous for the Ataxia Telangiectasia Mutation (ATM) have been reported to have more severe fibrosis following radiation.[82]

B5. Skin Telangiectasia and Atrophy

Telangiectasia or dilatations of the dermal vasculature that lie within a few millimeter of the epidermis can occur following radiation for breast cancer. Several studies examining post-mastectomy radiation have demonstrated that the incidence of telangiectasia is affected by total radiation dose,[84,85,87] larger fraction size,[81,84] and the occurrence of moist desquamation.[85–87]

The Gothenburg fractionation trials conducted during post-mastectomy radiation in Sweden in the 1970s examined the effect of radiation dose, fraction size, and dose-rate on the development of telangiectasia (as a measure of late skin reaction) following radiation with 12–13 MeV electrons.[83,84] These studies used patients as their own control comparing effects on the right versus left irradiated parasternal region. At greater than 5 years of follow-up, the frequency of mild, moderate, and severe telangiectasia was 79%, 49%, and 20%, respectively, for 2.61 Gy delivered daily 5 times per week for 21 fractions (54.81 Gy total dose) versus 100%, 79%, and 30%, respectively, for 5 Gy delivered twice weekly for 9 fractions (45 Gy total dose) ($P < 0.01$).[84] Another study in the Gothenburg series confirmed that the occurrence of telangiectasia were greater for 4 Gy delivered twice per week for 10, 11, and 12 fractions compared to 2 Gy delivered 5 times per week daily for 25, or 30 fractions. Within each fractionation schedule, the incidence of telangiectasia rose significantly with increasing total dose. Another study used four fractions of 7.2 Gy given once-a-week to compare the effect of delivering the dose per fraction over 4 minutes versus 32 minutes.[83] Prolongation of the treatment time resulted in a significant reduction in the incidence of telangiectasia: 85%, 65%, and 23%, respectively, for the minimal, distinct, and severe telangiectasia for the 4 minute treatment time versus 62%, 32% and 6%, respectively, for the prolonged treatment time of 32 minutes ($P < 0.01$). Bentzen et al. in the Aarhus fractionation studies described above,[81] also reported the effect of fraction size and the latency for development of telangiectasia. Like fibrosis, the incidence of telangiectasia increased over time. It was not until after 4.7 years of follow-up time that 90% of the telangiectasia was expressed. The incidence of moderate to severe telangiectasia was 81% in the 2 fractions per week schedule versus 62% in the 5 fractions per week schedule.

With the incorporation of these concepts into modern radiation practice, the incidence of telangiectasia is less frequent after post-mastectomy radiation. The overall incidence of telangiectasia was 59% at 5 years for 120 post-mastectomy patients whose chest wall was irradiated using 12 or 15 MeV electrons with 50–50.4 Gy over 25–28 fractions, 5 days-a-week. The use of a scar boost for 10–16 Gy with 9 MeV electrons was the only factor found to be predictive for the development of telangiectasia.[85]

The development of telangiectasia after breast conserving therapy is less common but still related to fraction size and total dose. The University of Hamburg study outlined above evaluating fibrosis, demonstrated the effect of dose and fraction size on subsequent development of telangiectasia.[79] Grades 2–3 telangiectasia developed in 29%, 17% and 6%, respectively, for 60 Gy delivered with 2.5 Gy fractionation 4 days-a-week, 55 Gy with 2.5 Gy fractionation 4 days-a-week, and 54 Gy with 2 Gy fractionation given 5 days-a-week with cobalt-60 teletherapy. Pezner et al. reported an overall 18% incidence of telangiectasia by 5–9 months following breast radiation that gradually increased to 30% by the second year of follow-up in 119 patients who underwent BCT and received 50–50.4 Gy at 1.8–2 Gy per fraction. On multivariate analysis, boost, patient age >60, and use of regional nodal fields was predictive for developing telangiectasia.[42] The incidence of telangiectasia was 7% for the no boost group ($n = 72$), compared to 36% for the 47 that were boosted ($P < 0.001$). An even lower rate of telangiectasia was reported in the women evaluated for cosmetic outcome on the Milan III trial where the incidence was 3% in the QUART versus 0% in the QUAD arms.[53]

The development of telangiectasia is also associated with the occurrence and severity of moist desquamation during the acute skin reaction.[86,87] From the Aarhus data, the estimated incidence of severe telangiectasia after 44 Gy in 22 fractions increases from 27% to 49% in patients who developed ≥grade 2 moist desquamation (10–49% of the field) as an early radiation reaction.[86]

Patients who are distressed by the appearance of the telangiectasia can be potentially treated with pulsed dye laser (PDL). PDL is an established treatment for cutaneous telangiectatic disorders and is considered both efficacious and safe.[88] A study of 8 patients with telangiectasia post-mastectomy demonstrated that in 7 who finished PDL treatment, there was 100% vessel clearance occurred in the treated areas.[89] Three patients required three treatments, 3 patients needed two treatments, and 1 patient was treated just once to obtain clearance.

B6. Collagen Vascular Diseases

These are a heterogeneous group of diseases that have been considered as a relative contraindication for breast conserving therapy with radiation because of sporadic reports of severe acute and late-treatment-related toxicity.[90,91] A study from Yale University specifically examined the incidence of acute and late toxicity after breast radiation for conservative therapy in the setting of CVD.[92] They identified 36 cases of CVD (17 rheumatoid arthritis (RA), 5 systemic or discoid lupus (S or DL), 4 scleroderma (SCD), 4 Raynaud's, 2 Sjögren's, 4 dermatomyositis/polymyositis) among the 1677 patients in their database who had undergone BCT, and matched each case to two control patients of similar age, tumor, and treatment factors. The breast was irradiated to a median dose of 48 Gy followed by a boost to the lumpectomy site to a total median dose of 64 Gy. There was no significant difference in acute toxicity for the CVD group overall compared to the controls. When analyzed by specific CVD, only the SCD subset was associated with an increased risk of acute toxicity. A significantly greater incidence of late toxicity was found between the CVD (17%) and control groups (3%) ($P = 0.0095$). Again, this was limited to the 4 SCD patients when this was analyzed by specific CVD. The late toxicities noted in 3 SCD patients were fibrosis-necrosis, ulceration-necrosis, and cord paralysis-dense fibrosis. The authors concluded that patients with SCD have higher rates of complications after breast irradiation, but that other CVD should not be considered contraindications.

Three other retrospective series have examined the relationship between CVD and radiation-induced complications. Two hundred nine patients with CVD with a variety of malignancies underwent irradiation to a median dose of 45 Gy (13–81 Gy) at Massachusetts General Hospital from 1960 to 1985.[93] Most patients, 131 (60%) had RA and the other 78 had non-RA CVD (28 patients had S or DLE, 17 polymyositis/dermatomyositis, 16 SCD, 8 ankylosing spondylitis, and four mixed connective tissue disorder). The patients in the RA group did not have higher rates of acute or late radiation toxicities. The non-RA CVD did not have higher acute toxicity rates, but had a significantly greater percentage of late complications, 21% versus 6% at 5 years ($P = 0.0002$).

Another series from the University of Iowa studied 61 patients with CVD who had been irradiated for various malignancies to matched-control groups of 61 irradiated patients without CVD.[94] Of the patients with CVD, 39 patients had RA, 13 had S or DLE, 4 had SCD, 4 had dermatomyositis, and 1 had polymyositis. Those with SLE had a non-significant higher rate of acute toxicity as compared to the control group (36% vs. 18%, P = n.s.). Patients with RA had a non-significant increase in late complications when compared to the control group (24% vs. 5%, P = n.s.). Among the late toxicities observed in the RA group were perforated sigmoid colon, small bowel obstruction, soft tissue necrosis, radiation pneumonitis, and fatal constrictive pericarditis. Patients with CVD treated with palliative doses of RT (<40 Gy) had acute and late complication rates equivalent to the controls.

Finally, another recent retrospective study from the University of Louisville compared acute and late toxicity from radiation for various malignancies in 38 patients with documented CVD to 38 matched-control cases.[95] There was not a significantly higher incidence of acute or late toxicity when the two groups were compared. However, the few SCD patients in this study had a higher rate of grade III acute and late complication following irradiation.

Breast cancer patients with CVD should be made aware of the potential for exaggerated acute and late toxicity related to radiation treatment, but should not be considered ineligible for breast conservation with radiation. From three retrospective studies so far, it appears that patients with SCD and other non-RA CVD may be at the highest risk for severe toxicities such that breast radiation in this group should be approached with caution.

B7. Lymphedema, Shoulder Immobility, and Brachial Plexopathy

These three toxicities are discussed together as they are all primarily consequences of supraclavicular and/or axillary irradiation in the treatment of breast cancer.

Lymphedema

Arm edema or lymphedema in breast cancer patients is caused by an interruption of the normal filtration process that occurs between capillaries, interstitial tissue, and lymphatic vessels in the arm. Under normal circumstances, capillary pressures force fluid into the interstitium and reabsorption pressures pull most of the fluid back into the capillary at the venous side. The remainder of the filtered fluid and protein are removed by lymphatic vessels. Without the functioning lymphatic system, protein, cells and non-reabsorbed fluid remain in the interstitial tissue. The stasis of fluid in the subcutaneous tissues of the arm leads to increased weight and girth of the extremity. Patients with arm edema secondary to breast cancer therapy can experience difficulty performing skills at home or work because of functional impairment, psychological distress as a result of the change of body image, and chronic pain, leading to significantly reduced QOL.[96,97,98] The primary treatment factors contributing to arm edema are the extent of axillary node dissection and nodal irradiation. There are multiple other clinical factors that have been associated with an increased subsequent risk of lymphedema, of these, infection[100,101] and obesity[116] are frequently reported.

Until recently, axillary node dissection was a standard part of the surgical management of invasive breast cancer regardless of tumor size or nodal involvement. The incidence of subsequent lymphedema in several studies is shown in Table 11 and averages about 13%. Studies with longer follow-up tend to show a greater incidence of arm edema. Increased rates of lymphedema have been reported with more extensive dissection,[103,104] greater number of nodes removed,[105,107,108] and splitting the pectoralis muscle.[107] Sentinel lymph node biopsy has resulted in significantly less morbidity with estimates of subsequent lymphedema being <1–3%.[110,111]

The addition of supraclavicular and/or axillary radiation following a dissection results in a higher incidence of lymphedema. The incidence of lymphedema following axillary node dissection and nodal irradiation ranges from 9% to 58% in the studies presented in Table 12. Increased rates of lymphedema have been described in association with both the British Columbia and the Danish Breast Cancer Cooperative Group (DBCG) 82B and 82C randomized trials that reported a survival advantage with the addition of chest wall and comprehensive nodal RT following mastectomy and chemotherapy. In the British Columbia trial, symptomatic lymphedema was reported in 9% of those irradiated versus 3% in the non-RT arm.[72] Hojris reported 14% lymphedema from

Table 11. Incidence of arm lymphedema after axillary dissection

Institution (author)	*N*	Measure	Nodal RT (%)	Lymphedema (%)
Johns Hopkins (Lin)[99]	283	Arm circumference >2 cm	6	16
Memorial Sloan Kettering, (Peterek)[100]	263	Arm circumference >2 cm	0	13
Wessex Radiotherapy (Ivens)[102]	126	Arm circumference, water displacement >200 cc	0	10

Table 12. Incidence of arm lymphedema after axillary dissection and nodal irradiation

Institution (author)	Year	*N*	Surgery	Measure	AND (%)	AND + RT (%)
Royal Marsden (Kissen)[104]	1986	200	BCS*35%	Limb volume >200 cc	0†	9.3†
					7.4‡	38.3‡
Odense University (Ryttov)[112]	1988	57	Mastectomy	Arm circumference >2.5 cm	11	46
Umea and Lund University (Segenstrom)[113]	1991	136	Mastectomy	Volume displacement >150 cc	21	58
Netherlands Cancer Inst. (Bijker)[114]	1998	691	Mastectomy	None given	6	28
Aarhus University (Hogris)[109]	2000	84	Mastectomy	Arm circumference/limb volume >200 cc	3	14
MD Anderson Cancer Center (Meric)[78]	2002	294	BCS¶	Arm circumference >3 cm	10	18
Massachusetts General Hosp. (Powell)[115]	2003	727§	BCS¶	Arm circumference "frequently" >2 cm	1.8	8.9

*BCS, breast conserving surgery.
†Axillary sampling.
‡Axillary clearance.
¶All patients received breast irradiation.
§No axillary dissection done in 14% of population.

irradiated versus 3% from non-RT in 84 women who had all been treated on the DCBG 82B and 82C trials at a single institution (Table 12). The extent of dissection prior to nodal irradiation impacts the rate of subsequent edema.[104] For instance, the risk of symptomatic edema in patients treated at JCRT/Harvard was 4% after RT alone without dissection, 6% after level I/II dissection plus axillary radiation versus 36% after a complete AND with axillary RT.[103] The incidence of arm edema following nodal irradiation in an un-dissected axilla ranges from 4% to 8%.[103,104]

Breast irradiation alone after lumpectomy and axillary node dissection seems to have a negligible effect on the incidence of lymphedema. The average incidence of lymphedema in the studies listed in Table 13 is 15%, which is similar to what is reported in the studies in Table 11 with axillary node dissection alone. The randomized trial from

Table 13. Incidence of arm lymphedema following breast conserving surgery, axillary node dissection, and breast irradiation

Institution	*N*	Measure	AND* (%)	Nodal RT (%)	Lymphedema (%)
Memorial Sloan Kettering (Werner)[116]	282	Arm circumference >2.5 cm	100	24	12.1
Northwestern University (Kiel)[105]	183	Arm circumference >2.0 cm	82	0.01	17.5
City of Hope (Pezner)[107]	37	Arm circumference >2.5 cm	86	0	14
Centro per lo Studio e la Prevenzione Onocologica (Herd-Smith)[108]	601	Arm circumference >5% difference	100	0	17.9

*Axillary node dissection.

the Uppsala-Orebro Breast Cancer Study that studied cancer recurrence from lumpectomy alone versus lumpectomy and breast irradiation in 381 women also evaluated arm morbidity.[117] Complete arm circumference data were available from 273 patients (117 in the RT group and 155 in the non-RT group). There was no associated difference between arm edema or any of the other arm symptoms evaluated (pain, numbness, impaired shoulder mobility) with the addition of breast irradiation. The number of nodes dissected was an important determinant of arm morbidity. At 3–12 months following treatment, arm symptoms were reported in 53.6% who had ≥10 lymph nodes found in the axillary specimen versus 33.6% who had <10 found. The frequency of arm symptoms reduced with time, such that at 13–36 months, the rate of arm symptoms was 33% and 19.5% for ≥10 versus <10 nodes found, respectively.

Radiation technique may influence the risk of lymphedema. Large fraction size and the inadvertent overlapping of fields have been associated with an increased incidence of arm edema.[118] Johansson et al. reported on 150 patients treated with RT in the mid-1960s following radical mastectomy. The patients were divided into three groups based on their fractionation: 4 Gy × 11 fractions delivered over 21 days; 4 Gy × 11 fractions delivered over 15 days; and 3 Gy × 14–15 fractions delivered over 20 days. With a follow-up of >30 years in surviving patients, the incidence of lymphedema was 70% and 69% from the two 4 Gy fractionation schedules versus 25% in the 3 Gy fractionation schedule ($P < 0.0001$). The patients in the 3 Gy fractionation group were treated with much smaller supraclavicular and internal mammary fields that may also have contributed to their lower rates of arm edema.

In the 1998–1999 Patterns of Care Study of post-mastectomy irradiation, the fractionation was ≤2 Gy in 97%, and 93% were prescribed a total dose between 45 and 50.4 Gy using 6 MV photons.[55] However, only 15% of the patients had CT-based treatment planning. A heterogeneous dose distribution can potentially lead to delivery of an unintentional larger fractions size and over-dosage in an area of the field that contains critical normal tissue. For instance, a 15–20% hot spot in a supraclavicular field dosed to 50.4 Gy over 25 fractions at a depth of 3 cm could lead close to 58–60 Gy being delivered with

2.2–2.3 Gy fractionation (Figure 1a). This is compounded with the use of an additional posterior axillary field that was used in 40% of the patients in the PCS post-mastectomy study.[55] This field was dosed most frequently to mid-axilla in the PCS study using 6 MV photons. When this field is used and dose prescribed at mid-axilla, it is important to watch the cumulative dose at $D = 3$ cm anteriorly, as the fractionation at this site with the combined supraclavicular field and exit from the posterior axillary field can become significantly higher than intended (Figure 1b). Omitting the posterior axillary field has resulted in lower rates of lymphedema in some retrospective studies. There was a 3% rate of lymphedema reported in 82 node-positive patients treated at the University of Michigan with supraclavicular irradiation only after a level I/II axillary dissection.[119]

Complete decongestive therapy (CDT) of complex physical therapy has become a commonly recommended therapy for management of lymphedema.[120,121] The goal of CDT is to reduce arm edema to a minimum level, maintain the results, and prevent infections. It has four main components: (1) manual lymph drainage, (2) skin and nail care, (3) compression bandaging and/or garments, and (4) therapeutic exercise. The efficacy of CDT was evaluated in a prospective trial of 20 breast cancer patients after diagnosis of lymphedema. Following CDT, there was a median decrease in girth of 1.5 cm and median volume reduction of 138 cc. During follow-up at 6 and 12 months, there was a mild increase in girth and volume but stabilized at less than 1 cm and 100 cc below study entry.[122] Other studies have demonstrated symptomatic and objective measures of response to CDT.[123]

Hyperbaric oxygen therapy (HBOT) has demonstrated effectiveness when studied for management of radiation associated sequelae of the mandible, bladder, soft tissue, as well as breast.[124] A recent Phase II trial from Royal Marsden Hospital evaluated HBOT in 21 patients with chronic lymphedema following nodal irradiation for breast cancer.[125] Only 3 of 19 patients achieved the primary treatment goal of a $\geq$20% relative reduction in volume. A larger percentage of patients (6/13) had evidence of improved clearance rate of radiotracer uptake on lymphoscintigraphy after HBOT. Twelve of 19 patients reported symptomatic improvement. Given these findings, HBOT deserves further study.

There have been several pharmacological agents studied for treatment of lymphedema. Two randomized trials have evaluated coumarin. An initial study in 31 breast cancer patients with arm edema and 21 patients with leg edema were randomized in a double-blind, crossover design to receive coumarin or placebo for 6 months. Each reported a >20% reduction in volume following coumarin therapy.[127] A second trial randomizing 140 women with arm edema following breast cancer treatment with the same double-blind cross over design failed to demonstrate any benefit from the coumarin and reported a 6% rate of hepatotoxicity.[126] Dafilon, a flavanoid, did not have an overall significant effect when evaluated in a randomized trial in 94 patients.[128] However, in 24 patients with severe edema there was a significant reduction in arm volume. Selenium for treatment of radiation-associated lymphedema has been prospectively studied in 12 breast cancer patients with arm edema and 36 patients with endolaryngeal edema.[129] Sodium selenite at 350 μg/kg for a total daily dose typically of 500 μg daily over 4–6 weeks was used. Ten of the 12 breast cancer patients demonstrated a significant reduction of arm circumference measures. Given this finding, further investigation is warranted.

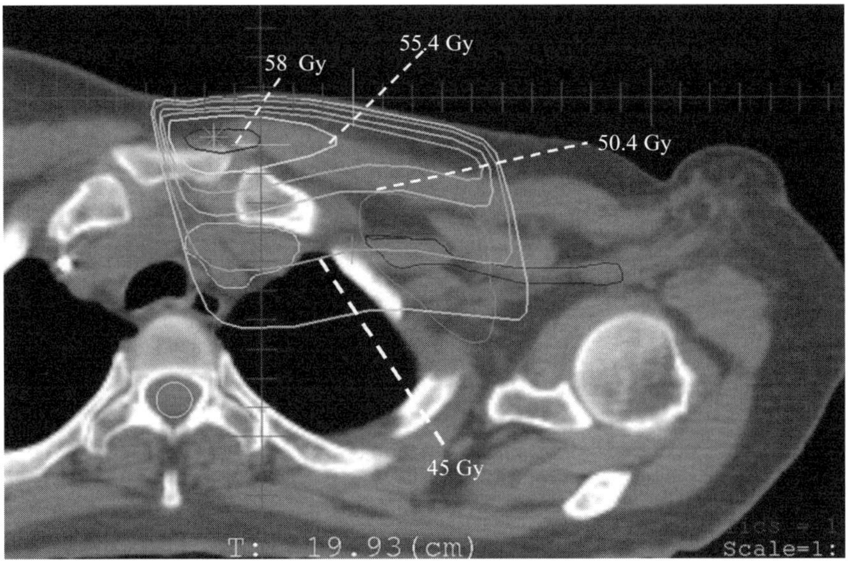

(a)

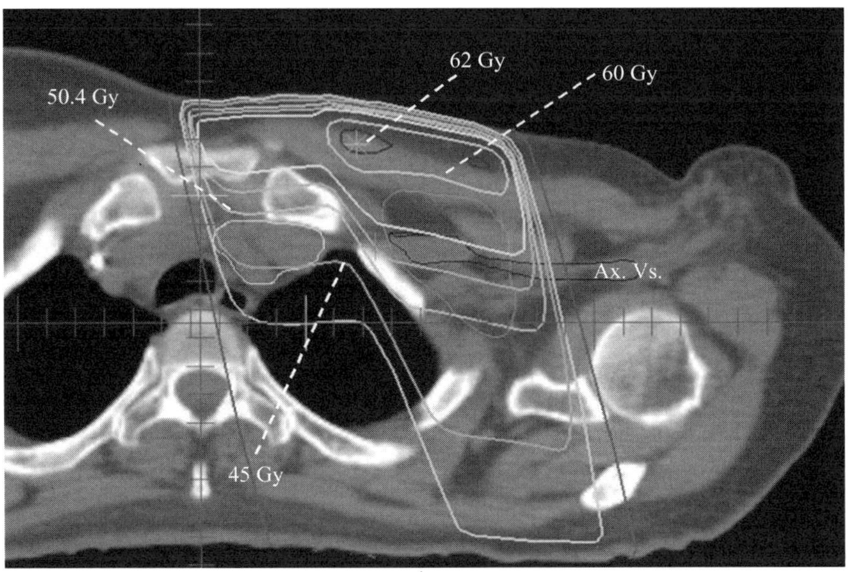

(b)

Figure 1. (a) Supraclavicular field. Isodose distribution from a prescription of 50.4 Gy to a depth of 3 cm with 6 MV photons and 1.8 Gy fractions. (b) Supraclavicular field with a posterior axillary boost (PAB). Isodose distribution for 50.4 Gy to a depth of 3 cm with 6 MV photons and 1.8 Gy fractions for the supraclavicular field. PAB dosed 10.6 Gy to mid-plane with 0.38 Gy fractions.

Shoulder Immobility

Impaired shoulder movement is primarily the consequence of axillary treatment. The type of surgical treatment and whether nodal irradiation is used influence the probability of subsequent shoulder consequences.

The cause of impaired shoulder motion following axillary node dissection and radiation is probably multifactorial. Damage to the pectoralis muscle is most likely an important factor for the development of shoulder dysfunction. Analysis of the Aarhus fractionation studies for post-mastectomy irradiation revealed that the occurrence of shoulder impairment post-treatment increased with increasing absorbed dose and the more hypofractionated schedule.[133] This gives credence to fibrosis of the pectoralis muscle and/or other chest-wall musculature as the main pathogenesis for impaired shoulder function post-irradiation. However, injury to ligaments, cartilage, joint capsule, vasculature, peripheral nerves, and lymphatic drainage may all contribute, directly or indirectly.

The impact of surgical procedure on shoulder movement was studied by Sugden et al. in 141 women treated for breast cancer in 1991 and assessed for arm function by a single observer 18 months post-treatment. Ninety-three women were assessed pre-RT and 18 months post, and the remaining 48 were only assessed post-treatment. Shoulder motion was measured for impairment in six movements: abduction, flexion, extension, both supination and/or pronation. The type of operation was the most important factor for the development of shoulder problems. Before RT, the incidence of a reduction in at least one shoulder movement was 78% for mastectomy patients and 43% in the lumpectomy group ($P < 0.01$).[130] Eighteen months post-treatment, the incidence of any reduced shoulder movement was 79% for the mastectomy patients and 35% in the lumpectomy group ($P < 0.01$).[130] Seventy-three percent had reduction in any of the shoulder movements measured following RT versus 35% who did not have axillary RT ($P \leq 0.001$). Patients with persistent shoulder dysfunction before RT had a 60% chance of persistent movement problems afterward, as compared to 24% with normal pre-RT shoulder movement ($P < 0.001$).

Review of Table 14 demonstrates three other studies with higher rates of shoulder impairment following post-mastectomy irradiation.[109,112,114] In these studies, impaired shoulder mobility ranged 2–6.8% following mastectomy alone versus 8–38% after the addition of irradiation. There has been less shoulder impairment reported after lumpectomy, axillary node dissection, and breast irradiation.[78,130,131] Deutsch reported a 1.5% rate of impaired shoulder motion in 232 post-lumpectomy patients and Meric et al. reported that 1.4% had decreased range of motion in 294 breast conservation patients. Arm mobility was among the arm symptoms that were not affected by the addition of breast RT following lumpectomy in the Upsala-Orebros randomized trial of lumpectomy and axillary node dissection ± breast irradiation described above.[117] Similarly, in the NIH randomized trial between MRM versus lumpectomy, node dissection, and irradiation, there was no significant difference in either treatment arm for shoulder range of motion at 1 year follow-up.[132]

Table 14. Incidence of impaired shoulder mobility after irradiation

Institution (author)	N	Surgery	Nodal RT (%)	Measure	Surgery (%)	Surgery + RT (%)
Netherlands Cancer Inst. (Bijker)[114]	691	Mastectomy	70	Patient self report	3.4	8* 18.9†
University of Oxford (Sugedn)[130]	39 102	Mastectomy Lumpectomy	35	Measured ROM‡	71¶ 31§	81¶ 59§
Aarhus Univ. Hosp. (Hogris)[109]	84	Mastectomy	100	Measured ROM	2	16
Odense University (Ryttov)[112]	57	Mastectomy	23	Measured ROM	6.8	38

*Axillary sampling.
†Axillary clearance.
‡ Range of Motion.
¶Mastectomy patients.
§Lumpectomy patients.

Brachial Plexopathy

Brachial plexopathy after radiation therapy is uncommon and typically seen only when regional nodal irradiation has been delivered. The clinical syndrome most frequently presents with paresthesias, and is associated with pain and/or weakness in the ipsilateral arm.[134,135] Weakness tends to be slowly progressive. The onset of symptoms can be seen within 6 months of completing radiation. While some studies document that most patients develop symptoms within 3 years,[134] others have demonstrated that the risk is progressive with time.[135,136] The entire brachial plexus is typically involved,[134,135] though some cases have documented involvement of just the upper or lower trunk. The mechanism of radiation-induced brachial plexopathy is not completely understood, but it is suspected that fibrosis of tissue around peripheral nerves occurs with injury to small vessels that leads to ischemia. Pathologic studies have shown loss of myelin, fibrosis and thickening of the neurolemma sheath, and obliteration of the vasonevum.[137]

The incidence of brachial plexopathy in reported series for breast conservation is very low. Pierce et al. from the Harvard group reported 20 (1.2%) of 1624 patients developed brachial plexopathy. The median time to occurrence was 10 months (range 1.5–77 months) and in 17 (85%), the symptoms had completely resolved by 1–2 years. Three women had severe, progressive symptoms for an overall rate of permanent brachial plexopathy of approximately 0.2%.[138] Supraclavicular/axillary radiation, axillary dose, and the use of chemotherapy were significantly associated with the development of brachial plexopathy. The 1117 patients treated with supraclavicular/axillary field developed brachial plexopathy in 1.8%, compared to none in the 507 patients treated to the breast alone ($P < 0.009$). Of those women who received nodal irradiation, higher rates of brachial plexopathy were seen with axillary doses >50 Gy (5.6% vs. 1.3%, $P = 0.004$), and the use chemotherapy (4.5% vs. 0.6%, $P < 0.001$). Other retrospective series of BCT from single institutions confirm that brachial plexopathy is very rare when just breast irradiation is delivered.[78,139,140]

Table 15. Hypofractionated supraclavicular/axillary irradiation and brachial plexopathy

Institution (author)	N	F/U (years)	Prescribed total dose (Gy)	Fraction size (Gy)	Fractions/ week	Energy	Brachial plexopathy (%)
Hamburg (Bajrovic)[141]	140	8	60	3.0	4	Co-60	14
Odense (Olsen)[142]	79	8	36.6	3.05	2	8–16 MV	35
Umea (Johansson)[136]	71	12	40	4	5	Co^{60}	63

Brachial plexopathy as a late morbidity from supraclavicular/axillary irradiation has been examined in older post-mastectomy series. In these studies, its incidence is associated with increasing fraction size and total dose (Table 15), similar to what is seen for late fibrosis. In the series from Hamburg University,[141] the 60 Gy in 3 Gy fractions was at a maximum depth of 0.5 cm. It is estimated that the dose to the brachial plexus at a depth of 3 cm was 52 Gy with a 2.6 Gy fraction. The rate of all brachial plexopathy grade 1 was 14% and all the damage was found to be progressive over the observation period, so that the percentage of patients with $\geq$3 plexopathy was 2% after 5 years, 5.5% after 10 years, 11.8% after 15 years, and 19.1% after 19 years, respectively.[141] In the report from Odense University by Olsen et al., patients had been treated according to the DBCG 77 protocol. Of the 35% rate of brachial plexopathy, 19% had mild symptoms of sensory disturbances and/or weakness, and 16% had severe symptoms that disabled her in daily life.[142] A very high rate of plexopathy was seen in the patients treated from 1963 to 1965 at the Umea University Hospital.[136] The prescription dose was 40 Gy in 11 fractions, but only 2 or 3 fields were treated per day so that the dose was given in 16–17 treatments over 3–4 weeks. Overlap occurred between the axillary and supraclavicular fields so that the given dose to the brachial plexus was much higher. A retrospective calculation showed that the dose to the brachial plexus was 54–57 Gy delivered over a complex combination of 1.8 Gy, 3.4 Gy, and 5.2 Gy fractions. The mean time for onset of BP was 4.2 years. There also was a progression of symptoms seen in this study over the entire follow-up period that was as long as 34 years. Of the 17% of women alive at 34 years follow-up, 92% had paralysis on their arm. A 5% rate of vocal cord paralysis that had onset at a mean of 19 years follow-up was also seen in this study. All of these occurred in left-sided lesions indicating recurrent nerve involvement.[136]

Subsequent post-mastectomy studies have demonstrated a lower rate of BP following nodal irradiation. One hundred and twenty-eight women irradiated on the DBCG 82B and 82C post-mastectomy studies were evaluated with thorough neurological exams to detect the presence of any neuropathy. The dose to the supraclavicular and axillary nodes was 50 Gy in 25 fractions on this study. After a median follow-up of 4.1 years, mild BP was noted in 9% and disabling symptoms in 5%. There was a higher incidence of plexopathy following radiation in patients who received chemotherapy ($P = 0.01$) and were younger than 47 years (0.04). Thirty three patients who did not receive radiation had no occurrence of plexopathy. These numbers represented a significant reduction in the incidence of BP when compared to the DBCG 77 trial.[135] Interestingly, Hogris et al. evaluated 84 patients for the presence of late morbidity that had been treated at his institution on the DBCG 82B and 82C trials. Paresthesias and weakness of the arm were more common in the irradiated patients than in the non-irradiated patients. Subjective complaints of paresthesia and weakness occurred in 7% and 28%, respectively, of the irradiated patients, and in none and 19%, respectively, of the non-irradiated patients. Objective examination revealed that 21% had paresthesias and 14% weakness in the irradiated group, and 7% and 2%, respectively, in the non-irradiated group. No patient had more than mild, grade I weakness measured.[109]

During the planning for supraclavicular or axillary nodal irradiation at our institution, the axillary vessels are contoured as a structure within the axilla to be a surrogate for the brachial plexus. It is our policy to not match over this structure to minimize the potential for inadvertent overlaps. The area of the contoured vessels is monitored to ensure that there are no dosimetric hotspots in or around the structure that would give an unintentional higher dose (Figure 1b).

B8. Cardiac Morbidity

Radiation of the breast or chest wall for left-sided breast cancers can inadvertently deliver significant doses to the heart. Radiation injury to the heart is seen most frequently in the pericardium. The parietal pericardium develops variable degrees of fibrosis that replaces the outer adipose tissue.[143] Although pericardial fibrosis can progress to constriction, this is uncommon and adhesions between the pericardium and epicardium are rarely seen. Accumulation of pericardial fluid is more commonly seen in this scenario. The occurrence of pericarditis associated with the radiation for breast conserving therapy is extremely uncommon. Pierce et al. reported 3 (0.4%) of 831 left-sided breast cancer patients developed chest pain requiring inpatient evaluation at 2, 2, and 11 months post-treatment.[138] Two of these patients had clinical syndromes consistent with pericarditis, and the third had evidence of a minor myocardial infraction. Other single institution series have reported no occurrence of pericarditis[139] or incidences $<1\%$.[140]

Pathologically, the myocardium is involved less frequently than the pericardium, but tends to develop a more serious lesion.[143] It is characterized by patches of diffuse fibrosis affecting usually the anterior wall of the left ventricle and, less frequently, the right ventricle. Myocardial fibrosis is thought to be a result of injury to endothelial cells of the myocardial capillaries. Lesions to the coronary arteries are also presumed to be as a result of endothelial cell injury. Injury to the intimal cells is followed by eventual replacement of the damaged intima by myofibroblasts, deposition of platelets, and all the other events that occur usually in atherosclerosis.

Radiation for left-sided breast cancer has been associated with increased morbidity and mortality from ischemic heart disease.[144–147] Older radiation therapy techniques, particularly those used for the initial post-mastectomy irradiation trials, included a significant portion of the heart. An initial meta-analysis of eight randomized post-mastectomy radiation trials that began before 1975 demonstrated that for long-term breast cancer survivors, patients who had received irradiation had higher subsequent mortality rates at 10–15 years follow-up.[144] A subsequent analysis was done that examined cause-specific mortality, included more post-mastectomy trials, and had longer follow-up revealing that there was not a significant difference in mortality after 10 years in those patients treated with irradiation. In fact, there was a trend for improved survival for those who were irradiated post-mastectomy. This modest survival benefit was offset by excess cardiac mortality in irradiated patients.[145] Most of the trials included in these initial overviews used radiation techniques with either orthovoltage or Co-60 that are now considered obsolete methods. These techniques compared to current ones with megavoltage radiation have been shown to deliver higher radiation doses to a larger percentage of the heart.

Cardiac mortality and the radiation treatment technique associated with it have been studied extensively in the Stockholm trial.[146–148] This trial included 960 breast cancer patients enrolled during 1971–1976 who were randomly allocated to preoperative RT, postoperative RT, or to mastectomy alone. There was no decrease in overall survival associated with radiation on this trial. Instead, there was a benefit with radiation (pre- and post-RT vs. surgical controls) during the entire follow-up period that was of borderline significance ($P = 0.09$). Each of the treatment techniques used in the trial were modeled with CT planning in four current breast cancer patients. The consistently largest irradiated heart volume was observed with left-sided tangential ^{60}CO fields. On the basis of this analysis, the different radiation techniques used on the trial were classified into three groups of low, intermediate, and high cardiac dose–volumes. When the records of the 960 patients in the Stockholm trial were linked with a Swedish registry of death certificates, mortality due to ischemic heart disease was significantly higher in the "high" dose–volume subgroup when compared to surgical control. In the low or intermediate dose–volume subgroups, the mortality due to ischemic heart disease was similar to surgical controls.[146] An update of this analysis in 1998 with 20 year median follow-up estimated a relative risk of myocardial infarction of 1.3 (95% CI 0.7–2.6) and cardiac mortality of 2.0 (95% CI 1.0–3.9, $P = 0.04$) in the high volume group only. No excess cardiac risk was observed in the lower dose–volume groups.[147]

This same group evaluated the proportion of heart volumes that was included in the 50% isodose (at least 25 Gy) from the dose–volume histogram (DVH) of 100 consecutive left-sided breast cancer patients irradiated following lumpectomy during 1994–1995 and compared it to the estimated heart volumes of patients treated on the Stockholm trial. The mean irradiated heart volume that received at least 25 Gy in the 1994–1995 cohort was 5.7% for the whole group and 11.9% in those with the highest volume.[148] The highest heart-volume group comprised 6% of the population. In comparison, the mean irradiated heart volume included in the 50% isodose for patients in the Stockholm Trial was 25%. This study demonstrates that the majority of left-sided breast cancer patients undergoing breast irradiation following lumpectomy do not receive irradiation to substantial heart volumes when modern radiation techniques are used.

A population-based study from Ontario, Canada, of patients receiving post-lumpectomy breast radiation during 1982–1987 demonstrated that 2% of women with left-sided RT had a fatal MI compared to 1% of women who had right-sided RT.[149] No data about radiation technique were available. Two other population-based studies, one from Sweden for patients treated during 1970–1985, and the other from SEER for patients treated in the US in 1973–1992, have reported a relationship between left-sided breast cancer treatment and subsequent late cardiac events and mortality.[150,151] In addition, the meta-analysis of 40 randomized trials of RT involving 20,000 breast cancer patients by the Early Breast Cancer Trialists Collaborative Group demonstrated that the addition of RT resulted in a reduction in breast cancer mortality, but was nearly offset by increased non-cancer mortality, particularly vascular.[152]

Three series from single institutions have not shown an increase in myocardial infarction (MI)[154] or cardiac-related mortality[153,155] after 9–12 years follow-up, respectively, in women radiated with more modern techniques as part of BCT.

Furthermore, no increase in morbidity or mortality from ischemic heart disease occurred in those patients receiving radiation compared to the non-radiation group in the DCBG 82B and 82C PMR trials that included 3083 women and have a median follow-up >10 years.[156] This is particularly important as all radiated patients enrolled in these trials received regional nodal treatment including the internal mammary chain. This underlies the importance of careful radiation treatment planning in order to minimize the amount of heart within the fields for left-sided breast cancer.

Multiple techniques have been described to reduce the amount of irradiated heart-volume during breast cancer treatment. These include adding a "heart block,"[157,158] 3-dimensional conformal therapy,[157] intensity-modulated radiation therapy,[157,158] and respiratory gating.[159,160] At our institution, the heart volume is contoured for all left-sided breast cancer with CT treatment planning using the definition of heart used by Geynes et al.[148] Our defined dose constraints are that the percent heart volume within the 50% isodose is kept ≦8% for breast only irradiation and ≦10% for when regional nodal irradiation is added. In some cases, we have used prone breast irradiation to reduce the amount of heart-volume irradiated for left-sided cancers.

B9. Radiation Pneumonitis

Symptomatic radiation pneumonitis is uncommon when only the breast is irradiated following breast conserving therapy. It typically onsets 2–3 months after completing treatment with a clinical syndrome of cough, fever, shortness of breath, and radiologic changes confined to the radiation therapy field.[161] Symptoms can persist for several weeks and in general are self-limiting. Pulmonary fibrosis typically follows in the effected portion of the lung.

Lingos et al. reported a 1% incidence of radiation pneumonitis in 1624 patients treated during 1968–1985 for breast conserving therapy. The incidence increased to 3% when nodal irradiation was added and 8.8% when nodal irradiation and chemotherapy was delivered.[162] Even higher incidences of radiation pneumonitis have been reported following regional nodal radiation depending on the treatment technique with and without chemotherapy.[163–165]

The incidence of pneumonitis based on irradiated lung volumes from different radiation therapy techniques used to treat breast cancer patients has been studied by Lind et al.[167] On the basis of the report of Graham et al., ≧20 Gy (V_{20}) was chosen as the ipsilateral lung tolerance level to document. The average irradiated ipsilateral lung volumes at ≧20 Gy (V_{20}) in 84 patients was: breast treatment only, 7%; breast + regional RT (without internal mammary nodes), 20%; breast + regional RT (with internal mammary nodes), 30%; post-mastectomy local regional RT (with internal mammary nodes), 35%. A positive correlation was found between the incidence of pulmonary complications and increasing ipsilateral lung volumes receiving >20 Gy ($P = 0.001$). The incidence of moderate symptomatic post-treatment pneumonitis (requiring steroid treatment) for the respective lung volumes was 0.5%, 7.5%, 11%, and 11.5%.

The dose constraints for lung at our institution are as follows. For breast irradiation alone, ≤10% of the ipsilateral lung should receive ≧20 Gy. For breast and/or chest wall and regional nodal irradiation ≤25% of the ipsilateral lung should receive ≧20 Gy.

B10. Secondary Malignancy

The overall survival of early stage breast cancer is good so that there are increasing numbers of long-term breast cancer survivors that need to be followed for the occurrence of secondary malignancies.

It is well established that patients treated for one breast cancer have a higher risk of subsequent contralateral breast cancer (CBC).[168–172] The risk for CBC averages between 1.1% and 1.5% per year. On the basis of the evidence from both randomized trials and population-based studies, it does not appear that breast radiation to one breast increases this risk for subsequent CBC. In the randomized trials evaluating breast conserving therapy, the rate of subsequent CBC was similar in either the mastectomy or radiation treatment arms. The Milan I trial that randomized 701 breast cancer patients to either radical mastectomy or quadrantectomy and radiation demonstrated 28 CBC in the mastectomy arm and 22 in the radiation group at up to 19 years follow-up.[170] Ten-year follow-up of the NCI randomized trial demonstrated 10 CBC in the 116 mastectomy patients and 7 in the 121 who underwent lumpectomy and radiation.[169] At 15-year follow-up of the Institut Gustave, Roussy, 13 CBC occurred in the 91 patients treated with mastectomy and 10 in the 88 patients who had radiation following tumorectomy.[168]

Multiple population-based studies have evaluated whether the incidence of CBC could be linked to radiotherapy for the first breast cancer. A study from the Connecticut Tumor Registry of 41,109 breast cancer patients treated between 1935 and 1982 revealed 655 CBC that were matched with 1189 controls did not demonstrate an overall increase in CBC after radiation treatment.[171] A non-significant trend for increase in CBC was seen in a subset of 45 women who were <45 years old at diagnosis and who were 10 years post-radiation treatments. A population-based study from Denmark looking at 529 breast cancer patients with CBC and 529 matched controls did not demonstrate an increased risk of CBC after radiation for a first breast cancer.[172] A 4.2% incidence of CBC was documented for 134,501 breast cancer cases treated between 1973 and 1996 in the SEER database.[173] In this study, a cox proportional hazards regression model demonstrated that radiation treatment for the first cancer was associated with an increased risk of CBC after 5 years of follow-up (RR = 1.14, 95% CI 1.03–1.26, $P = 0.001$). This study was limited by the unavailability of confounding information, such as tamoxifen use, that could affect the incidence of CBC. In conclusion, there has been no consistent evidence that the use of radiation for one breast cancer causes a second CBC. However, adherence to radiation techniques that reduce the contralateral breast dose is advised, especially in younger patients.

There is increasingly compelling evidence that breast cancer patients are at higher risk of subsequently developing lung cancer following radiation; especially for those who smoke. Data from SEER were used to assess the subsequent risk of lung cancer in breast cancer patients that were irradiated. A total of 122 lung cancers developed in 13,750 women who received radiation and 473 in the 41,196 who were not radiated (0.88% vs. 0.11%).[174] This risk was confined to the ipsilateral lung. A population-based study from the Danish Cancer Registry has also demonstrated a slightly elevated lung cancer risk after 10 years in radiated breast cancer patients.[176] A study from the Connecticut Tumor Registry with an analysis for smoking history demonstrated that the increased risk of subsequent lung cancer in the ipsilateral lung following radiation for breast cancer was much greater for smokers than non-smokers.[175] The relative risk for a subsequent ipsilateral lung cancer was 6.7 (95% CI 0.6–79.4) for non-smokers and 76.6 (95% CI 8.1–724) in smokers. No information was available in this study regarding radiation technique, volume of lung radiated, or extent of smoking history. This relationship between radiation for breast cancer, smoking, and secondary lung cancers was further evaluated in a study from MD Anderson Cancer Center using 280 lung cancer cases with a prior diagnosis of breast cancer matched to a group of 300 randomly selected breast cancer cases who did not develop lung cancer.[177] Smoking increased the odds of lung carcinoma in breast cancer patients who were not irradiated (OR 6.0, 95% CI 3.6–10.1). Irradiation did not increase the odds for developing lung cancer in non-smokers (OR 0.5, 95% CI 0.3–1.1). The odds ratio for both smoking and irradiation was 9.0 (95% CI 5.1–15.9). The volume of lung-irradiated during breast cancer treatment may be an important determinant for risk of secondary lung cancer. This was demonstrated in a study from the NSABP that found an increased risk of subsequent ipsilateral lung cancer in patients who underwent chest wall and regional nodal irradiation following mastectomy but non-breast irradiation alone after lumpectomy.[178] In summary, breast cancer patients who smoke should be strongly encouraged to quit. We find in our clinic that breast cancer patients are very receptive to and successful with smoking cessation interventions. The amount of lung irradiated in all patients should be minimized, but particular attention should be paid to smokers with low-risk breast cancer.

Second primary sarcomas occur in or near the treatment field in approximately 0.1–0.2% of patients at 10 years. At the Institut Gustave, Roussy, France, 6919 patients treated for breast cancer, 11 developed secondary soft tissue sarcoma at a mean latency time of 9.5 years.[179] Similarly, 19 soft tissue sarcomas were noted in a population of 13,490 women treated for breast cancer in Sweden between 1960 and 1980.[180] A higher incidence of angiosarcoma, in particular, was demonstrated after irradiation for breast cancer in 194,798 cases in the SEER database.[181] A total of 20 cases developed in 48,975 irradiated patients versus 7 in the 146,303 non-irradiated cohort. This emphasizes the importance of long-term follow-up for breast cancer patients who have been irradiated so that early diagnosis and intervention of this rare complication can be done.

REFERENCES

1. Podrock, D and L Kristjanson. 1999. Skin reactions during radiotherapy for breast cancer: the use and impact of topical agents and dressings. Eur J Cancer Care **8:**143–153.
2. Hopewell, JW. 1990. The skin: its structure and response to ionizing radiation. Int J Radiat Biol **57(4):**751–773.
3. Archanbeau, J, R Pezner, and T Wasserman. 1995. Pathophysiology of irradiated skin and breast. Int J Radiat Oncol Biol Phys **31(5):**1171–1185.
4. Cox, J, J Stetz, and T Pajak. 1995. Toxicity criteria of the Radiation Therapy Oncology Group (RTOG) and the European Organization for Research and Treatment of Cancer (EORTC). Int J Radiat Oncol Biol Phys **31(5):**1341–1346.
5. Collins, EE and C Collins. 1935. Roentgen dermatitis treated with fresh whole leaf of aloe vera. AJR **33:**396–397.
6. Roy, I, A Fortin, and M Larochelle. 2001. The impact of skin washing with water and soap during breast irradiation: a randomized study. Radiother Oncol **58:**333–339.
7. Lokkevik, E, E Slovlund, J Reitan, et al. 1996. Skin treatment with bepanthen cream versus no cream during radiotherapy. Acta Onocol **35(8):**1021–1026.
8. Maiche, AG, P Grohn, and H Maki-Hokkonen. 1991. Effect of chamomile cream and almond ointment on acute radiation skin reaction. Acta Oncol **30(3):**395–396.
9. Maiche, A, O Isokangas, and P Grohn. 1994. Skin protection by sucralfate cream during electron beam therapy. Acta Oncol **33(2):**210–203.
10. Liguori, V, C Guillemin, G Pesce, et al. 1997. Double-blind randomized clinical study comparing hyaluronic acid cream to placebo in patients treated with radiotherapy. Radiother Oncol **42:**155–161.
11. Williams, M, M Burk, C Loprinzi, et al. 1996. Phase III double-blind evaluation of an aloe vera gel as a prophylactic agent for radiation-induced skin toxicity. Int J Radiat Oncol Biol Phys **36(2):**345–349.
12. Heggie, S, G Bryant, L Tripcony, et al. 2002 A phase III study on the efficacy of topical aloe vera gel on irradiated breast tissue. Cancer Nurs **25(6):**442–451.
13. Olsen, D, W Raub, C Bradley, et al. 2001. The effect of aloe vera gel/mild soap versus mild soap alone in preventing skin reactions in patients undergoing radiation therapy. Oncol Nurs Forum **28(3):**543–547.
14. Bostrom, A, H Lindman, C Swartling, et al. 2001. Potent corticosteroid cream (mometasone furoate) significantly reduces acute radiation dermatitis: results from a double-blind, randomized study. Radiother Oncol **59:**257–265.
15. Schmuth, M, MA Wimmer, S Hofer, et al. 2002. Topical corticosteroid therapy for acute radiation dermatitis: a prospective, randomized double-blind study. Br J Dermatol **146:**983–991.
16. Potera, M, D Lookingbill, and J Stryker. 1982. Prophylaxis of radiation dermatitis with topical cortisone cream. Radiology **143:**775–777.
17. Fisher, J, C Scott, R Stevens, et al. 2000. Randomized phase III study comparing best supportive care to Biafine as a prophylactic agent for radiation-induced skin toxicity for women undergoing breast radiation: Radiation Therapy Oncology Group (RTOG) 97-13. Int J Radiat Oncol Biol Phys **48(5):**1307–1310.
18. Szumacher, E, A Wighton, E Franssen, et al. 2001 Phase II study assessing the effectiveness of Biafine cream as a prophylactic agent for radiation-induced acute skin toxicity to the breast in women undergoing radiotherapy with concomitant CMF chemotherapy. Int J Radiat Oncol Biol Phys **51(1):**81–86.
19. Fenig, E, B Brenner, A Katz, et al. 2001. Topical Biafine and Lipiderm for the preventions of radiation dermatitis: a randomized prospective trial. Oncol Rep **8:**305–309.
20. Pommier, P, F Gomez, A Sunyach, et al. 2004. Phase III randomized trial of *Calendula officinalis* compared with Trolamine for the prevention of acute dermatitis during irradiation of breast cancer. J Clin Oncol **22(8):**1447–1453.
21. Mallet, J, J Mulholland, D Laverty, et al. 1999. An integrated approach to wound management. Int J Palliat Nurs **5(3):**124–132.
22. Dobrzanski, S, CM Kelly, JI Gray, et al. 1990. Granuflex dressings in treatment of full thickness pressure sores. Prof Nurse **5(11):**594–599.
23. Shell, JA, F Stanutz, and J Grimm. 1986. Comparison of moisture vapor permeable dressings to conventional dressings for management of radiation skin reactions. Oncol Nurs Forum **13:**11–16.
24. Margolin, SG, JC Breneman, DL Denman, et al. 1990. Management of radiation induced moist skin desquamation using hydrocolloid dressing. Cancer Nurs **13(2):**71–80.
25. Mak, S, A Molassiotis, W Wan, et al. 2000 The effects of hydrocolloid dressing and gentian violet on radiation-induced moist desquamation wound healing. Cancer Nurs **23(3):**220–228.

26. Bentel, G, L Marks, C Whiddon, et al. 1999. Acute and late morbidity of using a breast positioning ring in women with large/pendulous breasts. Radiother Oncol **50:**277–281.
27. Grann, A, B McCormick, E Chabner, et al. 2000. Prone breast radiotherapy in early-stage breast cancer: a preliminary analysis. Int J Radiat Oncol Biol Phys **47(2):**319–325.
28. Mahe, MA, JM Classe, F Dravet, et al. 2002. Preliminary results for prone-position breast irradiation. Int J Radiat Oncol Biol Phys **52(1):**156–160.
29. Ellerbroek, N, S Martino, B Mautner, et al. 2003. Breast-conserving therapy with adjuvant paclitaxel and radiation therapy: feasibility of concurrent treatment. Breast J **9(2):**74–78.
30. Hanna, Y, K Baglan, J Stromberg, et al. 2002 Acute and subacute toxicity associated with concurrent adjuvant radiation therapy and paclitaxel in primary breast cancer therapy. Breast J **8(3):**149–153.
31. Formenti, S, M Volm, K Skinner, et al. 2003. Preoperative twice-weekly paclitaxel with concurrent radiation therapy followed by surgery and postoperative doxorubicin-based chemotherapy in locally advanced breast cancer: a phase I/II trial. J Clin Oncol **21(5):**864–870.
32. Bellon, J, K Lindsley, G Ellis, et al. 2000. Concurrent radiation therapy and paclitaxel or docetaxel chemotherapy in high-risk breast cancer. Int J Radiat Oncol Biol Phys **48(2):**393–397.
33. Issac, N, T Panzarella, A Lau, et al. 2002. Concurrent cyclophosphamide, methotrexate, and 5-fluorouracil chemotherapy and radiotherapy for breast carcinoma. Cancer **95(4):**696–703.
34. Fiets, WE, JWR van Helvoirt, I Nortier, et al. 2003. Acute toxicity of concurrent adjuvant radiotherapy and chemotherapy (CMF or AC) in breast cancer patients: a prospective, comparative, non-randomised study. Eur J Cancer **39:**1081–1088.
35. Greenberg, D, J Sawicka, S Eisenthal, et al. 1992. Fatigue syndrome due to localized radiation. J Pain Symptom Manage **7:** 38–45.
36. Barrere, C, P Trotta, and J Foster. 1993. The experience of fatigue in women undergoing radiation therapy for early stage breast cancer. Oncol Nurs Forum **20:**311.
37. Wratten, C, J Kilmurray, S Nash, et al. 2004. Fatigue during breast radiotherapy and its relationship to biological factors. Int J Radiat Oncol Biol Phys **59(1):**160–167.
38. Stone, P, M Richards, R Hern, et al. 2001. Fatigue in patients with cancer of the breast or prostate undergoing radical radiotherapy. J Pain Symptom Manage **22(6):**1007–1015.
39. Irvine, D, L Vincent, J Graydon, et al. 1998. Fatigue in women with breast cancer receiving radiation therapy. Cancer Nurs **21(2):**127–135.
40. Stasi, R, L Abriani, P Beccaglia, et al. 2003. Cancer-related fatigue. Cancer **98(9):**1786–1801.
41. Mock, V, K Hassey Dow, C Meares, et al. 1997. Effects of exercise on fatigue, physical functioning, and emotional distress during radiation therapy for breast cancer. Oncol Nurs Forum **24(6):**991–1000.
42. Pezner, R, M Patterson, J Lipsett, et al. 1991. Factors affecting cosmetic outcome in breast-conserving cancer treatment—objective quantitative assessment. Breast Cancer Res Treat **20:**85–92.
43. Ryoo, M, AR Kagan, M Wollin, et al. 1989. Prognostic factors for recurrence and cosmesis in 393 patients after radiation therapy for early mammary carcinoma. Radiology **172:**555–559.
44. De La Rochefordiere, A, A Abner, B Silver, et al. 1992. Are cosmetic results following conservative surgery and radiation therapy for early breast cancer dependent on technique? Int J Radiat Oncol Biol Phys **23(5):**925–931.
45. Taylor, M, C Perez, K Halverson, et al. 1995. Factors influencing cosmetic results after conservation therapy for breast cancer. Int J Radiat Oncol Biol Phys **31(4):**753–764.
46. Wazer, D, T Dipetrillo, R Schmidt-Ullirch, et al. 1992. Factors influencing cosmetic outcome and complication risk after conservative surgery and radiotherapy for early-stage breast carcinoma. J Clin Oncol **10(3):**356–363.
47. Tuamokumo, N, and B Haffty. 2003. Clinical outcome and cosmesis in African-American patients treated with conservative surgery and radiation therapy. Cancer J **9(4):**313–320.
48. Harris, JR, MB Levene, G Svensson, et al. 1979. Analysis of cosmetic results following primary radiation therapy for stage I and II carcinoma of the breast. Int J Radiat Oncol Biol Phys **5:**257–261.
49. Olivotto, IA, MA Rose, RT Osteen, et al. 1989. Late cosmetic outcome after conservative sugery and radiotherapy: analysis of causes of cosmetic failure. Int J Radiat Oncol Biol Phys **17(4):**747–753.
50. Sneeuw, KCA, NK Aaronson, JR Yarnold, et al. 1992. Cosmetic and functional outcomes of breast conserving treatment for early stage breast cancer. 1. Comparisons of patients' ratings, observers' ratings and objective assessments. Radiother Oncol **25:**153–159.
51. Vreilng, C, L Collette, A Fourquet, et al. 1999. The influence of the boost in breast-conserving therapy on cosmetic outcome in the EORTC "boost versus no boost" trial. Int J Radiat Oncol Biol Phys **45(3):**677–685.

52. Veronesi, U, E Marubini, V Galimberti, et al. 2001. Radiotherapy after breast-conserving surgery in small breast carcinoma: long term results of randomized trial. Ann Oncol **12(7):**997–1003.
53. Sacchini, V, A Luini, R Agresti, et al. 1995. The influence of radiotherapy on cosmetic outcome after breast conservative surgery. Int J Radiat Oncol Biol Phys **33(1):**59–64.
54. Pierce, LJ, J Moughan, J White, et al. 2004. 1998–1999 Patterns of Care Process Survey of National Practice Patterns Using Breast-Conserving Surgery and Radiotherapy in the Management of Stage I/II Breast Cancer. Int J Radiat Oncol Biol Phys. In press
55. White, J, J Moughan, LJ Pierce, et al. 2004. The status of post-mastectomy radiation therapy in the United States: A Patterns of Care Study. Int J Radiat Oncol Biol Phys **60(1):**77–85.
56. Romestaing, P, Y Lehingue, C Carrie, et al. 1997. Role of a 10 Gy boost in the conservative treatment of early breast cancer: results of a randomized clinical trial in Lyon, France. J Clin Oncol **15(3):**963–968.
57. Bartelink, H, JC Horiot, P Poortmans, et al. 2001. Recurrence rates after treatment of breast cancer with standard radiotherapy with or without additional radiation. NEJM **345(19):**1378–1387.
58. Victor, S, D Brown, E Horwitz, et al. 1998. Treatment outcome with radiation therapy after breast augmentation or reconstruction in patients with primary breast carcinoma. Cancer **82(7):**1303–1309.
59. Handel, N, B Lewinsky, J Jensen, et al. 1996. Breast conservation therapy after augmentation mammaplasty: is it appropriate? Plast Reconstr Surg **98(7):**1216–1224.
60. Ryu, J, J Yahalom, B Shank, et al. 1990. Radiation therapy after breast augmentation or reconstruction in early or recurrent breast cancer. Cancer **66:**844–847.
61. Chu, R, T Kaufmann, G Dawson, et al. 1992. Radiation therapy of cancer in prosthetically augmented or reconstructed breasts. Radiology **185:**429–433.
62. Mark, R, R Zimmerman, and J Greif. 1996. Capsular contracture after lumpectomy and radiation therapy in patients who have undergone uncomplicated bilateral augmentation mammoplasty. Radiology **200:**621–625.
63. Guenther, JM, KM Tokita, and AE Giuliano. 1994. Breast conserving surgery and radiation after augmentation mammoplasty. Cancer **73:**2613–2618.
64. Gabriel, SE, JE Woods, et al. 1997. Complications leading to surgery after breast implantation. N Engl J Med **336:**677–682.
65. Polednak, A. 2000. Geographic variation in postmastectomy breast reconstruction rates. Plast Reconstr Surg **106:**298–301.
66. Kuske, R, R Schuster, E Klein, et al. 1991. Radiotherapy and breast reconstruction: clinical results and dosimetry. Int J Radiat Oncol Biol Phys **21(2):**339–346.
67. Cordeiro, P, A Pusic, J Disa, et al. 2004. Irradiation after immediate tissue expander/implant breast reconstruction: outcomes, complications, aesthetic results, and satisfaction among 156 patients. Plast Reconstr Surg **113(3):**877–881.
68. Halpern, J, M McNeese, S Kroll, et al. 1990. Irradiation of prosthetically augmented breasts: a retrospective study on toxicity and cosmetic results. Int J Radiat Oncol Biol Phys **18(1):**189–191.
69. Zimmerman, R, R Mark, A Kim, et al. 1998. Radiation tolerance of transverse rectus abdominis myocutaneous-free flaps used in immediate breast reconstruction. Am J Clin Oncol **21(4):**381–385.
70. Williams, JK, GW Carlson, J Botswick III, et al. 1997 The effect of radiation treatment after TRAM flap breast reconstruction. Plast Reconstr Surg **100(50):**1153–1160.
71. Tran, N, D Chang, A Gupta, et al. 2001. Comparison of immediate and delayed free TRAM flap breast reconstruction in patients receiving postmastectomy radiation therapy. Plast Reconstr Surg **108(1):**78–82.
72. Ragaz, J, S Jackson, N Le, et al. 1997. Adjuvant radiotherapy and chemotherapy in node-positive premenopausal women with breast cancer. NEJM **337(14):**956–962.
73. Overgaard, M, P Hansen, J Overgaard, et al. 1997. Postoperative radiotherapy in high-risk premenopausal women with breast cancer who receive adjuvant chemotherapy. NEJM **337(14):**949–955.
74. Alderman, A, E Wilkins, H Kim, et al. 2002. Complications in postmastectomy breast reconstruction: two-year results of the Michigan Breast Reconstruction Outcome Study. Plast Reconstr Surg **109(7):**2265–2274.
75. Carpenter, J, M Andrykowski, P Sloan, et al. 1998. Postmastectomy/postlumpectomy pain in breast cancer survivors. J Clin Epidemiol **51(12):**1285–1292.
76. Ryan, G, L Dawson, A Bezjak, et al. 2003. Prospective comparison of breast pain in patients participating in a randomized trial of breast-conserving surgery and tamoxifen with or without radiotherapy. Int J Radiat Oncol Biol Phys **55(1):**154–161.
77. Whelan, T, M Levine, J Julian, et al. 2000. The effects of radiation therapy on quality of life of women with breast carcinoma. Cancer **88(10):**2260–2266.

78. Meric, F, T Buchholz, N Mirza, et al. 2002. Long-term complications associated with breast-conservation surgery and radiotherapy. Ann Surg Oncol **9(6):**543–549.
79. Fehlauer, F, S Tribius, U Holler, et al. 2003. Long-term radiation sequelae after breast-conserving therapy in women with early-stage breast cancer: an observational study using the LENT-SOMA scoring system. Int J Radiat Oncol Biol Phys **55(3):**651–658.
80. LENT-SOMA scales for all anatomical sites. 1995. Int J Radiat Oncol Biol Phys **31:**1049–1091.
81. Bentzen, S, H Thames, and M Overgaard. 1989. Latent-time estimation for late cutaneous and subcutaneous radiation reactions in a single follow-up clinical study. Radiother Oncol **15:**267–274.
82. Iannuzzi, C, D Atencio, S Green, et al. 2002. ATM mutations in female breast cancer patients predict for an increase in radiation-induced late effects. Int J Radiat Oncol Biol Phys **52(3):**606–613.
83. Turesson, I, G Notter, I Wickstrom, et al. 1984. The influence of irradiation time per treatment session on acute and late skin reactions: a study on human skin. Radiother Oncol **(2):**235–245.
84. Turesson, I, and G Notter. 1984. The influence of fraction size in radiotherapy on the late normal tissue reaction-II: comparison of the effects of daily and twice-a-week fractionation on human skin. Int J Radiat Oncol Biol Phys **10(5):**599–606.
85. Huang, EY, HC Chen, CJ Wang, et al. 2002. Predictive factors for skin telangiectasia following post-mastectomy electron beam irradiation. Br J Radiat Oncol **75:**444–447.
86. Bentzen, S and M Overgaard. 1991. Relationship between early and late normal-tissue injury after postmastectomy radiotherapy. Radiother Oncol **20:**159–165.
87. Turesson, I, J Nyman, E Holberg, et al. 1996. Prognostic factors for acute and late skin reaction in radiotherapy patients. Int J Radiat Oncol Biol Phys **36(5):**1065–1075.
88. Alora, MB and RR Anderson. 2000. Recent developments in cutaneous lasers. Lasers Surg Med **26:**108–118.
89. Lanigan, SW and T Joannides. 2003. Pulsed dye laser treatment of telangiectasia after radiotherapy for carcinoma of the breast. Br J Dermatol **148:**77–79.
90. Robertson, J, D Clarke, M Pevzner, et al. 1991. Breast conservation therapy. Severe breast fibrosis after radiation therapy in patients with collagen vascular disease. Cancer **68:**502–508.
91. Varga, J, UF Haustein, R Creech, et al. 1991. Exaggerated radiation-induced fibrosis in patients with systemic sclerosis. JAMA **265(24):**3292–3295.
92. Chen, A, E Obedian, and B Haffty. 2001. Breast-conserving therapy in the setting of collagen vascular disease. Cancer J **7(6):**480–491.
93. Morris, M, and S Powell. 1997. Irradiation in the setting of collagen vascular disease: acute and late complications. J Clin Oncol **15(7):**2728–2735.
94. Ross, J, D Hussey, N Mayr, et al. 1993. Acute and late reactions to radiation therapy in patients with collagen vascular diseases. Cancer **71:**744–752.
95. Phan, C, M Mindrum, C Silverman, et al. 2003. Matched-control retrospective study of the acute and late complications in patients with collagen vascular diseases treated with radiation therapy. Cancer J **9(6):**461–466.
96. Tobin, MB, HJ Lacey, L Meyer, and PS Mortimer. 1993. The psychological morbidity of breast cancer-related arm swelling. Cancer **72:**3248–3252.
97. Maunsell, E, J Brisson, and L Deshenes. 1993. Arm problems and psychological distress after surgery for breast cancer. Can J Surg **363:**15–320.
98. Ververs, J, R Roumen, A Vingerhoerts, et al. 2001. Risk, severity and predictors of physical and psychological morbidity after axillary lymph node dissection for breast cancer. Eur J Cancer **37:**991–999.
99. Lin, PP, DC Allison, J Wainstock, et al. 1993. Impact of axillary lymph node dissection on the therapy of breast cancer patients. J Clin Oncol **11(8):**1536–1544.
100. Petrek, J, R Senie, M Peters, et al. 2001. Lymphedema in a cohort of breast carcinoma survivors 20 years after diagnosis. Cancer **92(6):**1368–1377.
101. Petrek, J and M Heelan. 1998. Incidence of breast carcinoma-related lymphedema. Cancer Suppl **83(12):**2776–2781.
102. Ivens, D, AL Hoe, TJ Podd, et al. 1992. Assessment of morbidity from complete axillary dissection. Br J Cancer **66(1):**136–138.
103. Larson, D, M Weinstein, I Goldberg, et al. 1986. Edema of the arm as a function of the extent of axillary surgery in patients with stage I-II carcinoma of the breast treated with primary radiotherapy. Int J Radiat Oncol Biol Phys **12(9):**1575–1582.
104. Kissin, MW, G Querci della Rovere, D Easton, et al. 1986. Risk of lymphoedema following the treatment of breast cancer. Br J Surg **73(7):**580–584.

105. Kiel, K and A Rademacker. 1996. Early-stage breast cancer: arm edema after wide excision and breast irradiation. Radiology **198(1):**279–283.
106. Keramopoulos, A, C Tsionou, D Minaretzis, et al. 1993. Arm morbidity following treatment of breast cancer with total axillary dissection: a multivariated approach. Oncology **50:**445–449.
107. Pezner, R, M Patterson, LR Hill, et al. 1986. Arm lymphedema in patients treated conservatively for breast cancer: relationship to patient age and axillary node dissection technique. Int J Radiat Oncol Biol Phys **12(12):**2079–2083.
108. Herd-Smith, A, A Russo, M Grazia Muraca, et al. 2001. Prognostic factors for lymphedema after primary treatment of breast carcinoma. Cancer **92(7):**1783–1787.
109. Hojris, I, J Andersen, M Overgaard, et al. 2000. Late treatment-related morbidity in breast cancer patients randomized to postmastectomy radiotherapy and systemic treatment versus systemic treatment alone. Acta Oncol **39(3):**355–372.
110. Guiliano, AE, PI Haigh, MB Brennan, et al. 2000. Perspective observational study of sentinel lymphadenectomy without further axillary dissection in patients with sentinel node negative breast cancer. J Clin Oncol **18:**2553–2559.
111. Veronesi, U, G Paganelli, G Viale, et al. 2003. A randomized comparison of sentinel-node biopsy with routine axillary dissection in breast cancer. NEJM **349(6):**546–553.
112. Ryttov, N, NV Holm, N Qvist, et al. 1988. Influence of adjuvant irradiation on the development of late arm lymphedema and impaired shoulder mobility after mastectomy for carcinoma of the breast. Acta Oncol **27:**667–670.
113. Segerstrom, K, P Bjerle, S Graffman, et al. 1992. Factors that influence the incidence of brachial oedema after treatment of breast cancer. Scand J Plast Reconstr Hand Surg **26:**223–227.
114. Bijker, N, E Rutgers, J Peterse, et al. 1999. Low risk of locoregional recurrence of a primary breast carcinoma after treatment with a modification of the Halsted radical mastectomy and selective use of radiotherapy. Cancer **85(8):**1773–1781.
115. Powell, S, A Taghian, L Kachnic, et al. 2003. Risk of lymphedema after regional nodal irradiation with breast conservation therapy. Int J Radiat Oncol Biol Phys **55(5):**1209–1215.
116. Werner, R, B McCormick, J Petrek, et al. 1991. Arm edema in conservatively managed breast cancer: obesity is a major predictive factor. Radiology **180(1):**177–184.
117. Liljegren, G and L Holmberg. 1997. The Uppsala-Orebro Breast Cancer Study Group. Arm morbidity after sector resection and axillary dissection with or without postoperative radiotherapy in breast cancer Stage I. Results from a randomised trial. Eur J Cancer **33(2):**193–199.
118. Johansson, S, H Svensson and J Denekamp. 2002. Dose response and latency for radiation-induced fibrosis, edema, and neuropathy in breast cancer patients. Int J Radiat Oncol Biol Phys **52(5):**1207–1219.
119. Pierce, L, H Oberman, M Strawderman, et al. 1995. Microscopic extracapsular extension of the axilla: is this an indication for axillary radiotherapy? Int J Radiat Oncol Biol Phys **33(2):**253–259.
120. The diagnosis and treatment of peripheral edema: consensus development of the International Society of Lymphology Executive Committee. Lymphology 1998;**28:**113–113.
121. Brennan, MJ and LT Miller. 1998. Overview of treatment options and review of the current role of compression garments, intermittent pumps, and exercise programs in the management of lymphedema. Cancer **83(Suppl 12):**2821–2827.
122. Mondry, T, R Riffenburgh, P Johnstone, et al. 2004. Prospective trial of complete decongestive therapy for upper extremity lymphedema after breast cancer therapy. Cancer J **19(1):**42–48.
123. Erickson, V, M Pearson, P Ganz, et al. 2001. Arm edema in breast cancer patients. J Natl Cancer Instit **93(2):**96–111.
124. Carl, U, J Feldmeier, G Schmitt, et al. 2001. Hyperbaric oxygen therapy for late sequelae in women receiving radiation after breast conserving surgery. Int J Radiat Oncol Biol Phys **49(4):**1029–1031.
125. Gothard, L, A Stanton, J MacLaren, et al. 2001. Non-randomised phase II trial of hyperbaric oxygen therapy in patients with chronic arm lymphoedema and tissue fibrosis after radiotherapy for early breast cancer. Radiother Oncol **70:**217–224.
126. Loprinzi, C, J Kugler, J Sloan, et al. 1999. Lack of effect of coumarin in women with lymphedema after treatment for breast cancer. NEJM **340(5):**346–350.
127. Casley-Smith, JR, RG Morgan, and NB Piller. 1993. Treatment of lymphedema of the arms and legs with 5,6-benzo[α]-pyrone. NEJM **329:**1158–1163.
128. Pecking, AP, B Fevrier, C Wargon, et al. 1997. Efficacy of Daflon 500 mg in the treatment of lymphedema (secondary to conventional therapy of breast cancer). Angiology **48:**93–98.

129. Micke, O, F Bruns, R Mucke, et al. 2003. Selenium in the treatment of radiation-associated secondary lymphedema. Int J Radiat Oncol Biol Phys **56(1):**40–49.
130. Sugden, EM, M Rezvani, JM Harrison, et al. 1998. Shoulder movement after the treatment of early stage breast cancer. Clin Oncol **10:**173–181.
131. Deutsch, M and J Flickinger. 2001. Shoulder and arm problems after radiotherapy for primary breast cancer. Am J Clin Oncol **24(2):**172–176.
132. Gerber, A, M Lampert, C Wood, et al. 1992. Comparison of pain, motion, and edema after modified radical mastectomy versus local excision with axillary dissection and radiation. Cancer Res Treat **21:**139–145.
133. Bentzen, S, M Overgaard and H Thames. 1989. Fractionation sensitivity of a functional endpoint: impaired shoulder movement after post-mastectomy radiotherapy. Int J Radiat Oncol Biol Phys **17:**531–537.
134. Fathers, E, D Thrush, S Huson, et al. 2002. Radiation-induced brachial plexopathy in women treated for carcinoma of the breast. Clin Rehabil **16:**160–165.
135. Olsen, N, P Pfeiffer, L Johannsen, et al. 1993. Radiation-induced brachial plexopathy: neurological follow-up in 161 recurrence-free breast cancer patients. Int J Radiat Oncol Biol Phys **26(1):**43–49.
136. Johansson, S, H Svensson , and J Denekamp. 2000. Timescale of evolution of late radiation injury after postoperative radiotherapy of breast cancer patients. Int J Radiation Oncol Biol Phys **48(3):**745–750.
137. Rubin, D, P Schomberg, R Shepard, et al. 2001. Arteritis and brachial plexus neuropathy as delayed complications of radiation therapy. Mayo Clin Proc **76(8):**849–852.
138. Pierce, S, A Recht, T Lingos, et al. 1992. Long-term radiation complications following conservative surgery (CS) and radiation therapy (RT) in patients with early stage breast cancer. Int J Radiat Oncol Biol Phys **23(5):**915–923.
139. Kini, V, J White, E Horwitz, et al. 1998. Long term results with breast-conserving therapy for patients with early stage breast carcinoma in a community hospital setting. Cancer **82(1):**127–133.
140. Fowble, BL, LJ Solin, DJ Schultz, et al. 1991. Ten year results of conservative surgery and irradiation for stage I and II breast cancer. Int J Radiat Oncol Biol Phy **21:**269–277.
141. Bajrovic, A, D Rades, F Fehlauer, et al. 2004. Is there a life-long risk of brachial plexopathy after radiotherapy of supraclavicular lymph nodes in breast cancer patients? Radiother Oncol **71:**297–301.
142. Olsen, N, P Pfeiffer, K Mondrup et al. 1990. Radiation-induced brachial plexus neuropathy in breast cancer patients. Acta Oncol **29:**885–890.
143. Stewart, JR, L Fajardo, S Gillette, et al. 1995. Radiation injury to the heart. Int J Radiat Oncol Biol Phys **31(5):**1205–1211.
144. Cuzick, J, H Stewart, R Peto, et al. 1987. Overview of randomized trial of postoperative adjuvant radiotherapy in breast cancer. Cancer Treat Rep **71:**15–29.
145. Cuzick, J, H Stewart, L Rutqvist, et al. 1994. Cause-specific mortality in long-term survivors of breast cancer who participated in trials of radiotherapy. J Clin Oncol **12(3):**447–453.
146. Rutqvist, L, I Lax, T Fornander, et al. 1992. Cardiovascular mortality in a randomized trial of adjuvant radiation therapy versus surgery alone in primary breast cancer. Int J Radiat Oncol Biol Phys **22(5):**887–896.
147. Gyenes, G, L Rutqvist, A Liedberg, et al. 1998. Long-term cardiac morbidity and mortality in a randomized trial of pre- and postoperative radiation therapy versus surgery alone in primary breast cancer. Radiother Oncol **48:**185–190.
148. Gyenes, G, G Gagliardi, I Lax, et al. Evaluation of irradiated heart volumes in stage I breast cancer patients treated wit postoperative adjuvant radiotherapy.
149. Paszat, L, W Mackillop, P Groome, et al. 1999. Mortality from myocardial infarction following postlumpectomy radiotherapy for breast cancer: a population-based study in Ontario, Canada. Int J Radiat Oncol Biol Phys **43(4):**755–761.
150. Rutqvist, LE and H Johansson. 1990. Mortality by laterality of the primary tumour among 55,000 breast cancer patients from the Swedish Cancer Registry. Br J Cancer **61:**866–868.
151. Paszat, L, W Mackillop, P Groome, et al. 1998. Mortality from myocardial infarction after adjuvant radiotherapy for breast cancer in the surveillance, epidemiology, and end-results registries. J Clin Oncol **16:**2625–2631.
152. Early Breast Cancer Trialists' Collaborative Group. 2000. Favourable and unfavourable effects on long-term survival of radiotherapy for early breast cancer: an overview of the randomised trials. Lancet **355:**1757–1769.

153. Rutqvist, L, A Liedberg, N Hammar, et al. 1998. Myocardial infarction among women with early-stage breast cancer treated with conservative surgery and breast irradiation. Int J Radiat Oncol Biol Phys **40(2):**359–363.
154. Vallis, K, M Pintilie, N Chong, et al. 2002. Assessment of coronary heart disease morbidity and mortality after radiation therapy for early breast cancer. J Clin Oncol **20(4):**1036–1042.
155. Nixon, AJ, J Manola, R Gelman, et al. 1998. No long term increase in cardiac-related mortality after breast-conserving surgery and radiation therapy using modern techniques. J Clin Oncol **16:**1374–1379.
156. Hojris, J, M Overgaard, JJ Christensen, et al. 1999. Morbidity and mortality of ischaemic heart disease in high-risk breast-cancer patients after adjuvant postmastectomy systemic treatment with or without radiotherapy: Analysis of DBCG 82b and 82c randomised trials. Lancet **354:**1425–1430.
157. Hurkmans, C, BC Cho, E Damen, et al. 2002. Reduction of cardiac and lung complications probabilities after breast irradiation using conformal radiotherapy with or without intensity modulation. Radiother Oncol **62:**163–171.
158. Landau, D, E Adams, S Webb, et al. 2001. Cardiac avoidance in breast radiotherapy: a comparison of simple shielding techniques with intensity-modulated radiotherapy. Radiother Oncol **60:**247–255.
159. Chen, M, E Cash, P Danias, et al. 2002. Respiratory maneuvers decrease irradiated cardiac volume in patients with left-sided breast cancer. J Cardiovasc Magn Reson **4(2):**265–271.
160. Remouchamps, V, F Vicini, M Sharpe, et al. 2003. Significant reductions in heart and lung doses using deep inspiration breath hold with active breathing control and intensity-modulated radiation therapy for patients treated with locoregional breast irradiation. Int J Radiat Oncol Biol Phys **55(2):**392–406.
161. Movas, B, T Raffin, A Epstein, et al. 1997. Pulmonary radiation injury. Chest **111(4):**1061–1076.
162. Lingos, T, A Recht, F Vicini, et al. 1991. Radiation pneumonitis in breast cancer patients treated with conservative surgery and radiation therapy. Int J Radiat Oncol Biol Phys **21(2):**355–360.
163. Gagliardi, G, J Bjohle, I Lax, et al. 2000. Radiation pneumonitis after breast cancer irradiation: analysis of the complication probability using the relative seriality model. Int J Radiat Oncol Biol Phys **46(2):**373–381.
164. Lind, P, G Gagliardi, B Wennberg, et al. 1997. A descriptive study of pulmonary complications after postoperative radiation therapy in node-positive stage II breast cancer. Acta Oncol **36(5):**509–515.
165. Hernberg, M, P Virkkunen, P Maasilta, et al. 2002. Pulmonary toxicity after radiotherapy in primary breast cancer patients: results from a randomized chemotherapy study. Int J Radiat Oncol Biol Phys **52(1):**128–136.
166. Graham, M, J Purdy, B Emami, et al. 1999. Clinical dose–volume histogram analysis for pneumonitis after 3D treatment for non-small cell lung cancer (NSCLC). Int J Radiat Oncol Biol Phys **45(2):**323–329.
167. Lind, P, B Wennberg, G Gagliardi, et al. 2001. Pulmonary complications following different radiotherapy techniques for breast cancer, and the association to irradiated lung volume and dose. Breast Cancer Res Treat **68:**199–210.
168. Arriagada, R, MG Le, F Rochard, et al. 1996. Conservative treatment versus mastectomy in early breast cancer: Patterns of failure with 15 years of follow-up data. J Clin Oncol **14:**1558–1564.
169. Straus, K, A Lichter, M Lippman, et al. 1992. Results of the National Cancer Institute Early Breast Cancer Trial. J Natl Cancer Inst Monogr **11:**27–32.
170. Veronesi, U, A Luini, V Galimberti, et al. 1994. Conservation approaches for the management of stage I/II carcinoma of the breast: Milan Cancer Institute Trials. World J Surg **18:**70–75.
171. Boice, JD, EB Harvey, M Blettner, et al. 1992. Cancer in the contralateral breast after radiotherapy for breast cancer. N Eng J Med **326:**781–785.
172. Storm, HH, M Andersson and JD Boice 1992. Adjuvant radiotherapy and risk of contralateral breast cancer. J Natl Cancer Inst **84:**1245–1250.
173. Gao, X, S Fisher, and B Emami. 2003. Risk of second primary cancer in the contralateral breast in women treated for early-stage breast cancer: a population based study. Int J Radiat Oncol Biol Phys **56(4):**1038–1045.
174. Neugut, AI, E Robinson, and WC Lee. 1993. Lung cancer after radiation therapy for breast cancer. Cancer **71:**3054–3057.
175. Neugut, AI, T Murray, J Santos, et al. 1994. Increased risk of lung cancer after breast cancer radiation therapy in cigarette smokers. Cancer **73:**1615–1620.
176. Ewertz, M and Mouridsen HT. 1985. Second cancers following cancer of the female breast in Denmark. Natl Cancer Inst Monogr **68:**325–329.
177. Ford, M, A Sigurdson, E Petrulis, et al. 2003. Effects of smoking and radiotherapy on lung carcinoma in breast carcinoma survivors. Cancer **98:**1457–1464.

178. Deutsch, M, S Land, M Begovic, et al. 2003. The incidence of lung carcinoma after surgery for breast carcinoma with and without postoperative radiotherapy. Cancer **98:**1362–1368.
179. Taghian, A, F DeVathaire, and P Terrier. 1991. Long-term risk of sarcoma following radiation treatment for breast cancer. Int J Radiat Oncol Biol Phys **21:**361–367.
180. Karlsson, P, E Holmberg, and KA Johansson. 1996. Soft tissue sarcoma after treatment for breast cancer. Radiother Oncol **38:**25–31.
181. Huang, J and W Mackillop. 2001. Increased risk of soft tissue sarcoma after radiotherapy in women with breast carcinoma. Cancer **92:**172–80.

5. UPPER GASTROINTESTINAL TRACT

JOHANNA C. BENDELL, MD
CHRISTOPHER WILLETT, MD

Duke University Medical Center, Durham, NC

The upper gastrointestinal tract lies within the radiation field for most thoracic and abdominal cancers. Toxicity to the upper gastrointestinal tract often limits the radiation doses that can be given. Radiation therapy causes both acute and late effects. The acute effects of radiation include mucosal denudation, while late effects consist of fibrotic changes leading to decreased mobility and ischemia. Multifield and conformal radiation therapy, as well as patient positioning techniques, reduce the volume of normal tissue exposed to radiation and can decrease the potential toxicity. However, the treatment of radiation toxicity is mainly supportive. The increasing use of concurrent chemotherapy and radiation therapy has required enhanced awareness of potential effects and better methods to decrease toxicity, as this combination of treatments is associated with a higher rate of gastrointestinal toxicity. The first part of this chapter will review the pathologic changes of acute and chronic radiation effects, and the second part will discuss clinical effects, including radiation dosing and management of toxicities.

A. BIOLOGY OF RADIATION EFFECTS

A1. Esophagus

Pathologic studies of animal models have been used to describe and characterize the effects of radiation to the esophagus. Pathologic changes include an acute thinning of the squamous epithelial layer with vacuolization and absence of mitoses, followed by areas of complete denudation and areas of increased basal cell proliferation. Chronic changes include focal coagulation necrosis of the muscularis mucosa and deep muscle as well as inflammatory changes around the ganglion cells of the mesenteric plexus in the deep wall.[1,2] Physiologically, failure of the peristaltic wave and decreased relaxation of the lower esophageal sphincter are seen.

Studies of radiation therapy on the human esophagus have demonstrated similar acute and chronic effects. Studies of radiation therapy effects on the esophagus after radiation to the mediastinum and lung showed clinical and endoscopic evidence of esophagitis.[3,4] The acute pathologic findings from doses of 3000 to 4000 cGy and 6000 to 7500 cGy were similar to those seen in the mouse model of acute esophageal toxicity.[4] Studies by Lepke and Libshitz[5] and Goldstein et al.[6] found chronic changes of abnormal motility, aperistalsis, and failure to complete the primary peristaltic wave at 4–12 weeks after completion of radiation therapy at doses of 4500–6000 cGy. Areas of distal aperistalsis and resultant exposure of the lower esophagus to gastric acid were thought to be a cause of esophagitis in these patients. Human studies of chronic histologic changes after esophageal radiation show submucosal fibrosis and chronic inflammation of the lamina propria. Fibrosis was also prominent in the muscularis, especially around the muscle nerve plexus, and possibly the source of physiologic motility abnormalities and stricture. Rare chronic ulceration was also seen.[7,8]

A2. Stomach

Understanding of the pathologic response to radiation of the stomach is based mostly on animal models. Post-radiation changes included ulcerative and erosive gastritis at 2–3 weeks, stomach dilatation and gastroparesis at 4 weeks to 7 months, and gastric obstruction at 7 months in rats given doses between 1400 and 2300 cGy.[9] The rats were also found to have late changes of atrophic mucosa and intestinal metaplasia. Histologic changes include coagulation necrosis of the parietal and chief cells of the gastric mucosa.[10] In addition, there are mucosal sloughing and thinning and chronic inflammatory changes. A rabbit model also showed gastric ulceration between 23 and 58 days after first external radiation dose of 4000 cGy.[11]

A3. Small Intestine

Histologic damage to the small intestine is seen within hours after the radiation. The most sensitive cells to radiation therapy in the small intestine are the crypts of Langerhans.[12] The epithelial lining of the small intestine constantly undergoes shedding and replenishment, and damage to the actively proliferating cells results in an inability to replace cells that are naturally shed, causing a generalized mucosal sloughing.[13] With the sloughing, the villi shorten, and the area of absorption is decreased.[14] This damage is seen at doses as low as 2000 to 3000 cGy. In 2–4 weeks, there is an infiltration of leukocytes with crypt abscess formation. Ulceration may also occur. These effects peak within 3–4 weeks after radiation therapy and then subside.[13] Because of these effects, malabsorption of fat, carbohydrates, protein, bile salts, and vitamin B12 occurs.[15] There is also evidence of altered gut motility acutely after radiation.[16]

Late radiation effects occur at a median of 8–12 months following the radiation therapy, though they can appear as late as years later.[17] Progressive occlusive vasculitis with foam cell invasion of the intima and hyaline thickening of the arteriolar walls, as well as collagen deposition and fibrosis occurs. The small bowel becomes thickened with telengiectasia, while the vessel wall of small arterioles is obliterated,[18] causing ischemia of the small bowel. Lymphatic damage results in constriction of the lymphatic channels, which contributes to mucosal edema and inflammation.[19] The mucosa is atrophied, with atypical hyperplastic glands and intestinal wall fibrosis.[7] Mucosal ulceration is common, and can lead to perforation, fistulae, and abscesses. As the ulcers heal, there can be fibrosis with narrowing of the intestinal lumen with subsequent stricture formation. The bowel generally appears thickened and edematous. It should be noted that even if the gut appears normal, patients can still be at risk of spontaneous perforation.[20]

A4. Liver

Radiation-induced liver disease (RILD) is seen in 5–10% of patients when the whole liver radiation dose reaches 3000–3500 cGy.[21,22] The pathologic lesion in RILD is central vein thrombosis at the lobular level, or venoocclusive disease, which results in marked retrograde congestion leading to hemorrhage and secondary alterations in the surrounding hepatocytes.[23] Fibrin deposition in the central veins is thought to be the cause of the venoocclusive injury. It is unknown what stimulates the fibrin deposition, but there are hypotheses that suggest that TGFB is increased in the setting of exposure to radiation, and this in turn stimulates fibroblast migration to the site of injury, causing fibrin and collagen deposition. Foci of necrosis are found in the affected portion of the lobules.[24] Severe acute hepatic toxicity changes often progress to fibrosis, cirrhosis, and liver failure.

A5. Kidney

The major focus of injury after radiation therapy is on the arterial glomerular region rather than the tubular epithelium.[22] The cortical rather than the medullary tubules are involved, and this involvement usually follows, rather than proceeds, vascular alterations. Glomerular damage can be seen months before tubular changes. Microangiography dramatically shows glomerulosclerosis as a function of increasing dose, so that complete obliteration of glomeruli occurs at single doses of 500–2000 cGy. Animal experiments show that histological changes of toxicity with low doses of radiation (15 cGy) can occur 3 months after radiation.[25]

B. CLINICAL ISSUES

B1. Esophagus

Clinical radiation esophagitis presents as dysphagia or a substernal burning sensation, with acute esophagitis occurring approximately 2 weeks after the initiation of radiation therapy.[17] Patients may describe a sudden, sharp, severe chest pain radiating to the back. The symptoms may be confused with candidal esophagitis, which can occur in conjunction with radiation esophagitis. These symptoms typically resolve after 2 days without radiation treatment, but can last as long as 7–10 days. Perforation and bleeding are rare in the acute phase.[26] The occurrence of acute toxicity is not predictive of chronic toxicity. Chronic toxicity presents most commonly within 4–8 months after completion of radiation therapy, but can occur as long as years later.[27] The symptoms of chronic toxicity include dysphagia from stenosis of the esophagus, strictures, or motility abnormalities. Though rare, ulcerations can lead to hemorrhage and fistulas. Patients can also present with pseudodiverticula.[4] Patients with symptoms of chronic radiation effects should be evaluated with a barium swallow or upper endoscopy, as these patients are at risk for cancer recurrence or new primary cancer, which can present as esophageal stricture, ulceration, pseudodiverticula, and fistulas.

Much work has been done to investigate dose tolerance of the esophagus and additional factors that increase toxicity. Seaman and Ackerman treated patients at doses of 6000–7500 cGy.[3] Doses of 6500–7500 cGy did cause a severe esophagitis with stricture in some patients. Three patients with moderate esophagitis received over 6000 cGy. Their conclusion was that the upper limit of dose tolerance for patients was 6000 cGy given at 1000 cGy per week. Other studies treated patients with 6000 cGy and noted a late complication rate of 1.2–18%.[28] Using standard radiation therapy, doses of 4500–6000 cGy are associated with acceptable toxicity.

With the increased use of conformal radiation therapy and concurrent use of chemotherapy, further studies have been done to evaluate dose tolerance. Maguire et al. evaluated 91 patients treated with radiation therapy for non-small cell lung cancer and analyzed predictors of acute and late esophageal toxicity.[29] They found that the percent organ volume and surface area treated with over 5000 cGy predicted for late esophageal toxicity. Patients who had pre-existing gastroesophageal reflux disease and esophageal erosion secondary to tumor were at increased risk for late toxicity. Hyperfractionation was also associated with increased acute toxicity. Werner-Wasik et al. evaluated 277 patients treated with radiation therapy for non-small cell lung cancer.[30] In this study, the concurrent use of chemotherapy with either once daily or hyperfractionated radiation therapy was associated with a significantly high incidence and grade of acute esophagitis compared to radiation therapy alone. A study, by Singh et al., of patients with non-small cell lung cancer who received conformal daily radiation therapy with or without concurrent chemotherapy found a maximal esophageal point dose of 6900 cGy for patients treated with radiation therapy alone, and this was decreased to 5800 cGy for patients receiving concurrent chemotherapy.[31] Twenty-six percent of the patients receiving concurrent chemoradiotherapy developed grades 3–5 esophageal toxicity, while 1.3% of patients who received only radiation therapy developed grades 3–5 esophageal toxicity. The Radiation Therapy Oncology Group experience, using standard radiation therapy techniques, found grade 3 or higher esophageal toxicity in 34% of patients treated with concurrent hyperfractionated radiation therapy and chemotherapy, and in 1.3% of patients treated with standard thoracic radiotherapy.[32] From these data, the addition of chemotherapy does increases the incidence of esophageal toxicity.

Treatment and prevention of radiation-induced esophagitis have come under recent increased attention with the use of aggressive combination chemotherapy and radiation therapy regimens. Treatment of acute esophagitis is based on the grade of symptoms experienced by the patient (Table 1). Treatment interruptions of 1–3 days can ease the symptoms of acute esophagitis, but may result in compromise to the patient's treatment of cancer. Reassessment and modification of the treated fields may also help. Pharmacologic management includes systemic analgesics, with narcotic analgesics if necessary, and topical analgesics, such as viscous lidocaine. Dietary modification, including pureed or soft foods and soups, can help maintain food and liquid intake. A recent study of dietary modifications and pharmacological prophylaxis for radiation-induced esophagitis appeared to decrease toxicity and avoid treatment interruptions.[33] Dietary modification included avoidance of smoking, alcohol, coffee, spicy or acidic foods or liquids, chips, crackers, fatty, and indigestible foods. It was recommended to drink between meals, and eat six light meals per day, consisting of semi-solid food, soup, purees, puddings, milk, and soft breads.

Pharmacologic prophylaxis includes non-steroidal anti-inflammatory agents, antacids, and proton-pump inhibitors. There has been some suggestion that non-steroidal anti-inflammatory agents can help prevent esophagitis by decreasing inflammation.[34] Proton pump inhibitors have not specifically been studied in patients receiving radiation therapy, but large, placebo-controlled trials have shown that proton pump inhibitors can provide significant relief and protection against ulceration in patients receiving chemotherapy.[35] Promotility agents, such as metoclopramide, have been used to counteract the abnormal motility effects of radiation and lessen the degree of esophagitis. Some will also treat for possible candidal superinfection. Recently, amifostine has been studied as a protective agent to the esophagus during chemotherapy and radiation therapy. Amifostine, an organic thio-phosphate, is a scavenger of free radicals and serves as an alternative target to nucleic acids for alkylating or platinum agents.[36] In a randomized controlled trial of patients treated with chemotherapy and radiation therapy for non-small cell lung cancer, patients were randomized to receive amifostine or no drug. Patients who received amifostine had a significantly lower incidence of acute esophagitis.[37] Other trials have shown a similar protective effect,[38,39] while others have not.[40] Larger, randomized, placebo-controlled trials are planned.

Treatment of chronic esophagitis is also dependent on the degree of symptoms (Table 2) Patients should be treated with analgesics as necessary. The chronic changes to the esophagus are mainly fibrosis, and patients may require endoscopic dilatation, sometimes on a regular basis. Dilatation can allow patients to eat at least soft foods again.[41,42] Dilatations in advanced stricture can cause esophageal rupture and caution should be exercised. Tube feedings are required for patients with weight loss of 20% or greater, or for those who can only take liquids. Surgical intervention is needed for patients who develop perforation or fistula. Patients with strictures or ulcerations should also be evaluated to differentiate chronic radiation changes from cancer recurrence.

B2. Stomach

The clinical effect of gastric radiation in humans was originally described in the 1940s in patients with testicular cancer who received large doses of abdominal irradiation.[43] Patients developed abdominal pain, nausea, vomiting, and sometimes hematemesis. Gastritis and gastric ulcers were found within the radiation field. The healed ulcers could result in obstruction or perforation up to months after radiation therapy.[44] Sell and Jensen divided the post-radiation effects on the stomach into four categories: dyspepsia, occurring 6 months to 4 years after irradiation; gastritis, occurring 1–12 months after radiation; late ulceration, occurring 5 months after radiation; and acute ulceration, occurring shortly after completion of radiation.[45] Chronic gastric toxicity from necrosis of parietal cells included decreased stomach acid secretion. Multiple studies of patients treated with radiation for Hodgkin's disease, testicular cancer, gastric cancer, and cervical cancer have established dose tolerance limits for gastric radiation.[41,46–48] In these studies, doses of 4000–6000 cGy were given to patients. Patients who received over 5000 cGy experienced gastric ulceration and gastric ulcer associated with perforation at rates of 15% and 10%, respectively. If indicated, a recommended dose to the entire stomach with conventionally administered radiation therapy is to 4500–5000 cGy, with a 5–10% risk of severe radiation toxicity. If appropriate, reduced field boosts can be given to treat to doses up to 5500 cGy with acceptable toxicity.

The combination of chemotherapy and radiation therapy decreases the tolerance of the gastric mucosa to radiation. The most common combination of chemotherapy and radiation therapy is 5-fluorouracil (5-FU) and radiation therapy. This regimen is given as adjuvant therapy for gastric, pancreatic, and biliary cancers, and as neoadjuvant therapy or treatment for locally advanced pancreatic cancer. 5-FU is a radiation sensitizer, but has been given safely with radiation therapy at doses of 4500–5000 cGy without substantial increases in toxicity. Paclitaxel and radiation therapy have been studied as combination therapy for gastric cancer.[49] Weekly paclitaxel and 5040 cGy of external beam radiation therapy showed an incidence of grades 3 and 4 esophagitis and gastritis of 15% and 11%. Gemcitabine in combination with radiation therapy has shown more significant toxicity. Phase I studies of gemcitabine and concurrent radiation therapy for locally advanced pancreatic cancer have found significant dose-limiting toxicities of nausea, vomiting, dehydration, and gastric ulceration.[50,51] Lower gemcitabine doses are being studied in combination with radiation therapy to 4500–5040 cGy. The combination of 5-FU, gemcitabine, and radiation therapy has also been studied. In the phase I trial of this combination with radiation doses of 5940 cGy, significant occurrence of gastric ulcers was found.[52] This regimen remains under study with a radiation dose of 5040 cGy.

Treatment of nausea, vomiting, and dyspepsia is largely symptomatic. Antacids, H2 blockers, and anti-emetics are used. Anti-emetic regimens include 5HT3 inhibitors, phenothiazines, metoclopramide, corticosteroids, benzodiazepines, antihistamines, and anticholinergics. As with other side effects of radiation therapy, combined chemotherapy and radiation therapy result in worsened treatment-induced nausea and vomiting. Radiation-induced nausea and vomiting typically occur within the first 24 hours after treatment. The incidence of nausea and vomiting in patients receiving upper abdominal radiation is about 50–80%. Randomized trials of prophylactic 5HT3 inhibitors have shown efficacy compared to placebo in preventing radiation-induced nausea and vomiting.[53] Narcotic and non-narcotic agents are used for pain. Patients with bleeding ulceration require endoscopy. Argon laser coagulation has been used to temporarily control bleeding.[54] Local injections of epinephrine and vasoconstrictor agents are also used, but are also temporary measures. Repeat endoscopy and hemostasis can be attempted. Blood transfusions should be performed as needed. For patients with intractable bleeding, perforation, fistulae, or obstruction, surgery may be indicated.

B3. Small Intestine

The small intestine is highly radiosensitive, but the mobility of the small bowel protects it to some extent from the effects of radiation damage. Small bowel toxicity is often the dose-limiting toxicity for patients receiving pelvic irradiation. The first case of radiation enteropathy was described in 1897.[55] The small bowel can be within the field of treatment in stomach, pancreatic, rectal, and gynecologic cancers. Factors associated with small bowel toxicity during radiation include the use of concurrent chemotherapy with radiation therapy, previous abdominal or pelvic surgery, and cardiovascular diseases. Toxicity ranges from acute diarrhea and abdominal pain to chronic changes of small bowel ischemia, ulceration, and fibrosis.

Clinically, patients acutely experience diarrhea, abdominal pain, nausea and vomiting, anorexia, and malaise. The symptoms subside with the pathologic effects and, typically, spontaneously disappear 2–6 weeks after the completion of radiation therapy.[56] However, there is evidence to suggest that patients who develop acute small intestine toxicity may be at risk for chronic effects.[57] Chronic effects include malabsorption and diarrhea, with more rapid transit times occurring in the affected bowel. This chronic malnutrition may be severe, resulting in anemia and hypoalbuminemia. There can be bleeding from ulceration and pain and bloating from strictures, as well as fevers from abscess. The clinical syndrome is progressive with worsening symptoms and effects with time.

Certain factors have been found to predispose patients to radiation toxicity to the small intestine. Women, older patients, and thin patients have a larger amount of small bowel in the pelvic cul-de-sac, which can increase the probability of radiation effect.[58] Patients with a history of pelvic inflammatory disease or endometriosis appear to be at higher risk of complications.[59,60] Patients who have had previous abdominal surgery can have adhesions that decrease the mobility of the small bowel, allowing it to be consistently exposed to fractionated radiation therapy.[61,62] In addition, patients with prior pelvic surgery can have an increase in the amount of small bowel within the pelvis, allowing increased exposure of small bowel during pelvis irradiation. Patients with diabetes, hypertension, and cardiovascular disease have an increased risk of pre-existing vascular damage or occlusion.[63] These baseline changes are compounded by the pathologic changes of chronic radiation injury, which include vasculitis obliterans and ischemia, making patients with pre-existing vascular disease predisposed to small bowel toxicity from radiation. Patients with collagen vascular disease and inflammatory bowel disease also have a high risk of both acute and chronic radiation-induced injury. Collagen vascular diseases, such as rheumatoid arthritis, systemic lupus erythematosis, and polymyositis, and inflammatory bowel diseases have pathologic changes that include transmural fibrosis, collagen deposition, and inflammatory infiltration of the mucosa. The late effects induced by the radiation therapy to the small bowel are additive to pre-existing injury from collagen vascular disease and inflammatory bowel disease, and studies have shown that these patients have a lower gastrointestinal tolerance to radiation therapy.[28,64,65] Patients whose disease is quiescent or well-controlled do better than patients with active disease.

Studies have addressed the effect of radiation dose and occurrence of small bowel toxicity. Volume of the treatment field, total radiation dose, fraction size, treatment time, and treatment technique all affect small bowel damage. Patients can receive 4500–5000 cGy in 180–200 cGy daily fractions to a pelvic field without significant incidence of toxicity.[66] For postoperative patients, radiation to 4500–5000 cGy in 5 weeks is associated with a 5% incidence of small bowel obstruction requiring surgery, while at doses over 5000 cGy, the incidence rises to 25–50%.[56] Doses of >200 cGy per fraction in the postoperative setting also increase risk of toxicity. At radiation doses of 7000 cGy or greater, the incidence of toxicity rises precipitously.[67] A study of different treatment techniques to minimize the effect of pelvic radiation on the small bowel showed that a smaller volume of irradiated bowel yielded less toxicity.[68] In addition, treating patients in the prone position with external compression and bladder distension decreased side effects, likely from exclusion of portions of the small bowel from the radiation field. Another study treating patients postoperatively with radiation to the pelvis noted a decrease in toxicity to the small bowel by placing patients in the decubitus position.[69]

The combination of radiation and chemotherapy is known to increase the risk of small bowel toxicity. Most of the combination regimens of chemotherapy and radiation use 5-FU. In a GITSG trial of postoperative bolus 5-FU at 500 mg/m^2 and radiation at 4000–4800 cGy using parallel, opposed fields for patients with rectal cancer, the incidence of severe small bowel complications was significantly higher in patients who received both chemotherapy and radiation therapy than in patients who received radiation therapy alone. The combination arm had two treatment-related deaths, which translated into a 4% mortality rate.[70,71] In additional trials where multiple field radiation techniques were used, bolus 5-FU and radiation therapy showed no increase in chronic toxicity when chemotherapy and radiation therapy were combined. There was, however, a mild increase in acute diarrheal symptoms.[68,72] The use of continuous infusional 5-FU with radiation therapy has also been studied. Continuous infusional 5-FU with radiation to 5040 cGy in 180 cGy fractions was associated with more acute diarrhea, but no significant increase in chronic or severe small bowel toxicity.[73] Capecitabine also appears to enhance acute diarrhea, but not late effects, when combined with radiation.[74]

Treatment of small bowel radiation toxicity varies with the symptoms. Acute toxicity, including diarrhea, nausea, vomiting, and abdominal cramping is treated symptomatically. Anti-diarrheals such as loperamide, diphenoxylate with atropine, anti-cholinergic agents, and opiates can be used. Anti-emetic agents are also used. A low fat, lactose-free diet may also improve symptoms. A study of oral sulcralfate in patients receiving pelvic irradiation noted a decrease in frequency and improvement in consistency of bowel movements. In this study, not only acute effects were improved, but also chronic effects at a year after completion of radiation seemed to be improved.[75] Cholestyramine to treat bile acid malabsorption has also shown some effect.[76] Treatment with anti-inflammatory agents such as buffered aspirin have also decreased some symptoms.[77] Chronic effects of diarrhea can be treated symptomatically as above. However, in the setting of malnutrition, total parenteral nutrition (TPN) can improve clinical outcome, and methylprednisolone adds to the effects of TPN.[78] Endoscopic control is used for bleeding ulcers that can be reached by endoscopy. Significant bleeding not controlled by endoscopy may be managed surgically. Small bowel obstruction is generally managed conservatively with bowel rest. If the obstruction is severe or chronic, surgical resection or lysis of adhesions may be used. Perforations and fistulae are managed surgically. It should be noted that many of these patients with chronic small bowel radiation toxicity are nutritionally depleted and are more susceptible to anastomotic leakage and dehiscence after surgery. The postoperative mortality of these patients is significant and must be taken into consideration before a decision to proceed with surgery is made.

B4. Liver

Radiation-induced liver disease is a clinical syndrome of anicteric hepatomegaly, ascites, and elevated liver enzymes, particularly alkaline phosphatase. Alkaline phosphatase levels are often elevated out of proportion to transaminases or bilirubin. The RILD occurs typically between 2 weeks and 4 months after completion of radiation therapy. Patients note fatigue, weight gain, increased abdominal girth, and occasionally right upper quadrant pain. Abdominal imaging with CT scan or MRI can be used in diagnosis. The RILD can progress to a chronic phase, where patients can develop increased fibrosis and liver failure.

Recent studies have emphasized the effect of volume addition to dose.[24] Although radiation hepatopathy can occur within doses of 3500 and 4000 cGy to the entire liver, significantly higher doses can be given with few clinical complications if sufficient normal tissue is spared. Studies by Lawrence and colleagues report that if less than 25% of the normal liver is treated with radiation therapy, there may be no upper limit on dose associated with radiation hepatopathy.[23] Estimates of the liver doses associated with a 5% risk of RILD for uniform irradiation of one-third, two-thirds, and the whole liver are 9000, 4700, and 3100 cGy, respectively. Combination of chemotherapy and radiation can increase liver damage if the chemotherapeutic agents are hepatotoxic. Such is the case with chlorambucil, busulfan, and platinum drugs, used with radiation in bone marrow transplantation. In contrast, fluoropyrimidines do not seem to increase radiation-related hepatotoxicity.[21,79]

B5. Kidney

The original paper describing radiation toxicity to the kidneys was from Luxton and Kunkler and Farr and Luxton in the early 1950s. They followed the outcomes of seminoma patients who were treated with abdominal bath radiotherapy.[80,81] They described an initial acute radiation nephritis, appearing 6–12 months after radiation treatment, including headache, vomiting, hypertension, fatigue, and edema. Patients could be found to have proteinuria and microscopic hematuria. These acute effects resolved in some patients, but in others it progressed into chronic radiation nephropathy. Chronic radiation nephropathy ranged from benign hypertension to malignant hypertension, which could be fatal.[82]

Investigators have described the response and tolerance of both the kidneys to fractionated radiation therapy.[24] When both the kidneys are irradiated, renal tolerance is defined at 2000 cGy. A dose–response curve shows an approximate threshold dose of 1500 cGy (conventional fractionation) and a plateau at 4000 cGy. There is a 6–12 month latency period before the expression of radiation nephropathy. Chronic radiation nephropathy and hypertension do not develop until 12–18 months after treatment. Because renal damage may not manifest for years after treatment, long-term follow up is important

Table 1. RTOG Acute Radiation Morbidity Scoring Criteria, Esophagus

Score	Symptoms	Treatment
0	No change over baseline	None
1	Mild dysphagia or odynophagia	May require topical anesthetic or non-narcotic analgesics/May require soft diet
2	Moderate dysphagia or odynophagia	May require narcotic analgesics/May require pureed or liquid diet
3	Severe dysphagia or odynophagia with dehydration or weight loss(>15% from pre-treatment baseline)	Requires NG feeding tube, IV fluids, or hyperalimentation
4	Complete ulceration, obstruction, perforation, fistula	Tube feedings, possible surgical intervention

as the latency period may be greater than 10 years. Because of the recognition of the limited tolerance of this organ to fractionated radiation therapy, radiation nephropathy is an uncommon toxicity.

Recent literature has examined the biochemical, radiologic, and clinical sequelae of unilateral kidney irradiation.[83] Available data suggest that irradiation of one-half or less of a kidney is well-tolerated without serious long-term complications. Investigators have also examined the outcome of patients receiving irradiation to 50% or more of one kidney to doses of at least 2000 cGy and have reported a limited risk of renal nephropathy. If justified during the treatment of upper abdominal malignancies and if the contralateral kidney is functioning normally, this should not be considered a dose or volume-limiting tissue.

Treatment of radiation nephrotoxicity is supportive. Patients can be given a low protein diet and fluid and salt restriction in an effort to decrease the renal work load. Anemia is treated with erythropoietin. In the setting of renal failure, dialysis and renal transplantation can be considered.

Table 2. RTOG Chronic Radiation Morbidity Scoring Criteria, Esophagus

Score	Symptoms	Treatment
0	No change over baseline	None
1	Mild fibrosis and slight difficulty swallowing solids No pain on swallowing	Diet modification, antacids
2	Unable to take solid food Normally swallowing semi-solid food	Dilatation may be needed Dietary modification
3	Severe fibrosis, able to swallow only liquids, may have pain on swallowing	Dilatation required May require tube feedings Analgesics
4	Complete ulceration, obstruction, perforation, fistula	Tube feedings, possible surgical intervention

REFERENCES

1. Philips, TL and G Ross. 1974. Time–dose relationships in the mouse esophagus. Radiology **113:**435–440.
2. Northway, MG, HI Libshitz, JJ West, et al. 1979. The opossum as an animal model for studying radiation esophagitis. Radiology **131:**731–735.
3. Seaman, WB and LV Ackerman. 1957. The effect of radiation on the esophagus. Radiology **68:**534–540.
4. Mascarenhas, F, ME Silvestre, M da Costa, et al. 1989. Acute secondary effects in the esophagus in patients undergoing radiotherapy for carcinoma of the lung. Am J Clin Oncol **12:**34–40.
5. Lepke, RA and HI Libshitz. 1983. Radiation-induced injury of the esophagus. Radiology **148:**375–378.
6. Goldstein, HM, LF Rogers, GH Fletcher, et al. 1975. Radiological manifestations of radiation-induced injury to the normal upper gastrointestinal tract. Radiology **117:**135–140.
7. Berthrong, M and LF Fajardo. 1981. Radiation injury in surgical pathology. II. Alimentary tract. Am J Surg Pathol **5:**153–178.
8. Papazian, A, JP Capron, JP Ducroix, et al. 1983. Mucosal bridges of the upper esophagus after radiotherapy for Hodgkin's disease. Gastroenterology **84:**1028–1031.
9. Breiter, N, KR Trott, and T Sassy. 1989. Effect of x-irradiation on the stomach of a rat. Int J Radiat Oncol Biol Phys **17:**779–784.
10. Goldgraber, MB, CE Rubin, WL Palmer, et al. 1954. The early gastric response to irradiation. A serial biopsy study. Gastroenterology **27:**1–20.
11. Schultz-Hector, S, Dorr W Brechenmacher, et al. 1996. Complications of combined intraoperative radiation (IORT) and external radiation (ERT) of the upper abdomen: an experimental model. Radiother Oncol **38:**205–214.
12. Hagemann, RF, CP Sigdestad, and S Lesher. Intestinal crypt survival and total and per crypt levels of proliferative cellularity following irradiation: single x-ray exposures. Radiat Res **46:**533–546.
13. Sher, ME and J Bauer. 1990. Radiation-induced enteropathy. Am J Gastroenterol **85:**121–128.
14. Shamblin, JR, RE Symmonds, WG Sauer, et al. 1964. Bowel obstruction after pelvis and abdominal radiation. Ann Surg **160:**81–89.
15. Galland, RB and J Spencer. 1987. Natural history and surgical management of radiation enteritis. Br J Surg **74:**742–747.
16. Erickson, BA, MF Otterson, JE Moulder, et al. 1994. Altered motility causes the early gastrointestinal toxicity of irradiation. In J Radiat Oncol Biol Phys **28:**905–912.
17. Coia, LR, RJ Myerson, and JE Tepper. 1995. Late effects of radiation therapy on the gastrointestinal tract. Int J Rad Oncol Biol Phys **31:**1213–1236.
18. Shofield, PF, ND Carr, and D Holden. 1986. Pathogenesis and treatment of radiation bowel disease. J R Soc Med **79:**30–32.
19. Greenberger, NJ and KJ Isselbacher. 1964. Malabsorption following radiation injury to the gastrointestinal tract. Am J Med **36:**450–456.
20. Galland, RB and J Spencer. 1985. Spontaneous postoperative perforation of previously asymptomatic irradiated bowel. Br J Surg **72:**285.
21. Lawrence, TS, JM Robertson, MS Anscher, et al. 1995. Hepatic toxicity resulting from cancer treatment. Int J Radiat Oncol Biol Phys **31:**1237–1248.
22. Constine, LS, JP Williams, M Morris, et al. 2004. Late effects of cancer treatment on normal tissue. In: Perez, Brady, Halperin, and Schmidt-Ullrich, eds. Principles and Practice of Radiation Oncology, 4th ed. Lippincott, pp 357–390.
23. Dawson, L, R Ten Haken, and TS Lawrence. 2001. Partial irradiation of the liver. Sem Rad Oncol **11:**240–245.
24. Ogata, K, K Kizawa, M Yosida, et al. 1963. Hepatic injury following irradiation—a morphologic study. J Exp Med **9:**240–251.
25. Glatstein, E, L Fajardo, and M Brown. 1977. Radiation injury in mouse kidney—sequential light microscopy study. Int J Rad Oncol Biol Phys **2:**933–943.
26. Chowan, NM. 1990. Injurious effects of radiation on the esophagus. Am J Gastroenterol **85:**115–120.
27. Seeman, H, JA Gates, M Traube. 1992. Esophageal motor dysfunction years after radiation therapy. Dig Dis Sci **37:**303–306.
28. Willett, CG, CJ Gooi, AL Zietman, et al. 2000. Acute and late toxicity of patients with inflammatory bowel disease undergoing irradiation for abdominal and pelvic neoplasms. Int J Radiat Oncol Biol Phys **46:**995–998.

29. Maguire, PD, GS Sibley, SM Zhou, et al. 1999. Clinical and dosimetric predictors of radiation-induced esophageal toxicity. Int J Radiat Oncol Biol Phys **45:**97–103.
30. Werner-Wasik, M, E Pequignot, D Leeper, et al. 2000. Predictors of severe esophagitis include the use of concurrent chemotherapy, but not the length of irradiated esophagus: a multivariate analysis of patients with lung cancer treated with nonoperative therapy. Int J Radiat Oncol Biol Phys **48:**689–696.
31. Singh, AK, MA Lockett, and JD Bradley. 2003. Predictors of radiation-induced esophageal toxicity in patients with non-small cell lung cancer treated with three-dimensional conformal radiotherapy. Int J Radiat Oncol Biol Phys **55:**337–341.
32. Byhardt, RW, C Scott, WT Sause, et al. 1998. Response, toxicity, failure patterns, and survival in five RTOG trials of sequential and/or concurrent chemotherapy and radiotherapy for locally advanced non-small cell carcinoma of the lung. Int J Radiat Oncol Biol Phys **42:**469–478.
33. Sasso, FS, G Sasso, HR Marsigiglia, et al. 2001. Pharmacological and dietary prophylaxis and treatment of acute actinic esophagitis during mediastinal radiotherapy. Dig Dis Sci **46:**746–749.
34. Tochner, Z, M Barnes, JB Mitchell, et al. 1990. Protection by indomethacin against acute radiation esophagitis. Digestion **47:**81–87.
35. Steer, CB and PG Harper. 2002. Gastro-oesophageal complications in patients receiving cancer therapy: the role of proton pump inhibitors. Eur J Gastroenterol Hepatol **14(suppl 1):**S17–S21.
36. Capizzi, RL and W Oster. 2000. Chemoprotective and radioprotective effects of amifostine: an update of clinical trials. Int J Hematol **72:**425–435.
37. Komaki, R, JS Lee, L Milas, et al. 2004. Effects of amifostine on acute toxicity from concurrent chemotherapy and radiotherapy for inoperable non-small cell lung cancer: report of a randomized comparative trial. Int J Radiat Oncol Biol Phys **58:**1369–1377.
38. Antonadou, D, N Throuvalas, A Petridis, et al. 2003. Effect of amifostine on toxicities associated with radiochemotherapy in patients with locally advanced non-small cell lung cancer. Int J Radiat Oncol Biol Phys **57:**402–408.
39. Werner-Wasik, M, RS Axelrod, DP Friedland, et al. 2002. Phase II: trial of twice weekly amifostine in patients with non-small cell lung cancer treated with chemoradiotherapy. Semin Radiat Oncol **12(suppl 1):**34–39.
40. Arquette, M, T Wasserman, R Govindan, et al. 2002. Phase II evaluation of amifostine as an esophageal mucosal protectant in the treatment of limited-stage small cell lung cancer with chemotherapy and twice-daily radiation. Semin Radiat Oncol **12(suppl 1):**59–61.
41. Pearson, JG. 1977. The present status and future potential of radiotherapy in the management of esophageal cancer. Cancer **39:**882–890.
42. O'Rourke, IC, K Tiver, C Bull, et al. 1988. Swallowing performance after radiation therapy for carcinoma of the esophagus. Cancer **61:**2022–2026.
43. Friedman, M. 1952. Calculated risks of radiation therapy of normal tissue in the treatment of cancer of the testis. In: Proceedings of the Second National Cancer Conference, New York, The American Cancer Society. National Cancer Institute, USPHS Federal Science Agency, pp 390–400.
44. Hamilton, FE. 1947. Gastric ulcer following radiation. Arch Surg **55:**394–399.
45. Sell, A and T Jensen. 1966. Acute gastric ulcers induced by radiation. Acta Radiol **4:**289–297.
46. Cosset, J, M Henry-Amar, J Burgers, et al. 1988. Late radiation injuries of the gastrointestinal tract in the H2 and H5 EORTC Hodgkin's disease trials: emphasis on the role of exploratory laparotomy and fractionation. Radiother Oncol **13:**61–68.
47. Hamilton, C, A Horwich, J Bliss, et al. 1987. Gastrointestinal Morbidity of adjuvant radiotherapy in stage I malignant teratoma of the testis. Radiother Oncol 10L85–10L90.
48. Gunderson, LL, RB Hoskins, AC Cohen, et al. 1983. Combined modality treatment of gastric cancer. Int J Radiat Oncol Biol Phys **9:**965.
49. Safran, H, HJ Wanebo, PJ Hesketh, et al. 2000. Paclitaxel and concurrent radiation for gastric cancer. Int J Radiat Oncol Biol Phys **46:**889–894.
50. Blackstock, AW, AB Stephen, F Richards, et al. 1999. Phase I trial of twice-weekly gemcitabine and concurrent radiation in patients with advanced pancreatic cancer. J Clin Oncol **17:**2208–2212.
51. McGinn, C, D Smith, C Szarka, et al. 1998. A phase I study of preoperative gemcitabine in combination with radiation therapy in patients with localized, unresectable pancreatic cancer. Proc Am Soc Clin Oncol **17:**264a.
52. Talamonti, MS, PJ Catalano, DJ Vaughn, et al. 2000. Eastern Cooperative Oncology Group phase I trial of protracted venous infusion fluorouracil plus weekly gemcitabine with concurrent radiation therapy in patients with locally advanced pancreas cancer: a regimen with unexpected early toxicity. J Clin Oncol **18:**3384–3389.

53. Horiot, JC and M Aapro. 2004. Treatment implications for radiation-induced nausea and vomiting in specific patient groups. Eur J Cancer **40:**979–987.
54. Morrow, JB, JA Dumot, JJ Vargo, II. 2000. Radiation-induced hemorrhagic carditis treated with argon plasma coagulator. Gastrointest Endosc **51:**498–499.
55. Walsh, D. 1987. Deep tissue traumatism from roentgen ray exposure. Br Med J **2:**272–273.
56. Hauer-Jensen. 1990. Late radiation injury of the small intestine: clinical, pathophysiologic, and radiobiologic aspects. A review. Acta Oncol **29:**401–415.
57. Buchler, DA, JC Kline, BM Peckham, et al. 1971. Radiation reactions in cervical cancer therapy. Am J Obstet Gynecol **111:**745–750.
58. Green, N, G Iba and WR Smith. 1975. Measures to minimize small intestine injury in the irradiated pelvis. Cancer **35:**1633–1640.
59. Letschert, GJ, JV Lebesque, BMP Aleman, et al. 1994. The volume effect in radiation-related late small bowel complications: results of a clinical study of the EORTC Radiotherapy Cooperative Group in patients treated for rectal carcinoma. Radiother Oncol **32:**116–123.
60. Stockbrine, MF, JE Hancock, and GH Fletcher. 1970. Complications in 831 patients with squamous cell carcinoma of the intact uterine cervix treated with 3000 rads or more whole pelvis radiation. Am J Roentgenol **108:**283–304.
61. Louidice, T, D Baxter, and J Balint. 1977. Effects of abdominal surgery on the development of radiation enteropathy. Gastroenterology **73:**1093–1097.
62. Green, N. 1983. The avoidance of small intestine injury in gynecologic cancer. Int J Radiat Oncol Biol Phys **9:**1385–1390.
63. DeCosse, JJ, RS Rhodes, WB Wentz, et al. 1969. The natural history and management of radiation induced injury of the gastrointestinal tract. Ann Surg **170:**369–384.
64. Chon, BH and JS Loeffler. 2002. The effect of nonmalignant systemic disease on tolerance to radiation therapy. Oncologist **7:**136–173.
65. Song, DY, WT Lawrie, RA Abrams, et al. 2001. Acute and late radiotherapy toxicity in patients with inflammatory bowel disease. Int J Radiat Oncol Biol Phys **51:**455–459.
66. Kao, MS. 1995. Intestinal complications of radiotherapy in gynecologic malignancy—clinical presentation and management. Int J Obstet Gynecol **49(suppl):**S69–S75.
67. Perez, CB, S Breaux, H Madoc-Jones, et al. 1984. Radiation therapy alone in the treatment of carcinoma of the uterine cervix: analysis of complications. Cancer **54:**235.
68. Gallagher, MJ, HD Brereton, RA Rostock, et al. 1986. A prospective study of treatment techniques to minimize the volume of pelvic small bowel with reduction of acute and late effects associated with pelvic irradiation. Int J Radiat Oncol Biol Phys **12:**1565–1573.
69. Duttenhaver, JR, RB Hoskins, LL Gunderson, et al. 1986. Adjuvant postoperative radiation therapy in cancer of the colon. Cancer **57:**955.
70. Gastrointestinal Tumor Study Group. 1985. Prolongation of the disease-free interval in surgically resected rectal cancer. N Engl J Med **312:**1465.
71. Douglass, HO, CG Moertel, RJ Mayer, et al. 1986. Survival after postoperative treatment of rectal cancer. N Engl J Med **315:**1294–1295.
72. Krook, JE, CG Moertel, LL Gunderson, et al. 1991. Effective surgical adjuvant therapy for high-risk rectal cancer. N Engl J Med **324:**709.
73. O'Connell, MJ, JA Martenson, HS Weiand, et al. 1994. Improving adjuvant therapy by combining protracted infusion fluorouracil with radiation therapy after curative surgery. N Engl J Med **331:**502–507.
74. Dunst J, T Reese, T Sutter, et al. 2002. Phase I trial evaluating the concurrent combination of radiotherapy and capecitabine in rectal cancer. J Clin Oncol **20:**3983–3991.
75. Henriksson, R, L Franzen, and B Littbrand. 1992. Effects of sucralfate on acute and late bowel discomfort following radiotherapy of pelvic cancer. J Clin Oncol **10:**969–975.
76. Berk, RN and DG Seay. 1972. Cholerheic enteropathy as a cause of diarrhea and death in radiation enteritis and its prevention with cholestyramine. Radiology **104:**153–156.
77. Mennie, AT, VM Dalley, LC Dinneen, et al. 1975. Treatment of radiation-induced gastrointestinal distress with acetylsalicylate. Lancet **2:**942–943.
78. Loudice, TA and JA Lang. 1983. Treatment of radiation enteritis: a comparison study. Am J Gastroenterol **78:**481–487.
79. Lawrence, TS, RK Ten Haken, ML Kessler, et al. 1992. The use of 3-D dose volume analysis to predict radiation hepatitis. Int J Rad Oncol Biol Phys **23:**781–788.

80. Kunkler, PB, RF Farr, and RW Luxton. 1952. The limit of renal tolerance to x-rays. Br J Radiol **25:**190–201.
81. Luxton, RW. 1953. Radiation nephritis. Q J Med **22:**215–242.
82. Cassaday, JR. 1995. Clinical radiation nephropathy. Int J Rad Oncol Biol Phys **31:**1249–1256.
83. Willett, CG, JE Tepper, BA Orlow, et al. 1986. Renal complications secondary to radiation treatment of upper abdominal malignancies. Int J Radiat Oncol Biol Phys **12:**1601–1604.

6. RADIATION COMPLICATIONS OF THE PELVIS

KATHRYN MCCONNELL GREVEN, M.D.

Comprehensive Cancer Center of Wake Forest University Medical Center, Winston Salem, NC

TATJANA PAUNESKU, Ph.D.

Feinberg School of Medicine, Northwestern University, Chicago, IL

INTRODUCTION

Radiation is used with or without chemotherapy to treat malignancies in the pelvis that occur in gynecologic, genitourinary, and gastrointestinal organs. One of the most sensitive organs in the pelvis can be the small bowel which is discussed in a separate chapter (upper GI). Radiation can cause functional effects on other organs including the rectum, anus, bone and bone marrow, bladder, urethra, ureter, vulva, vagina, uterus, ovaries, testicles, and sexual organs. This chapter will discuss the pathologic and clinical effects that can result during treatment and shortly thereafter. Long-term sequelae can be seen at variable intervals following radiation. Prevention and management issues will be discussed.

A. COMPLICATIONS RELATED TO GI EFFECTS

A1. Rectum

Pathogenesis

The mucosa of the large intestine is composed of a single layer of epithelial cells which rest upon a basement membrane that lies on the lamina propria. These epithelial cells are predominantly mucin-producing goblet cells, with interspersed absorptive cells. Their undifferentiated progenitor cells, located in the bases of the crypts of Lieberkuhn, have a turnover rate of 4–8 days. Both the rates of regeneration and maturation of these cells and the rate of repair of non-lethally injured cells determine the tolerance dose for radiation treatment.[1,2]

Early injury at the cellular level is characterized by mucosal cell loss, acute inflammation, eosinophilic crypt abscesses, and endothelial swelling in the arterioles can be seen following radiation to the rectum.[3] A thickened and edematous lamina propria with patchy fibroblastic proliferation and decreased mitotic rate within the mucosa are seen.[4] At doses of 10 Gy mucosal production is decreased and mitosis of the crypt cells is decreased.[3] At 50 Gy doses (administered in 20 fractions over 1 month) in addition to mucosal cell injury and crypt shortening, infiltration of inflammatory cells occurs,[5] accompanied by the accumulation of eosinophils and the degranulation of mast cells. The pathogenesis of the early lesions depends on injury to the mucosal cells, enhanced by ischemia due to endothelial cell injury and fibrin–platelet thrombi accumulation. Cytokines secreted by the endothelial cells such as tumor necrosis factor α and transforming growth factor β contribute significantly to the development of the early injury.[6] For example, tumor necrosis factor α contributes to repression of thrombomodulin which is usually induced by irradiation; this leads to an increase of thrombin which in turn activates such injurious pathways as the activation of proteases, fibrin deposition, etc. Recently, it was found in an experimental mouse model that radiation-induced crypt damage can be minimized by avoidance of endothelial cell apoptosis either by basic fibroblast growth factor (bFGF) administration or by deletion of the sphingomyelinase gene.[7] Expression and activity of the tumor suppressor gene p53 are also of major importance in preventing mitotic catastrophe in irradiated epithelial cells,[8] while over-expression of the transcription factor NF-κB may also serve a radioprotective role.

The development of delayed tissue injury starts to be apparent as early as at 6 months posttreatment and may gradually worsen. This delayed colorectal injury is a result of lesions in the slowly responding cells of connective tissues and blood vessels.[6] The pathogenesis of the delayed injury is a result of the development of fibrosis in the stroma and in the blood vessels, causing ischemia. On the other hand, there is a belief that fibrosis may be initially caused by ischemia due to vascular deficiency,[9] or, alternatively, by fibroblast dysfunction.[10] Fibrogenic induction by cytokines mentioned above in regard to early injury can result in protracted and/or irreversible gene expression changes (e.g., thrombomodulin expression can be repressed for years posttreatment) and tissue remodeling—fibrin deposition and collagen accumulation. Therefore, late changes include subsequent fibrosis of connective tissue and endarteritis of the arterioles.[11] This fibrosis can lead to relative ischemia, and mucosal capillaries that attempt to compensate for this develop telangiectasia with friable vessels that are prone to bleeding.[12] More severe ischemia can lead to ulceration, perforation fistula, or abscess formation.

Clinical Aspects

Radiation fields may include the entire rectum as when treating patients with external beam for adjuvant radiation following resection of rectal cancer. Treatment may also include a combination of external radiation and brachytherapy resulting in high doses of radiation to a more localized area as when treating for intact cervical cancer. The last decade has seen increasing interest in limiting the volume of rectum exposed to radiation, particularly when treating for non-rectal cancers, as when treating with conformal beams shaped around the prostate or with prostate brachytherapy alone. Common observations among all these treatments have included the correlation of higher doses and increased volumes of rectum being directly proportional to chronic complications.

Acute symptoms of the rectum can be seen early in the course of radiation therapy for cancers in the pelvic region. Symptoms usually begin following 20 Gy of standard fractionation. Early symptoms may include tenesmus, bleeding, and diarrhea. One report that documented acute rectal symptoms demonstrated acute grade 2 rectal complications in 18% of prostate cancer patients at a mean dose of 38 Gy. Patients without diarrhea had a mean rectal volume receiving a dose of at least 70 Gy–8.5 cm^3. Patients with grade 2 diarrhea had a volume of 16.5 cm^3.[13] Although radiobiological doctrine has been that acute symptoms are caused by an unrelated mechanism to late symptoms, other authors have suggested that late complications may be related to the development of acute complications.[14] O'Brien et al. found that the presence of acute proctitis was the only factor to predict any of the late rectal symptoms of urgency, frequency, and diarrhea.[15]

Late pathological changes result in rectal tissue ischemia, leading to mucosal friability, bleeding, ulcers, strictures, and fistulae. Patients typically present with painless rectal bleeding. Other symptoms include evacuation difficulties, frequent elimination, fecal incontinence, and urgency which may also develop from alterations in anorectal function as discussed in the section on anal complications. At sigmoidoscopy, a spectrum of mucosal changes can be seen including mucosal pallor or erythema, prominent telangiectasia, friability, or fistulae.[16] The onset of radiation proctitis is typically 12–18 months following treatment. Patient-related factors that may increase the risk of proctitis include hypertension, diabetes, and cerebrovascular disease that can all affect the vascular supply in the radiated field.

A recent report correlated the dose–volume histograms (DVH) of the rectum to the probability of rectal bleeding following radiation in a group of men treated with either conventional or conformal radiation for prostate cancer.[17] The analysis of relative DVH of the rectal wall (with and without the anal region) showed a significant ($P < 0.01$) relationship between the irradiated volume and the probability of rectal blood loss within 3 years for dose levels between 25 and 60 Gy. Similarly, another report showed that the average percent volume DVH for the rectal wall of patients with bleeding was significantly higher than those of patients without bleeding[18] (Figures 1 and 2). One report compared a group of men treated with MRI-guided brachytherapy alone or with supplemental external beam radiation.[19] The addition of external beam radiation increased the incidence of grade 3 rectal bleeding from 8% to 30% ($P = 0.0001$).

Treatment for cervical cancer includes EBRT with brachytherapy. A rectal point is chosen for dose calculations based on ICRU guidelines.[20] Cumulative dose to this rectal point of >75 Gy with low dose rate brachytherapy using tandem and ovoids has been demonstrated to increase the risk of serious late rectal sequelae.[21] There did not seem to be a dose threshold for less severe complications. Patients treated with cylinders or line

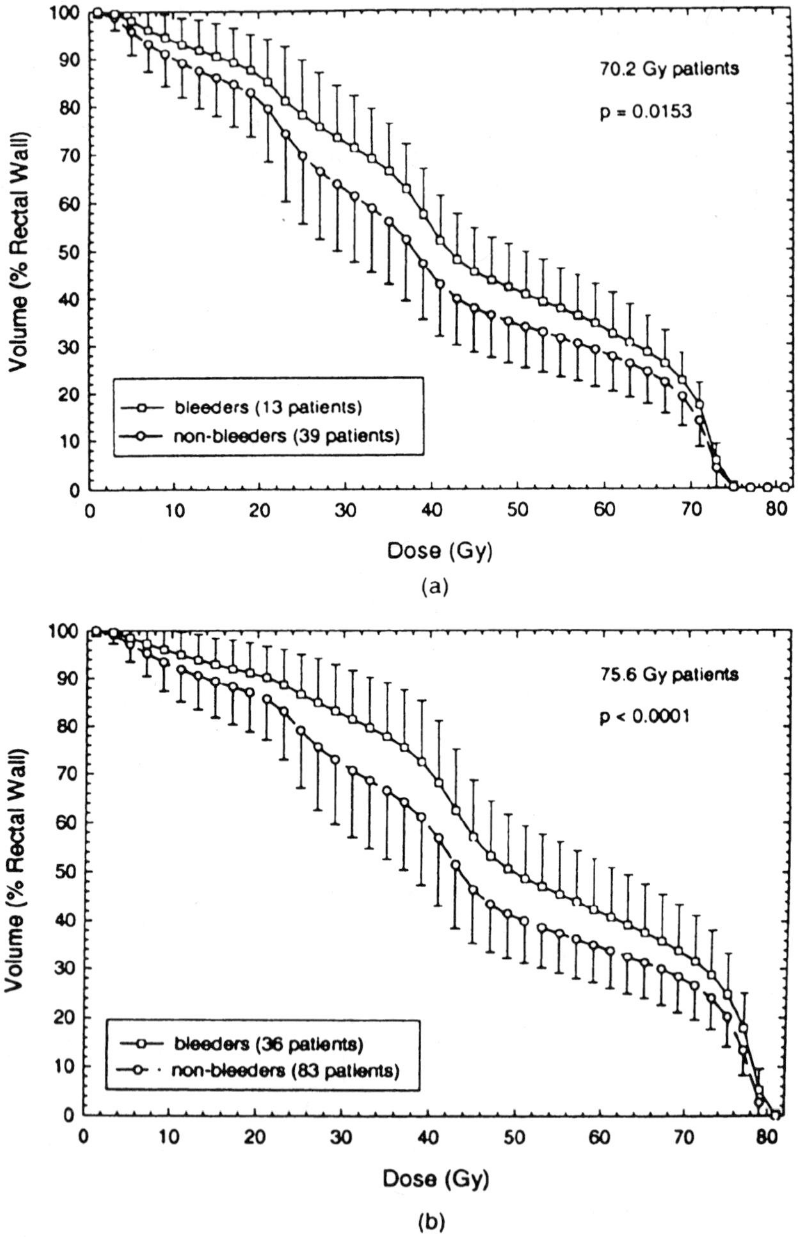

Figure 1. These two figures represent the average percent volume DVHs for patients with and without bleeding. The solid curves with squares show the results for patients with bleeding, the dashed curves with circles show the results for patients without bleeding. Reproduced with permission from Elsevier.[18]

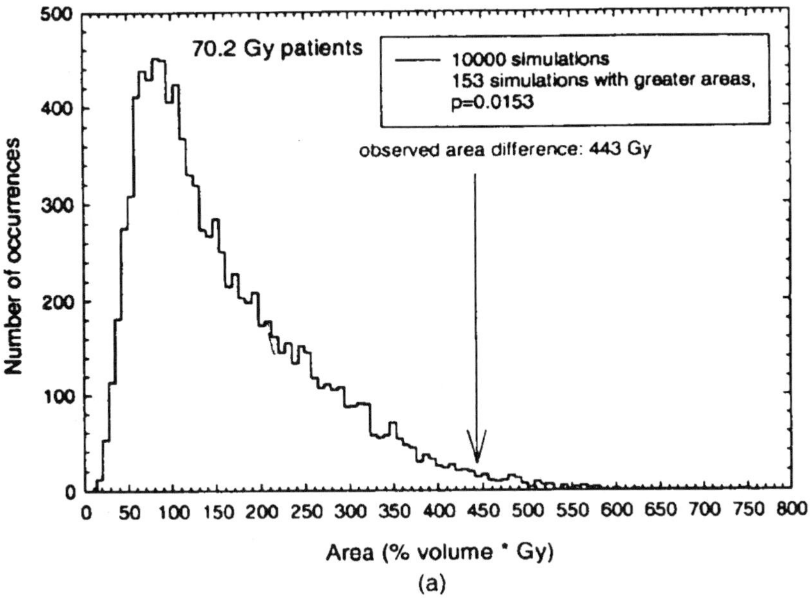

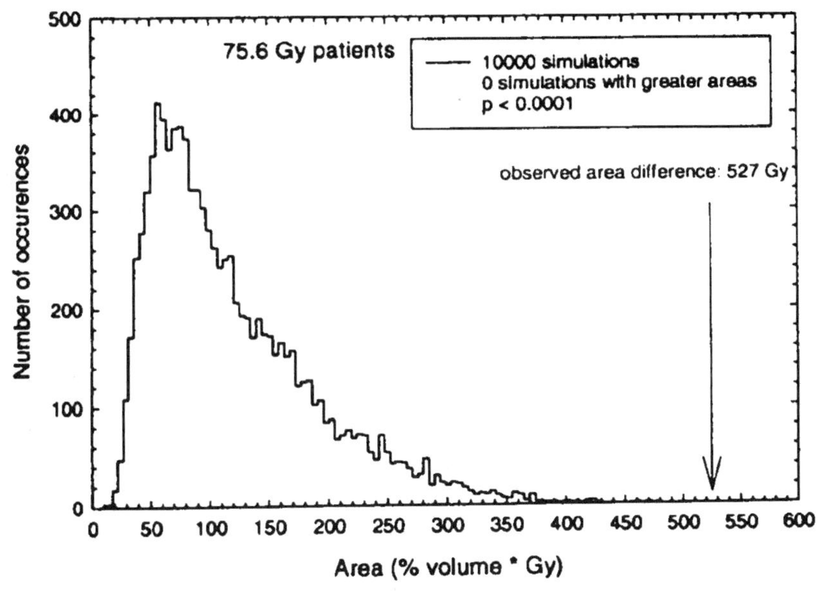

Figure 2. The distributions of the 10,000 simulated differences in area between the average histograms for bleeding and non-bleeding patients with simulated outcomes. The vertical arrows show the observed values of the area differences in the data.[18]

sources that would treat a larger volume of rectum had an increased risk of moderate to severe sequelae.[21] Typically, cumulative doses to the ICRU rectal point are limited to 65–70 Gy from tandem and ovoids. There is no indication that concurrent chemotherapy increases the risk of late rectal complications. Following treatment for cervix cancer with chemotherapy and radiation or radiation alone, grades 3–5 rectal complications occurred in 9% of patients in both the groups.[22] High dose rate brachytherapy requires careful fractionation in order not to increase the risk of rectal complications.[23] In order to stay within the same biologically effective dose range, dose to the rectal point should be limited to 60–70% of the prescribed dose to Point A.

Management

Acute symptoms of urgency and tenesmus can be treated with an antispasmodic such as Lomotil or Imodium. Pain is treated systemically with a narcotic or non-narcotic preparation titrated to the patient's level of discomfort.

Chronic radiation proctitis typically includes bleeding, stricture formation, and/or fistula. Biopsy of mucosal changes should be discouraged if they occur in an area that likely received a high dose of radiation such as the anterior rectal wall. Biopsy may cause persistent inflammation, decrease healing, and precipitate fistula formation. Interventions include low residue diets and pain control. The patient's hematocrit should be monitored so that transfusion can be given as indicated. Some patients will have sequelae that resolve in a few months with little intervention, while other patients will have a longer course that may involve 1–2 years of rectal bleeding. Non-surgical therapies include steroid enemas or Proctofoam with cortisone which is used to decrease inflammation. Mesalazine can be used as an enema, delayed absorbing capsule, or rectal suppository. This agent works as an anti-inflammatory agent directly on the bowel mucosa. Bleeding from telangiectasias has been treated with thermal coagulation or formalin application. Oral and rectal administrations of sucralfate have been described as a method of preventing proctitis. Sucralfate is an aluminum hydroxide complex of sulfated sucrose which has been used to heal ulcers in the esophagus. It is postulated to reduce the extent of microvascular injury. One study that compared rectal sucralfate to a combination of oral sulfasalazine and rectal steroids demonstrated clinical improvement in 16/17 patients compared to 8/15 patients in the steroid group. No endoscopic improvement was noted between the two groups and follow-up in this study was only for 4 weeks.[24] Another prospective study of rectal sucralfate described a benefit in 3 patients for a minimum of 3 years.[25] It can be seen that there is no report that demonstrates a superior approach for individual patients. Patients have variable presentations and degrees of sequelae. Most reports in the literature represent small single institutional experiences with incomplete follow-up. Quality-of-life data is limited.

Surgical treatment can be used if there is a failure of medical treatment, obstruction caused by a stricture, or other serious complications such as perforation, abscess, or fistula. Surgical options include diversion without resection, resection without anastomosis, and resection with anastomosis. Because of the high morbidity and mortality in these patients the simplest operation is preferred by most surgeons.[26]

A2. Anus

Pathogenesis

Mucosa above the anal orifice is made of stratified squamous epithelial cells which show a rapid turnover and hence are very radiosensitive; this mucosa is involved in the pathology of the early radiation injury in this region. Creation of microvascular thrombi also contributes to early injury. Injury sustained by muscle, stromal, and vascular cells which respond slowly to irradiation are the cause of the delayed anal radiation injury. The pathogenesis of the late injury is linked with injury of fibroblasts and miofibroblasts, leading to the development of severe fibrosis.[6] Histologically, pelvic irradiation has been found to result in damage to the myenteric plexus of the internal anal sphincter of patients with rectal cancer and these alterations seemed to be time-dependent. A trend toward increased collagen deposition following irradiation has also been observed.[27]

Tolerance dose of the normal tissue is considered to be a little above 65 Gy. When external beam therapy is given alone, doses of 60–65 Gy are prescribed, close to the tolerance dose in 1.8–2 Gy fractions over 6–7 weeks.[28]

Acute grade 3 toxicity with 2-Gy fractions is 40%, while it is 75% with 2.5-Gy fractions. Late radiation-related complications are observed in 15% of the patients, and are more common when fractions higher than 2 Gy are used.[29]

Clinical Aspects

Radiation effects on anorectal function have been increasingly recognized. Acute effects on the anus include epithelial discomfort which may be aggravated by radiation-induced diarrhea. Epithelial effects follow a sequential progression from erythema to desquamation. Shallow erosions and ulcerations can develop which can lead to tenesmus. Direct radiation to the anus can result in severe acute reactions that are exacerbated with the use of chemotherapy.

Injury to the anal sphincter complex after pelvic radiotherapy has been reported. There is limited information available on sphincter continence following radiation with or without chemotherapy for anal carcinoma. Evaluation of the sphincter is complicated by the fact that the sphincter may have been damaged by the disease process itself. The reported rates of colostomy following EBRT for complications range from 0% to 7%.[29–31] Strictures of the anus or ulceration are the most commonly reported reasons for intervention. Actual data reporting subjective and objective measurements of function are limited. One report found complete continence in 56%, liquid soiling in 26%, solid soiling in 17%, and complete incontinence in 6% of colostomy free survivors of anal cancer.[32] Manometry measurements on these patients demonstrated that both resting pressures and maximum squeeze pressures were decreased.

There have been inconsistent outcomes of anorectal studies after pelvic radiotherapy not directed to the anus. The most common changes include decreased resting anal canal pressures and decreased rectal volumes which are consistent with fibrosis.[33] The reported effects have been conflicting because of the mixture of retrospective and prospective investigations, different radiotherapeutic regimens, as well as the variance in pretreatment sphincter function, rectal capacity, and bowel activity. In addition, the intra- and inter-individual reproducibility of anorectal manometry values, even under standard conditions in healthy volunteers, is low.[34]

A recent report from Yeoh et al. evaluated 35 patients following radiation for prostate carcinoma.[35] One year following EBRT, 56% of patients had an increase in frequency of defecation while 26% reported incontinence. Objective measurements made 1 year after radiation revealed that volumes of rectal distension associated with perception of the stimulus and desire to defecate were lower compared with baseline volumes, reflecting a heightened rectal sensitivity in the patients.[35] This may cause symptoms of urgency that cause patients to limit their activities in order to remain near a bathroom.[36] A similar study involving a group of patients with cervical cancer demonstrated that 33% of patients had late symptoms related to anorectal dysfunction.[37]

Management

If direct radiation to the anus is not necessary as in prostate cancer, cervix cancer, or rectal cancer, it may be possible to exclude at least a portion of the anus from the treatment fields. This requires marking the sphincter with a radio opaque marker or identifying it at CT simulation. Blocking this region from high dose radiation may decrease acute and chronic complications.

If it is necessary to include the anus in the treatment field, aggressive skin care is very important. In addition, a planned treatment break may actually shorten the overall treatment time by improving the tolerance of the proposed regimen. Therapeutic interventions usually include antidiarrheal medications such as loperamide or codeine. Care of the skin includes cleansing with gentle cleansers. Application of aloe, gentian violet, and/or lidocaine can help manage symptoms.

Biopsy of the anus following high dose radiation can result in non-healing ulceration. Avoidance of this procedure is preferred but if a non-healing ulceration develops, conservative management is generally used initially. This involves stool softeners, sitz baths, and wound care. There have been reports of the use of hyperbaric oxygen in the management of these complications.[38] There are limited therapeutic interventions for incontinence with the primary treatment being colostomy.

B. GU EFFECTS

B1. Bladder

Pathogenesis

The urinary bladder and ureters are covered by urothelium—mucosa made of transitional epithelium of several layers of cells (from 3–4 in full to 5–7 in the empty bladder). These cells are replenished by undifferentiated basal cells that divide so slowly that their mitotic index cannot be measured.[39] The surface layer of urothelium is made of large polyploid cells connected by tight junctions and covered by a monomolecular film of sulfonated polysaccharides or glycosaminoglycan that serves the need for internal impermeability of the bladder.

Following radiation treatment, the initial injury to bladder is mild, and the early response linked with the urothelium occurs at 6–12 months. Therefore, mucosal cell injury (loss of the surface layer of epithelial cells, resulting in the loss of bladder impermeability) becomes evident approximately at the same time when the late response occurs, caused by injury of stroma and blood vessels.[6] Radiotherapy results in urothelial cell enlargement, multinucleation, and vacuolization, although nuclear to cytoplasmic ratios remain low.[40] Enlarged nuclei may have large nucleoli, but degenerative nuclear features are usually present. A reactive, tumor-like epithelial proliferation associated with hemorrhage, fibrin deposits, fibroid vascular changes, and multinucleated stromal cells is seen in chronic cases. The adjacent tissue is hemorrhagic with deposits of fibrin and, deeper within the stroma, mesenchymal cells are often large and multinucleated.[41] The transitional epithelium becomes thin and numerous dilated submucosal capillaries create a telangiectatic appearance. Bladder contracture can develop with muscle fiber replacement.[42] This late phase of radiation cystitis can occur months to years after ionizing radiation.

Clinical Aspects

Radiation effects on the bladder have been documented following treatment for various pelvic malignancies including cervical cancers, prostate cancers, and bladder cancers. In these instances, however, the function of the bladder may have been impaired by the disease itself and separating radiation effects from disease effects may be difficult. Also, dose to the bladder can vary with treatment to encompass a substantial portion of the organ with external beam RT as in bladder cancer or for high dose delivered to a small volume of the bladder as in cervical or prostate cancer where at least a portion of the treatment may be delivered with brachytherapy.

Acute sequelae during radiation commonly include frequency and dysuria. These symptoms typically occur following more than 20 Gy to the bladder with conventional fractionation. Following completion of radiation, resolution of symptoms is seen in 2–3 weeks.

The tolerance doses (TD 5/5) for the whole bladder have been estimated to be 65 Gy. The tolerance increases if only two-thirds of the bladder is treated to 80 Gy.[43] Another analysis of bladder complications demonstrates that complication rates appear to be dependent on both the whole bladder dose (i.e., from external beam radiation) and the maximum bladder dose (i.e., from brachytherapy)[44] (Table 1). Long-term sequelae include persistent dysuria, severe pain, contracted bladder, vesicovaginal fistula, and varying degrees of hematuria. Median onset of late complications after radiation is 13–20 months.[44]

Lajer et al. followed 177 consecutive patients treated for cervical cancer prospectively and documented subjective and objective urologic morbidity at regular follow-up intervals.[45] Doses to the bladder were 46 Gy in 2-Gy fractions with additional dose delivered to at least part of the bladder from brachytherapy. The cumulative incidence of morbidity was found to increase throughout the study period until the 48-month follow-up interval. The 5-year incidences of severe morbidity were 5%, moderate morbidity

Table 1. Bladder complication summary in patients with or without chemotherapy.[44]

Disease treated	Approximate dose to ≥ 50% of the bladder (Gy)	Approximate maximum bladder dose (Gy)	Approximate clinical complication rate (%)
Prostate	40	60–65	5
Bladder	50–65	50–65	6–20†
Cervix	40	65–75	5–10
	40	≥80	10–20
Rectal	40–50	40–50	0

*These results are in patients treated with or without chemotherapy.
†Many of these symptoms may be due to the cancer.

27%, and mild morbidity was 25%. A subsequent study evaluated 36 patients who were treated with curative intent with radiotherapy for cervical cancer.[46] Urodynamic examinations were performed on admission and at regular intervals after RT. Detrusor instability and frequent small voiding did develop in 15–20% of patients during follow-up. However, there was no control group for comparison which would have helped to control for an unknown incidence of urologic morbidity which exists in the general population.[47] Hemorrhagic cystitis can occur from 6 months to 10 years following pelvic irradiation.[48] Levenback et al. reported a 6.5% incidence seen in 1784 patients treated with radiotherapy for stage IB cervical cancer.[49] Patients treated for cervical cancer with combined external beam radiation and brachytherapy have a 5–10% incidence of radiation cystitis with doses of 75 Gy to the bladder but the incidence increases with higher doses.[50] Recent reports using conformal radiation to the prostate have reported the incidence of moderate to severe hematuria in a range of 3–5%.[51] Notably, bladder complications may be less dose-dependent than rectal complications as seen in Table 2.

Management

Patients with mild to moderate urinary frequency may be treated symptomatically. Phenazopyridine hydrochloride is frequently used to relieve these symptoms. It acts as an analgesic on the bladder mucosa. Oxybutynin chloride is an antispasmodic that relaxes the bladder smooth muscle and may relieve the symptoms of frequency and

Table 2. Distribution of patients by late complication grade according to dose. Data presented as the percentage of patients, with the number in parentheses.[51]

Group	Grade 0	Grade 1	Grade 2	Grade 3	p^*
Rectal complications					
70-Gy arm	53 (78)	36 (53)	11 (16)	1 (1)	
78-Gy arm	46 (69)	28 (42)	19 (28)	7 (10)	0.006
Bladder complications					
70-Gy arm	72 (106)	20 (29)	7 (11)	1 (2)	
78-Gy arm	66 (98)	22 (32)	10 (15)	3 (4)	0.63

urgency. Pharmaceuticals used to increase bladder outlet resistance include ephedrine hydrochloride, pseudoephedrine hydrochloride, and phenylpropanolamine.

The primary treatment modality for hematuria is bladder irrigation. Intravesical treatments with silver nitrate, prostaglandins, or formalin have also been used. More serious interventions can include embolization of the hypogastric arteries or urinary diversion and cystectomy. Treatment with hyperbaric oxygen has also been tried with some success. One report of 62 patients demonstrated complete resolution or marked improvement in 86% of the treated patients.[52] Another study with 40 patients treated with HBO demonstrated good response in 30 (75%) patients. Failure of the treatment was seen only in patients with very severe hemorrhagic cystitis.[53]

B2. Urethra

Clinical Aspects

Urethral injury usually consists of stricture formation. For patients undergoing radiation to the prostate, most reports have documented increased risk of stricture in patients who have had prior transurethral resections of the prostate. Following therapeutic doses of radiation ranging from 60 to 70 Gy, patients with prior TURP demonstrated stricture rates of 6–16% compared to patients without prior TURP who had stricture rates ranging from 0% to 5%.[54]

Incontinence can also result following radiation to the urethra. Following radiation to the prostate, incontinence rates have been reported as 1–2%.[55] Patients who have had a transurethral prostate resection may have an increased risk of incontinence. One study reported incontinence in 5.4% of patients who had a TURP compared to 1% of patients who had not.[45] Incontinence following pelvic radiation in women is poorly documented. Following radiation for cervical cancer, Parkin et al. reported that 45% of women responding to a mailed questionnaire complained of incontinence.[56] Pourquier et al. documented that 11% of urinary complications were incontinence.[57] Most modern series do not report incontinence as a frequent complication. It is the author's experience that women who are treated with interstitial brachytherapy to the periurethral area have frequent incontinence following treatment which might be attributed to the high doses of radiation to the sphincter that probably result in fibrosis. Incontinence following radiation and chemotherapy for bladder cancer has been described. Of 71 patients with intact bladders, a questionnaire showed that flow symptoms occurred in 6%, urgency in 15%, and control problems in 19%. Of all women 11% wore pads. Urodynamic studies demonstrated incontinence in 2 out of 32 patients.[58]

Unfortunately, the mechanism of incontinence is poorly understood. Many variables can affect incontinence in addition to damage to the urethral sphincter including age, prior childbearing history, weight, comorbid medical conditions, bladder irritability, and pelvic floor weakening. Urodynamics may be done on patients who suffer from incontinence symptoms to better define the source of the problem.

Management

Intervention needs to be tailored to the individual patient.

B3. Ureter

Clinical Aspects

Acute effects from radiation on the ureters are not clinically observed in patients. The most frequent cause of ureteral injury after treatment for cancer is a progressive disease. However, ureteral damage including stenoses, necrosis, and reflux from radiation has been described.[59] This complication is typically seen in patients treated with external RT and brachytherapy for cervical cancer. In one series, the majority of ureteral complications were seen with marked signs of radiation cystitis as well.[59] The mean latency time between RT and the manifestation of severe ureteral complications was 19.4 years with a range of 0.5–41.5 years. Two other reports documented the incidence of ureteral stricture. One report had an actual incidence of 1.5%,[60] while the second had an actuarial estimate of 1.2% at 10 years and 2.5% at 20 years.[61] Because the occurrence is rare, correlation with factors that increase the frequency of the damage is difficult. The use of a midline block during external beam,[61] deviation of the uterine tandem,[62] combination of radical surgery and RT which may further compromise the vascular supply of tissue,[63] and transvaginal radiation[61] have all been implicated as factors responsible for increasing the risk of stricture. There are no dose response data for development of this complication.

Management

Management of ureteral stenosis is individualized. An increased index of suspicion is necessary for physicians following these patients since ureteral injury may not be manifested for many years. Mild stenosis may be treated by placement of a ureteral stent. Reimplantation of the ureters with an ureteroneocystostomy or ureteroileocystotomy was successful in 5 out of 8 patients in one series.[61] Other procedures to divert the urinary stream may be used including placement of ileal conduits. Nephrectomy may be required with recurrent urinary tract infections and a non-functional kidney.

B4. Lymphatics

Pathogenesis

The lymphatics of the lower extremity can be disrupted by either surgery or radiation to the groin or pelvis. Evaluation of patients with lymphangiography following radiotherapy demonstrates obstruction of the lymphatics with extravasation of the radiopaque material from the lymphatics.[64] Microscopic examination of lymph nodes following radiation has demonstrated thickening of the fibrous capsule and a decrease in the number of lymphocytes and reticulum cells with sparse germinal centers.[64]

Clinical Aspects

Certainly, in patients who have both surgery and radiation the incidence of lymphedema is usually increased.[65] Lymphedema is underreported in the literature and may only be called to the attention of the physician once the patient has difficulty finding shoes or pants that fit or pain with standing or ambulation. Lymphedema causes effects on mobility, self-image, finances, and appearance. Edema may be unilateral or bilateral. It can occur in as short a time as 3 months following treatment and may be mild or severe. Cellulitis or infection in the extremity may precipitate the occurrence of lymphedema. Edema usually begins as soft and pitting but may progress to become hard and brawny.

One recent series documented edema following hysterectomy with or without adjuvant radiation. The incidence of lymphedema of the leg was 11% which was similar in the surgery alone group.[65] Another study retrospectively investigated the prevalence of leg edema in gynecologic survivors. The diagnosis of lower limb lymphedema was made in 18% of the total sample: 53% of these were diagnosed within 3 months of treatment, 18% within 6 months, 13% within 12 months, and the remaining 16% up to 5 years following treatment.[66] Women most at risk for developing lower extremity lymphedema were those who had treatment for vulvar cancer with removal of lymph nodes and adjuvant radiotherapy. In this group, the prevalence was 47%. It is important for all health care providers to include care and assessment of the legs particularly during the immediate pre- and postoperative period. Another report of patients treated with surgery and radiation for cervical cancer found patients (41%) had a unilateral increase in volume of 5% or more in one leg compared with 15 healthy controls in whom the difference between limbs did not exceed 4%.[67] Of the 54 patients, 15 (28%) had a slight swelling (>5% volume increase); 3 (6%) had moderate swelling (>10% volume increase); and 4 (7%) had severe swelling (>15% volume increase), which was interpreted as treatment-induced lymphedema. Twelve (22%) of the patients had lymphoedema that was severe enough to cause symptoms.

Management

Management includes patient education of the causes and conditions that may exacerbate their edema. No optimal management exists for treatment of this problem. Precautions regarding skin care, avoidance of trauma, and checking for signs of infection in the leg or foot should be discussed. Compression should be offered as soon as edema becomes apparent. Early treatment is more likely to result in successful management. Compression hose, wrapping the leg, and static compression devices have been used. Some patients have been taught self-massage, while others have professionally administered lymphatic massage. Once edema develops, it will be a lifelong situation with which the patient will have to coexist.

B5. Skin-Vulva

Pathogenesis

The vulva is covered by stratified squamous epithelium, overlying connective tissue with elastic fibers, mucus-forming glands, sweat and sebaceous glands. The clitoris has a cavernous vascular structure.[68]

Radiation induces early vulvar lesions including gross erythema and edema. Basal epithelial cells die due to injury or endothelial cell injury leading to microvascular occlusions. Late injury includes loss of vulvar hair, depigmentation, atrophy of the epithelium, and fibrotic induration.[69]

Clinical Aspects

The skin over the pelvis has a similar tolerance to radiation of skin elsewhere in the body. However, the vulvar tissues are very sensitive to radiation. Even mild erythema can cause significant symptoms for the patient. Generally, erythema occurs around 20 Gy with routine fractionation and can progress to moist desquamation fairly quickly after that. Because of the anatomy certain structures in the vulva can self-bolus and cause early reactions. Because of the early and painful reactions induced by vulvar radiation, many treatment regimens for the anus and/or vulva have a planned treatment break included to improve the acute tolerance of the treatment. As a matter of fact, acute reaction, moist desquamation, is expected in 100% of the patients, while late effects such as fibrosis and telangiectasia occur in 37% of the patients treated with 45–70 Gy; however, these effects are minimized when dose is fractionated at 1.65–1.7 Gy.[69,70]

Management

Good skin hygiene with cleansers will improve the skin tolerance. Utilizing Aquaphor and aloe products will moisturize the skin and improve re-epithelization. The overuse of sitz baths is discouraged because excess moisture will soften the skin and make it more likely to macerate. Areas of moist desquamation may be painted with Gentian Violet that works as an antibacterial agent and a skin barrier to moisture. The use of topical 2% lidocaine gel may enable less discomfort if used prior to urinating or defecating.

Following completion of radiation, the skin of the vulva can become atrophic and thin. Telangiectasias can occur and cause bleeding with minor trauma. Soft tissue necrosis can result and may require lengthy healing times. In order to minimize long-term radiation complications to the pelvis, radiation fractionation schemes have used doses per fraction of less than 180 cGy/fraction.

B6. Vagina

Pathogenesis

The lining of the vagina is made of stratified squamous epithelium over a connective tissue lamina propria and longitudinal muscle fibers and elastic fibers.[68] Radiosensitivity of the squamous epithelium is significant and early vaginal injury is marked by acute epithelial denudation with endothelial injury that may lead to thrombosis, edema, and smooth muscle necrosis. Delayed injury involves severe fibrosis that may obliterate portions of the muscle and vasculature potentially resulting in vaginal stenosis and ulceration.[6]

Clinical Aspects

Vaginal mucosa is reasonably tolerant to radiation. An irradiation tolerance level of the proximal vagina was suggested by Hintz in 1980.[71] None of the patients treated to a maximum dose of 140 Gy developed severe complications or necrosis of the upper vagina. The distal vagina (introitus) and posterior wall are more sensitive to radiation. Hintz suggested doses to the distal vagina not to be greater than 98 Gy. A recent report of 274 patients with cervical carcinoma treated from 1987 to 1997 led to an estimated

TD 5/5 of 175 Gy for combined external and brachytherapy.[72] Serious complications include mucosal necrosis or fistula formation. Less serious complications included vaginal stenosis or shortening, formation of telangiectasia (which can lead to bleeding) or thinning of the vaginal mucosa, and dryness. One study documented a decrease in vaginal length following treatment with intracavitary radiation[73] for patients with cervical or endometrial cancer. Shortening occurred with a mean value of 1.5 cm compared to pretreatment values. Another study of patients who were asked to document changes 1 year following radiation reported that 48% of patients felt their vaginal dimensions were decreased following radiation for cervical cancer.[74]

Management

Treatment issues for vaginal toxicity depend on the level of suspicion for a recurrence. If soft tissue necrosis is observed, symptomatic management with antibiotics, estrogen cream, and gentle irrigation may heal the area. Overzealous biopsy may contribute to the formation of a fistula. But biopsy may be necessary if recurrent tumor is suspected. The strategy for prevention of vaginal stenosis or shortening has been to encourage sexual intercourse or use of vaginal dilators. Estrogen cream or systemic estrogen may also aid in the rejuvenation of cells and increase the elasticity of the vagina. Early intervention is necessary because once shortening and stenosis occur it is difficult if not impossible to reverse. It has been suggested that psychoeducational intervention may increase the compliance rate of some patients for vaginal dilatation and may reduce the sexual fears of many patients.[75] No optimal approach to vaginal dilatation is recognized. Recommendations range from every day dilatation to twice weekly. Appropriate frequency and satisfactory outcome probably depend on the patient's age, surgical procedure, radiation dose, tumor stage, and motivation. Hopefully, investigation will yield more information regarding this topic in the future.

B7. Ovaries

Pathogenesis

Radiation to the ovaries can damage oocytes and result in premature menopause because of ovarian failure of estrogen production. Primary germ cells, oocytes, are surrounded by a single layer of granulosal cells embedded in the stroma to form ovaries. Enlargement of oocytes and the proliferation of granulosal cells into Graafian follicles occur monthly during the reproductive period of life, as well as proliferation of stromal cells in the cortex. After menopause, arteries and veins develop endarteritis oblitrans and ovaries are partially atrophied. A single layer of cells (germinal epithelium) from which oocytes originated covers mature ovaries.[6]

Oocytes undergo meiosis and are relatively radioresistant (single dose LD50 is 4 Gy); however, proliferating granulosal cells are very radiosensitive and their demise leaves oocytes without support and Graafian follicles cannot be formed. Therefore, a total dose of 24 Gy (fractionated in 2-Gy single doses) leads to ablation of ovaries due to the loss of granulosa cells.[76] Early radiation injury then comprises of necrotic changes in proliferating granulosa cells, while other early changes include microvascular thrombi and endothelial cell swelling.[76] Nevertheless, if the dose is sufficiently low, the primordial follicles with non-dividing cells may survive and later develop normally. Late radiation effects include atrophy and fibrosis, with thick walled and hyaline arterioles and venules.[6] The effects on the ovary are dependent on the age of the patient and total dose to the ovary. Low doses of radiation (4–7 Gy in 1–4 fractions) can result in permanent menopause in women over 40 years of age.[77] However, permanent sterility in young women may not result until a total dose of 20 Gy is given.

Management

Radiation-induced ovarian dysfunction should be considered following not only direct pelvic radiation, but also irradiation from inverted Y fields of Hodgkin's disease treatment or craniospinal irradiation. Estrogen replacement may be given to the patient if desired.

B8. Uterus

Pathogenesis

The uterus has four smooth muscle layers creating the myometrium, and is covered with peritoneum and connective tissue adventia. The lamina propria has specialized connective tissue cells, and the endometrium is made of columnar epithelium. The lower uterus and cervix at the vaginal surface are covered by stratified squamous epithelium. The cervical channel is covered by columnar mucus-forming glands. After menopause the blood vessels develop endarteritis oblitrans.[68]

The endometrial glands and stroma (lamina propria) are proliferating only when stimulated by estrogen (and are therefore most radiosensitive at that stage). Henceforth, early radiation injury of uterus is not dramatic. At 6–8 weeks post-intracavity irradiation, cells of the endometrium and stroma are often enlarged and have bizarre nuclei, the stroma is infiltrated by leukocytes, and fibrosis develops in all tissue layers. Delayed injury resembles the postmenopausal uterus, and post-intracavity radiation endometrium and adjacent myometrium show hyaline collagen scars (though fewer deep lesions than post-external beam therapy).[16]

When HDR intracavity brachytherapy was used for intrauterine therapy in four 8.5-Gy doses, not more than 4.6% patients experience severe complications at 5 years.[78] External beam therapy if used without brachytherapy is prescribed near to the tolerance dose, as total external beam dose of 45–50 Gy; in combination with brachytherapy it is used usually at 20–40 Gy.[28]

Radiation to the uterus can result in impaired uterine growth and blood flow that lead to early pregnancy loss and premature labor if pregnancy is achieved.[79] Uterine volume correlates with the age at which radiation was received. Radiation at a young age results in decreased volume. One study examined women who had received total body irradiation (14.4 Gy). Four of 6 women with ovarian failure had reduced uterine volume, undetectable blood supply, and absent endometrium at baseline assessment. After 3 months of sex steroid replacement treatment, uterine blood supply and endometrial response were not significantly different from controls. Uterine volume improved but remained significantly smaller than controls.[80] Another study of patients treated with low radiation doses to the uterus for benign disease examined 1817 women treated with intrauterine radium for uterine bleeding. The radiation dose to the uterus was at least 24 Gy. Three hundred and eleven patients were less than 40 years of age. Nineteen patients became pregnant with 33 conceptions but only 6 live births resulted.[81]

In the cervix, delayed injury may include the presence of atrophic squamous epithelial cells often with such nuclei as to suggest dysplasia.[6]

B9. Testicles

Pathogenesis

The walls of the seminiferous tubules are made of a basement membrane over lamina propria containing fibromyocytes and elastic fibers. Inside the tubules are postmitotic Sertoli cells surrounded by spermatogonia A, spermatogonia B, primary and secondary spermatocytes, spermatids, and spermazoa. In the stroma are blood and lymphatic vessels and nerves, and cells of different types: fibroblasts, macrophages, mast cells, and Leydig cells.[82]

Of these cells, in the postpuberty testis, spermatogonia B and then spermatocytes are the most radiosensitive, followed by non-dividing spermatogonia A, with postmitotic cells—spermatids and spermazoa being least sensitive. The Sertoli and Leydig cells are comparatively radioresistant, surviving doses causing sterility. In the prepubescent testis, Sertoli cells are the dominant cell type in seminiferous tubules, are still dividing, and are therefore radiosensitive.[6] Therefore in prepuberal boys, irradiation can cause hormonal imbalance and arrested entry into puberty.[83]

Death of spermatogonia B and spermatocytes can be caused by cGy doses of irradiation, and follows an apoptotic pattern of cell death. This is accompanied by gene induction of apoptosis-regulating genes such as p53 and myc, and cytokines such as tumor necrosis factor alpha.[84] Due to the fact that spermatogonia B are recruited from the pool of less radiosensitive spermatogonia A, fractionated radiation may cause a more severe oligospermia. A high dose of radiation, such as 30 Gy, causes significant cell death of most cell types in testis, including Leydig cells, resulting in a decrease in testosterone.[85] A late effect of irradiation is testicular atrophy, and this could probably be best attributed to ischemia, by extrapolation from other tissues.[6]

Clinical Aspects

The testis is one of the most radiosensitive tissues in the body with a radiation dose as low as 15 cGy causing a significant depression in the sperm count.[77] The testis may be directly in the radiation field or receive scatter dose from a nearby field. Irradiation of the testis during radiation usually involves fractionated doses that may cause more stem cell killing than single-dose treatments.

Low doses of radiation kill spermatogonia which are differentiating into spermatocytes. Therefore, low doses of radiation deplete the stem cells of these developing sperm which result in decreased sperm production during the first 50–60 days after irradiation. Temporary oligo- or azoospermia result. Complete recovery takes place within 9–18 months after less than 1 Gy, 30 months for 2–3 Gy, and 5 or more years after

4–6 Gy.[77] One study of 11 cancer patients who received 118–223 cGy delivered in 24–35 fractions demonstrated temporary aspermia in all patients beginning about 3 months after RT.[86] Recovery of spermatogenesis was first noted between 10 and 18 months in 5 patients. Another group of patients who received fractionated doses of 19–178 cGy to the remaining testis following unilateral orchiectomy had azoospermia in 10–14 patients who received over 65 CGy to the testis. Sperm reappeared in the semen with 30–80 weeks after the start of treatment.[87]

Direct testicular irradiation of 24 Gy results in ablation of the germinal epithelium (responsible for sperm development) and Leydig cell function (responsible for testosterone) is seriously affected in most patients. Tsatsoulis et al. evaluated Leydig and Sertoli cell function in 18 men who had undergone unilateral orchidectomy for a testicular seminoma followed by 30 Gy in 20 fractions.[88] The median testosterone level was significantly less than in normal controls and 6 men had levels below the normal adult male range. Leydig cell damage was suggested by the decreased testosterone/LH ratio. Similarly, 10 of 12 boys demonstrated Leydig cell dysfunction 1–8 years after testicular irradiation (24 Gy) for acute lymphoblastic leukemia.[89] Lower doses of 3–9 Gy received as a scatter dose to the testes in childhood in fractionated doses resulted in oligo- or azoospermia many years later. LH and testosterone levels were normal indicating normal Leydig cell function. Also, another report demonstrated that low doses of testicular irradiation (12–15 Gy) did not result in abnormal pubertal development in 12 of 13 boys, although 7 boys who were tested demonstrated azoospermia.[90]

Management

Androgen replacement therapy to enable normal puberal development and future sexual function is required for patients with deficient testosterone production.

B10. Sexual Function

Women

Sexual function in women following radiation has been poorly evaluated. Most studies focus on vaginal stenosis because it can be quantitated. However, measurement of vaginal anatomy may not correlate well with overall sexual function.[91] Other factors including dyspareunia, bleeding or concern of bleeding, and lubrication changes can also occur.[92]

Jensen et al. evaluate 118 patients following radiation with a self-assessment questionnaire. Approximately 85% had low or no sexual interest, 35% had moderate to severe lack of lubrication, 55% had mild to severe dyspareunia, and 30% were dissatisfied with their sexual life.[74]

Emotional distress after a cancer diagnosis and treatment can certainly cause disruption in sexual function. Radiation following surgery has the potential for causing more sexual dysfunction than radiation alone.[93]

Management

Intervention strategies have focused on vaginal dilatation. Robinson et al. found increased compliance with the use of vaginal dilators and reduction of sexual fears in women following careful counseling about potential sexual difficulties and suggestions on alternate sexual practices in addition to careful instruction in the use of a vaginal dilator.[75] Use of topical or systemic estrogens may decrease vaginal irritation and improve lubrication. However, hormone replacement therapy may not be an option for many patients who have hormone-sensitive tumors or other contraindications.

It is obvious that sexual dysfunction affects a high proportion of women receiving radiation to the pelvis. Counseling of patients and their partners regarding potential problems that may affect sexual function following RT should help patients to understand anatomic changes and allay fears. More information is needed regarding intervention strategies for dealing with various issues.

Men

Erectile dysfunction is a common sequela following curative local treatment for early-stage carcinoma of the prostate. Most reports focus on erectile function although additional symptoms that affect sexual function can develop after either prostate brachytherapy or external beam radiation to that area of the body. Reported symptoms after brachytherapy have included hematospermia, pain at orgasm, and alteration in the intensity of orgasm.[94] After EBRT symptoms have included a lack of ejaculation in 2–56% of patients, dissatisfaction with sex life in 25–60%, decreased libido in 8–53%, and decreased sexual desire in 12–58%.[94]

The etiology of erectile dysfunction has been attributed to changes in the arteriolar system supplying the corporal muscles. Goldstein et al. documented abnormal vascularity by penile Doppler ultrasonography in all patients who had altered erectile function after EBRT.[95] Similarly, Zelefsky and Eid documented abnormal distensibility of the cavernosal arteries in patients with erectile dysfunction.[96] Merrick et al. found no significant difference in the mean dose to the neurovascular bundles between potent and impotent men following brachytherapy.[97] Approximately 50% of patients develop erectile dysfunction within 5 years of prostate radiation. Factors related to the likelihood of this occurrence include pretreatment potency, patient age, use of supplemental external beam irradiation, radiation dose to the prostate, radiation dose to the bulb of the penis, time since radiotherapy, and diabetes mellitus.[97] Radiation dose to the bulb of the penis seems to correlate with the risk of erectile dysfunction after EBRT and after BT.[98,99] In the past, men who received brachytherapy for treatment have been believed to have improved potency rates than patients treated with EBRT. However, selection bias can favor these patients who may have a lower age, better performance status, and more motivation to maintain potency.[100] Another study investigated the erectile function and satisfaction of men treated for prostate cancer with 3D conformal radiation or transperineal prostate brachytherapy.[101] This report of 128 men suggested that either treatment had a similar impact on erectile function and overall satisfaction. Another report of 201 men treated with MRI-guided brachytherapy with or without external beam irradiation found that all patients (82–93%) experienced some degree of erectile dysfunction compared with baseline function within 4 years after therapy.[19]

Management

When sildenafil citrate was used at least two-thirds of patients reported rates of erectile function comparable to or superior to baseline function.[102] Intracavernosal injection of prostaglandins can also be effective. Vacuum pumps and penile prosthesis can be used. There is no doubt that better understanding of quality-of-life issues that may lead to sexual counseling have the potential to improve sexual function. Radiation strategies that limit radiation dose to the bulb of the penis may also improve sexual outcomes.[103]

B11. Bone Effects

Pathogenesis

Radiation can affect the microvasculature of the mature bone. This injury causes decreased blood supply to the periosteum which compromises osteoblastic function and can result in an insufficiency fracture (IF). Insufficiency fractures of bone occur as a result of physiological stress on bones with deficient elastic resistance. Irradiation can damage osteoblasts, osteocytes, and osteoclasts and leave an acellular matrix that appears radiographically normal. Such radiation-induced atrophy reduces the number of functional and structural components of a tissue. These two processes can result in clinically and radiographically significant bone atrophy. In addition, previously irradiated atrophic bone is at risk for fracture, second malignancy, or infection, leading to true necrosis.[104] Resulting injuries include atraumatic femoral neck fracture, and osteonecrosis of the femoral head or of the acetabulum.

When bone marrow is irradiated, permanent ablation or hypoplasia can occur. This was demonstrated by failure of bone marrow to regenerate in-field after 30–40 Gy mantle irradiation for Hodgkin's disease.[105] However, marrow recovery has been demonstrated to occur over extended periods depending on the volume irradiated.[106] Irreversible injury after greater than 50 Gy is a consequence of irreparable damage to the microvasculature manifested by irreversible bone marrow fibrosis.

Clinical Aspects

Insufficiency fractures have been described in postmenopausal women with osteoporosis, in patients treated with high doses of corticosteroids, and in patients following radiation exposure. Osseous complications are usually considered uncommon after radiation with megavoltage radiation because of decreased absorption in bone compared to lower energy machines of the past. However, they are important to recognize because the differential diagnosis includes pelvic bone metastases.

In a retrospective study of scintigrams of 80 patients, Abe et al. reported that asymptomatic IF was found in 34% of postmenopausal patients treated with adjuvant postoperative radiation for endometrial cancer.[107] The incidence of symptomatic pelvic fractures in several series of women treated for gynecologic malignancies ranges from 1.7% to 6% following doses of 46–50 Gy to the whole pelvis.[108–112] At least one report suggested increased incidence of IF in women receiving brachytherapy in addition to EBRT.[109] Pain in the pelvic area is the initial complaint of patients. The average time to onset of symptoms is usually 11–12 months after radiation therapy. CT scans can reveal radiological findings of IF, although MRI is currently the most sensitive modality for detecting these lesions. Radionuclide bone scans reliably and non-invasively screen for bony abnormalities in the pelvis and elsewhere. Increased radionuclide uptake at the fracture site is informative, and a characteristic H-shaped pattern of uptake across the sacrum and sacroiliac joints often corresponds to horizontal and vertical fractures.[113] Most IF is multiple and the most common location for them is in the sacrum and pubic bones.

Femoral head/acetabular damage. The tolerance doses for the femoral head have been estimated to be 52 Gy for the TD 5/5 and 65 Gy for the TD 50/5.[42] One review from Mallinckrodt reported that the cumulative actuarial incidence of femoral neck fracture was 11% at 5 years and 15% at 10 years for patients who were treated APPA to the pelvis with 18 MV photons.[114] No fracture occurred below doses of 42 Gy. Multivariate analysis demonstrated that independent prognostic variables for increasing the risk included cigarette use and radiographic evidence of osteoporosis.

Bone marrow sequelae. The bone marrow is one of the most radiosensitive organs in the pelvis. Approximately 40% of the total body bone marrow reserve lies within the pelvic bones as seen in Figure 3.[115] Hematologic toxicity can be seen acutely during radiation and exposure to radiation can result in long-term myelotoxicity. The radiation dose, dose rate, and volume all affect the acute response of the bone marrow to therapy. When small bone marrow volumes are irradiated, bone marrow in unexposed areas of the body responds by increasing its population of progenitor cells meeting the demands for hematopoiesis. Therefore, acute effects are not seen unless a substantial portion of the marrow is exposed. With exposure to large bone marrow volumes, neutropenia occurs in 2–3 weeks followed by thrombocytopenia and then anemia in 2–3 months.[114] This is represented in Figure 4. The majority of chemotherapeutic agents affect the bone marrow in a similar way. Therefore, the combination of the two modalities can be additive. Many patients receiving radiation are now treated with either sequential or concomitant systemic chemotherapy and myelotoxicity can be a significant problem.

Management

Biopsy is not recommended because of the risk of trauma-inducing radiation necrosis and also because of the low diagnostic efficiency. Histologic changes of hemorrhage, fibrosis, necrotic bone fragments, trabecular bone, and cartilage growth can result in misinterpretation by the pathologist.[109] Treatment of these lesions is usually conservative with pain management, rehabilitation exercises, and restriction of weight bearing. Most series report improvement and complete resolution in symptoms by 6–12 months.

Treatment for bone fractures following radiation has included Provera, Premarin, calcium supplements, and pamidronate. One report reported a trend toward earlier healing with drug treatment.[119]

Treatment planning in the pelvis should consider the volume of the boney pelvis that is included in the radiation field. Techniques that reduce the bone volume and avoid high dose areas in the bone should help to keep IF at a minimum level.

The management of patients with bone marrow toxicity can be divided into those that are supportive and those that are preventative. Growth factor administration is now a common supportive measure in patients with white cell deficiencies. Erythropoietin is now approved for use in patients with depressed hemoglobin levels. Transfusion is typically reserved for patients with hemoglobin levels below 8 g/dL or those that are symptomatic from low levels with the goal of ameliorating physiologic responses more quickly. Erythropoietin is typically used if hemoglobin levels are below 12 g/dL in order to improve tolerance to therapy[118] or improve "cancer-related fatigue" symptoms.[119]

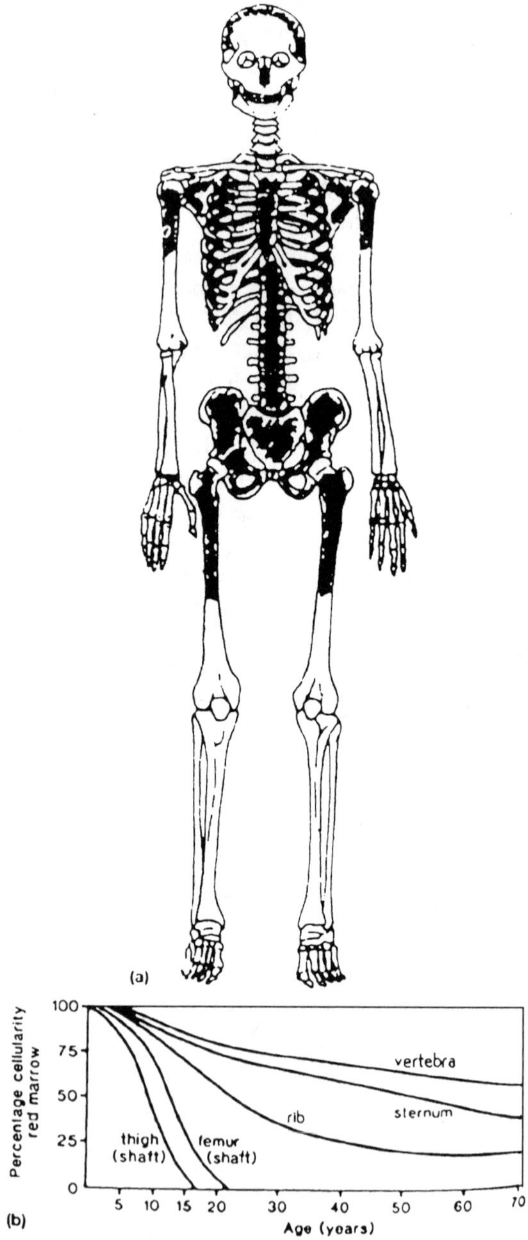

Figure 3. Bone marrow distribution in adult humans as determined by autopsy finding: active areas are shaded. The relative amount of red bone marrow in difference anatomic sites as a function of age.[114]

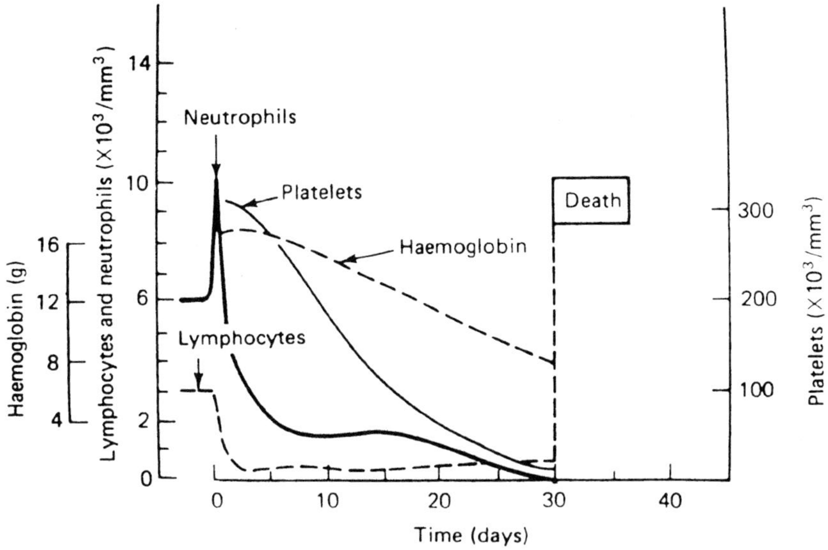

Figure 4. Temporal sequence of changes in numbers of neutrophils, platelets, and lymphocytes, and hemoglobin after lethal total body irradiation.[114]

There is increased interest in prevention of bone marrow toxicity using bone marrow sparing techniques with intensity-modulated radiation therapy. Brixey et al. evaluated 36 patients with uterine or cervical cancer who received treatment with IM-WPRT and compared them to 88 patients treated to the same target volume and total dose with conventional four-field WPRT as seen in Table 3.[120] The comparison of pelvic BM dose–volume histograms revealed that IM-WPRT planning resulted in significantly less BM volume being irradiated compared with WPRT planning, particularly within the iliac crests as seen in Figure 5. Administration of chemotherapy was held more often in the WPRT group and patients treated with chemotherapy and WPRT experienced more acute WBC toxicity. This report suggests that IMRT may be important for bone marrow sparing when pelvic radiation is required and may improve the tolerance for treatment that combines radiation with systemic chemotherapy.

Table 3. Comparison of doses to iliac crest bone marrow irradiated between whole pelvic radiation and intensity-modulated radiation.[120]

Dose (Gy)	WPRT (% vol)	IM-WPRT (% vol)	p
10	94.9	97.3	0.007
20	88.8	78.1	<0.001
30	54.9	52.9	0.167
40	42.4	26.2	<0.001
45	32.1	15.1	<0.001
50	0	0.46	0.012

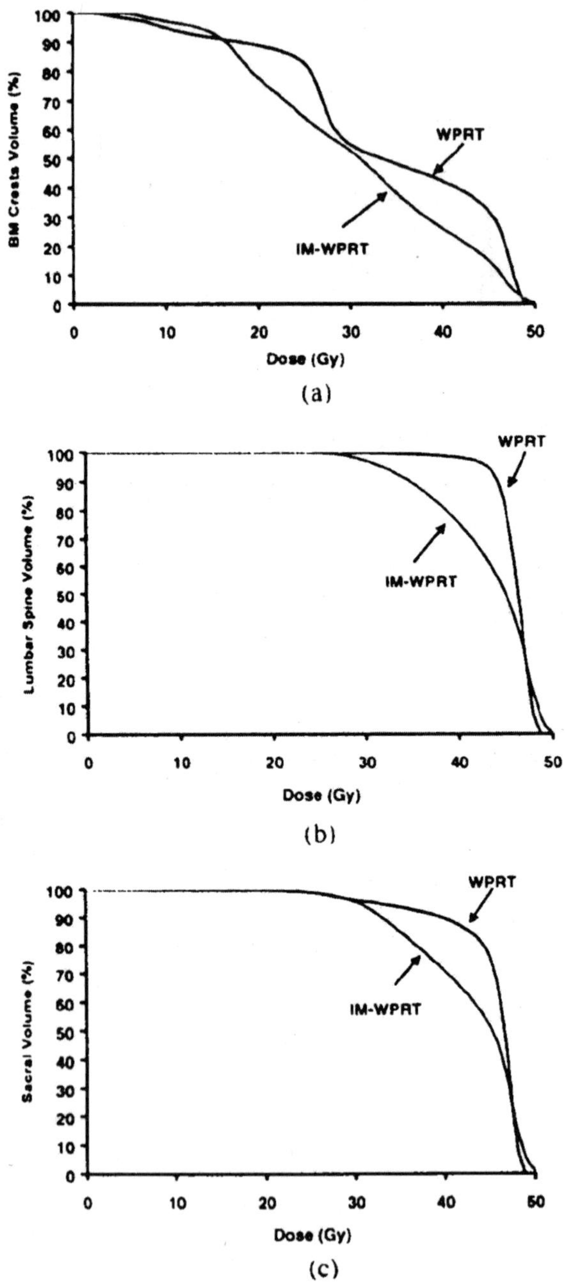

Figure 5. Comparison of the average bone marrow dose–volume histograms of 10 patients with treatment planned using both conventional whole pelvic radiation therapy and intensity-modulated pelvic radiation therapy.[120]

REFERENCES

1. Williamson, RCN. 1978. Intestinal adaptation—structural, functional, and cytokinetic changes. N Engl J Med **298:**1393–1402.
2. Withers, HR and KA Mason. 1974. The kinetics of recovery in irradiated colonic mucosa of the mouse. Cancer **34(Suppl):**896–903.
3. Gelfand, MD, M Tepper, LA Katz, HJ Binder, R Yesner, and MH Floch. 1968. Acute radiation proctitis in man. Gastroenterology **54:**401–411.
4. Haboubi, NY, PF Schofield, and PL Rowland. 1988. The light and electron microscopic features of early and late phase radiation-induced proctitis. Am J Gastroenterol **83:**1140–1144.
5. Sedgwick, DM, DCG Howard, and A Ferguson. 1994. Pathogenesis of acute radiation injury to the rectum. A prospective study in patients. J Colorect Dis **9:**23–30.
6. Fajardo, LF, M Berthrong, and RE Anderson. 2001. Radiation Pathology. New York, NY: Oxford University Press, Inc.
7. Paris, F, Z Fuks, A Kang, P Capodieci P, G Juan, D Ehleiter, A Haimovitz-Friedman, C Cordon-Cardo, and R Kolesnick. 2001. Endothelial apoptosis as the primary lesion initiating intestinal radiation damage in mice. Science **293(5528):**293–297.
8. Gudkov, AV and EA Komarova. 2003. The role of p53 in determining sensitivity to radiotherapy. Nat Rev Cancer **3(2):**117–129.
9. Anderson, R, M Berthrong, and LF Fajardo. 1996. Radiation injury. In: Damjanov, I and Linder, J, eds. Anderson's Pathology, 10th ed. Philadelphia, PA: Mosby.
10. Withers, HR, LJ Peters, and HS Kogelnik. 1980. The pathobiology of late effects of irradiation. In: Meyn, RE and Withers, HR, eds. Radiation Biology in Cancer Research. New York, NY: Raven Press.
11. Anseline, PF, IC Lavery, VW Fazio, DG Jagelman, and FL Weakley. 1981. Radiation injury to the rectum. Ann Surg **194:**716–724.
12. Haaselton, PS, N Carr, and PF Schofield. 1985. Vascular changes in radiation bowel disease. Histopathology **9:**517–534.
13. Nuyttens, JJ, S Milito, PF Rust, and AT Turrisi. 2002. Dose–volume relationship for acute side effects during high dose conformal radiotherapy for prostate cancer. Radiother Oncol **64:**209–214.
14. Schultheiss, TE, WR Lee, MA Hunt, AL Halon, RS Peter, and GE Hanks. 1997. Late GI and GU complications in the treatment of prostate cancer. Int J Radiat Oncol Biol Phys **54(1):**3–11.
15. O'Brien, PC, CI Franklin, MG Poulsen, DJ Joseph, NS Spry, and JW Denham. 2002. Acute symptoms, not rectally administered sucralfate, predict for late radiation proctitis: longer term follow-up of a phase III trial—Trans-Tasman Radiation Oncology Group. Int J Radiat Oncol Biol Phys **54:**442–449.
16. Gilinsky, NH, DG Burns, GO Barbezat, W Levin, HS Myers, and IN Marks. 1983. The natural history of radiation-induced proctosigmoiditis: an analysis of 88 patients. Q J Med **52:**40–53.
17. Koper, PC, WD Heemsbergen, MS Hoogeman, PP Jansen, GA Hart, AJ Wijnmaalen, M van Os, LJ Boersma, JV Lebesque, and P Levendag. 2004. Impact of volume and location of irradiated rectum wall on rectal blood loss after radiotherapy of prostate cancer. Int J Radiat Oncol Biol Phys **58:**1072–1082.
18. Jackson, A, MW Skwarchuk, MJ Zelefsky, DM Cowen, ES Venkatraman, S Levegrun, CM Burman, CJ Kutcher, Z Fuks, SA Liebel, and CC Ling. 2001. Late rectal bleeding after conformal radiotherapy of prostate cancer. II. Volume effects and dose–volume histograms. Int J Radiat Oncol Biol Phys **49:**685–698.
19. Albert, M, CM Tempany, D Schultz, MH Chen, RA Cormack, S Kumar, MD Hurwitz, C Beard, K Tuncali, M O'Leary, GP Topulos, K Valentine, L Lopes, A Kanan, D Kacher, J Rosato, H Kooy, F Jolesz, DL Carr-Locke, JP Richie, and AV D'Amico. 2003. Late genitourinary and gastrointestinal toxicity after magnetic resonance image-guided prostate brachytherapy with or without neoadjuvant external beam radiation therapy. Cancer **98:**949–954.
20. International Commission on Radiation Units and Measurements. 1985. Report 38: Dose and volume specification for reporting intracavitary therapy in gynecology. Bethesda: International Commission on Radiation Units and Measurements.
21. Esche, B, J Crook, and J Horiot. 1987. Dosimetric methods in the optimization of radiotherapy for carcinoma of the uterine cervix. Int J Radiat Oncol Biol Phys **13:**1183–1192.
22. Eifel, PJ, K Winter, M Morris, C Levenback, PW Grigsby, J Cooper, M Rotman, D Gershenson, DG Mutch. 2004. Pelvic irradiation with concurrent chemotherapy versus pelvic and para-aortic irradiation for high-risk cervical cancer: an update of radiation therapy oncology group trial (RTOG) 90-01. J Clin Oncol **22:**872–880.

23. Chen, SW, JA Liang, SN Yang, RT Liu, and FJ Lin. 2000. The prediction of late rectal complications following the treatment of uterine cervical cancer by high-dose rate brachytherapy. Int J Radiat Oncol Biol Phys **47:**955–961.
24. Kochlar, R, F Patel, A Dhar, SC Sharma, S Ayyagari, R Aggarwal, MK Goenka, BD Gupta, and SK Mehta. 1991. Radiation induced proctosigmoiditis: prospective, randomized, double-blind controlled trial of oral sulfasalazine plus rectal steroids verus rectal sucralfate. Dig dis Sci **36:**103–107.
25. Kochhar, R, SK Mehta, R Aggarwal, A Dhar, and F Patel. 1990. Sucralfate enema in ulcerative rectosigmoid lesions. Disease of the Colon and Rectum **33:**49–51.
26. Johnston, MJ, GJ Robertson, and FA Frizelle. 2003. Management of late complications of pelvic radiation in the rectum and anus. Dis Coln Rectum **46:**247–259.
27. Da Silva, GJ, M Berho, SD Wexner, J Efron, EG Weiss, JJ Nogueras, AM Vernava, JT Connor, and P Gervaz. 2003. Histologic analysis of the irradiated anal sphincter. Dis Colon Rectum **46:**1492–1497.
28. Cummings, BJ and JD Brierley. 2004. In: Perez, CA, Brady, LW, Halperin, EC, and Schmidt-Ullrich, RK, eds. Principles and Practice of Radiation Oncology, 4th ed. Philadelphia, PA: Lippincott, Williams and Wilkins.
29. Cummings, B, TJ Keane, B O'Sullivan, CS Wong, and CN Catton. 1991. Epidermoid anal cancer: treatment by radiation alone or by radiation and 5-Fluorouracil with and without mitomycin C. Int J Radiat Oncol Biol Phys **21:**1115–1125.
30. Myerson, R, SJ Shapiro, D Lacey, M Lopez, E Birnbaum, J Fleshman, R Fry, and I Kodner. 1995. Carcinoma of the anal canal. Am J Clin Onc **18:**32–29.
31. Tanum, G, K Tveit, KO Karlsen, and M Hauer-Jensen. 1991 Chemotherapy and radiation therapy for anal carcinoma. Cancer **67:**2462–2466.
32. Dirk, V, S Marco, F Michael, T Arnulf, and K Oliver. 1999. Curative-intent radiation therapy in anal carcinoma: quality of life and sphincter function. Radiother Oncol **52:**239–243.
33. Hayne, D, CJ Vaizey, and PB Boulos. 2001. Anorectal injury following pelvic radiotherapy. Br J Surg **88:**1037–1048.
34. Freys, SM, KH Fuchs, M Fein, J Heimbucher, M Sailer, and A Thiede. 1998. Inter-and intraindividual reproducibility of anorectal manometry. Langenbecks Arch Surg **383:**325–329.
35. Yeoh, EE, R Botten, A Russo, R McGowan, R Fraser, D Roos, M Penniment, M Borg, and W Sun. 2000. Chronic effects of therapeutic irradiation for localized prostatic carcinoma on anorectal function. Int J Radiat Oncol Biol Phy **47:**915–924.
36. Vordermark, D, M Sailer, M Flentje, A Thiede, and O Kolbl. 2002. Impaired sphincter function and good quality of life in anal carcinoma patients after radiotherapy: a paradox? Front Radiat Ther Oncol **37:**132–139.
37. Iwamoto, T, S Nakahara, R Mibu, M Hotokezaka, H Nakano, and M Tanaka. 1997. Effect of radiotherapy on anorectal function in patients with cervical cancer. Dis Colon Rectum **40:**693–697.
38. Bern, J, S Bern, and A Sign. 2000. Use hyperbaric oxygen chamber in the management of radiation-related complications of the anorectal region. Dis Colon Rectum **43:**1435–1438.
39. Stewart, FA. 1986. Mechanisms of bladder damage and repair after treatment with radiation and cytostatic drugs. Br J Cancer **53(Suppl):**280–291.
40. Lopez-Beltran, A, RJ Luque, R Mazzucchelli, M Scarpelli, and R Montironi. 2002. Changes produced in the urothelium by traditional and newer therapeutic procedures for bladder cancer. J Clin Path **55:**641–647.
41. Fajardo, LF and M Berthrong. 1978. Radiation injury in surgical pathology. Am J Surg Pathol **2:**159–199.
42. Radiation Biology and Radiation Pathology Syllabus. 1975. Editor Philip Rubin. The American College of Radiology.
43. Emami, B, J Lyman, A Brown, L Coia, M Goitein, JE Munzenrider, B Shank, LJ Solin, and M Wesson. 1991. Tolerance of normal tissue to therapeutic irradiation. Int J Radiat Oncol Biol Phy **21:**109–122.
44. Marks, LB, PR Carroll, TC Dugan, and MS Anscher. 1995. The response of the urinary bladder, urethra and ureter to radiation and chemotherapy. Int J Radiat Oncol Biol Phys **31:**1257–1280.
45. Lajer, H, IR Thranov, P Bagi, and S Aage Engelholm. 2002. Evaluation of urologic morbidity after radiotherapy for cervical carcinoma by urodynamic examinations and patient voiding schemes; a prospective study. Int J Radiat Oncol Biol Phy **54:**1362–1368.
46. Lajer, H, IR Thranov, LT Skovgaard, and SA Engelholm. 2002. Late urologic morbidity in 177 consecutive patients after radiotherapy for cervical carcinoma: a longitudinal study. Int J Radiat Oncol Biol Phys **54:**1356–1361.
47. Moller, LA, G Lose, and T Jorgensen. 2000. Incidence and remission rates of lower urinary tract symptoms at one year in women aged 40–60; Longitudinal study. BMJ **320:**1429–1432.

48. Eifel, P, C Levenback, JT Wharton, and MJ Oswald. 1995. Time course and incidence of late complications in patients treated with radiation therapy for FIGO stage IB carcinoma of the uterine cervix. Int J Radiat Oncol Biol Phys **32:**1289–1300.
49. Levenback, C, PJ Eifel, TW Burke, M Morris, and DM Gershenson. 1994. Hemorrhagic cystitis following radiotherapy for stage IB cancer of the cervix. Gynecologic Oncol **55:**206–210.
50. Montana, G and W Fowler. 1989. Carcinoma of the cervix: analysis of bladder and rectal radiation dose and complications. Int J Radiat Oncol Biol Phys **16:**95–100.
51. Pollack, A, GK Zagars, G Starkschall, JA Antolak, JJ Lee, E Huang, AC von Eschenback, DA Kuban, and I Rosen. 2002. Prostate cancer radiation dose response: results of the M.D. Anderson phase III randomized trial. Int J Radiat Oncol Biol Phys **1**(**53**)**:**1097–1105.
52. Corman, JM, D McClure, R Pritchett, P Kozlowski, and NB Hampson. 2003. Treatment of radiation induced hemorrhagic cystitis with hyperbaric oxygen. J Urol **169:**220–222.
53. Bevers, RFM, DJ Bakker, and KH Kurth. 1995. Hyperbaric oxygen treatment for haemorrhagic radiation cystitis. Lancet **346:**803–805.
54. Seymore, CH, AM el-Mahdi, and PF Schellhammer. 1986. The effect of prior transurethral resection of the prostate on post radiation urethral strictures and bladder neck contractures. Int J Radiat Oncol Biol Phys **12:**1597–1600.
55. Green, N, D Treible, and H Wallack. 1990. Prostate cancer: postirradiation incontinence. J Urol **144:**307–309.
56. Parkin, DE, JA Davis, and RP Symonds. 1987. Long term bladder symptomatology following radiotherapy for cervical carcinoma. Radiother Oncol **9:**193–199.
57. Pourquier, H, R Delar, D Archille, N Daly, J Horiot, R Keiling, J Pigneux, R Rozan, S Schraub, and C Vrousos. 1987. A quantified approach to the analysis and prevention of urinary complications in radiotherapeutic treatment of cancer of the cervix. Int J Radiat Oncol Biol Phys **13:**1025–1033.
58. Zietman, AL, D Sacco, U Skowronski, P Gromery, DS Kaufman, JA Clark, JA Talcott, and WU Shipley. 2003. Organ conservation in invasive bladder cancer by transurethral resection, chemotherapy and radiation; results of a urodynamic and quality of life study on long-term survivors. J Urol **170:**1772–1776.
59. Gellrich, J, OW Hakenberg, S Oehlschlager, and MP Wirth. 2003. Manifestation, latency and management of late urological complications after curative radiotherapy for cervical carcinoma. Onkologie **26:**334–340.
60. Perez, CA, PW Grigsby, MA Lockett, KS Chao, and J Williamson. 1999. Radiation therapy morbidity in carcinoma of the uterine cervix: dosimetric and clinical correlation. Int J Radiat Oncol Biol Phys **44:**855–866.
61. McIntyre, JF, PJ Eifel, C Levenback, and MR Oswald. 1995. Ureteral stricture as a late complication of radiotherapy for stage IB carcinoma of the uterine cervix. Cancer **75:**836–843.
62. Unal, A, AD Hamberger, JC Seski, and GH Fletcher. 1981. An analysis of the severe complications of irradiation of carcinoma of the uterine cervix: treatment with intracavitary radium and parametrial irradiation. Int J Radiat Oncol Biol Phys **7:**999–1004.
63. Rotman, M, MJ John, SH Moon, KN Choi, SM Stowe, A Abitbol, T Herskovic, and S Sall. 1979. Limitations of adjunctive surgery in carcinoma of the cervix. Int J Radiat Oncol Biol Phys **5:**327–332.
64. Averette, HE and JH Ferguson. 1963. Lymphographic alterations of pelvic lymphatics after radiotherapy. JAMA **186:**554–557.
65. Snijders-Keilhoz, A, BW Hellebrekers, AH Zinderman, MJ van de Vijver, and JB Trimbos. 1999. Adjuvant radiotherapy following radical hysterectomy for patients with early stage cervical carcinoma. Radiother Oncol **51:**161–167.
66. Ryan, M, MC Stainton, EK Slaytor, C Jaconelli, S Watts, and P Mackenzie. 2003. Aetiology and prevalence of lower limb lymphoedema following treatment for gynaecological cancer. P. Aust N Z J Obste Gynael **43:**148–151.
67. Werngren-Elgstrom, M and D Lidman. 1994. Lymphoedema of the lower extremitites after surgery and radiotherapy for cancer of the cervix. Scan J Plast Reconstr Surg Han Surg **28:**289–293.
68. Junqueira LC, J Carneiro, and O Kelley. 1992. Basic Histology. Norwalk, CT: Appleton and Lange.
69. Thomas, GM, AJ Dembo, SC Bryson, R Osborne, and AD DePetrillo. 1991.Changing concepts in the management of vulvar cancer. Gynecol Oncol **42(1):**9–21.
70. Perez, CA, PW Grigsby, A Galakatos, R Swanson, HM Camel, M Kao, and MA Lockett. 1993. Radiation therapy in management of carcinoma of the vulva with emphasis on conservation therapy. Cancer **71:**3707–3716.

71. Hintz, BL, AR Kagan, P Chan, HA Gilbert, H Nussbaum, AR Rao, and M Wollin. 1980. Radiation tolerance of the vaginal mucosa. Int J Radiat Oncol Biol Phys **6:**711–716.
72. Au, SP and PW Grigsby. 2003. The irradiation tolerance dose of the proximal vagina. Radiother Oncol **67:**77–85.
73. Bruner, DW, R Lanciano, M Keegan, B Corn, E Martin, and GE Hanks. 1993. Vaginal stenosis and sexual function following intracavitary radiation for the treatment of cervical and endometrial carcinoma. Int J Radiat Oncol Biol Phys **27:**825–830.
74. Jensen, PT, M Groenvold, MC Klee, I Thranov, MA Petersen, and D Machin. 2003. Longitudinal study of sexual function and vaginal changes after radiotherapy for cervical cancer. Int J Radiat Oncol Biol Phys **56:**937–949.
75. Robinson, JW, PD Faris, and CB Scott. 2000. Psychoeducational group increases vaginal dilation for younger women and reduces sexual fears for women of all ages with gynecological carcinoma treated with radiotherapy. Int J Radiat Oncol Biol Phys **46:**1077–1078.
76. Grigsby, PW, A Russel, D Brunner, P Eifel, W-J Koh, W Spanos, J Stetz, JA Stitt, and I Sullivan. 1995. Late injury of cancer therapy of the female reproductive tract. Int J Radiat Oncol Biol Phys **31:**1281–1299.
77. Ash, P. 1980. The influence of radiation on fertility in man. Br J Radiol **53:**271–278.
78. Kucera, H, TH Knocke, E Kucera, and R Potter. 1998. Treatment of endometrial carcinoma with high-dose-rate brachytherapy alone in medically inoperable stage I patients. Acta Obstet Gynecol Scand **77(10):**1008–1012.
79. Critchley, H, W Wallace, S Shalet, H Mamtora, J Higginson, and D Anderson. 1992. Abdominal irradiation in childhood; the potential for pregnancy. Br J Obestetr Gynecol **99:**392–394.
80. Bath, LE, H Critchley, S Chambers, R Anerson, C Kelnar, and W Wallace. 1999. Ovarian and uterine characteristics after total body irradiation in childhood and adolescence: response to sex and steroid replacement. Br J Obstetr Gynecol **106:**1265–1272.
81. Dickson, RJ. 1969. The late results of radium treatment for benign uterine hemorrhage. Br J Radiol **42:**582–594.
82. Trainier, TD. 1992. Testis and excretory duct system. In: Sternberg, SS, ed. Histology for Pathologists. New York, NY: Raven Press.
83. Kagan, AR. 1989. Bladder, testicle, and prostate irradiation injury. Front Rad Ther Oncol **23:**323–337.
84. Withers, HR and WH McBride. 1998. Biological basis of radiation therapy. In: Perez, CA and Brady, LW, eds. Principles and Practice of Radiation Oncology, 3rd ed. Philadelphia, PA: JB Lippincott.
85. Shalet, SM, A Tsatsoulis, E Whitehead, and G Read. 1989. Vulnerability of the human Leydig cell to radiation damage is dependent upon age. J Endocrinol **120:**161–165.
86. Hahn, EW, SM Feingold, and L Nisce. 1976. Aspermia and recovery of spermatogenesis in cancer patients following incidental gonadal irradiation during treatment: a progress report. Radiology **119:**223–225.
87. Hahn, EW, SM Feingold, L Simpson, and M Batala. 1982. Recovery from aspermia induced by low-dose radiation in seminoma patients. Cancer **50:**337–340.
88. Tsatsoulis, A, AM Shalet, ID Morris, and D deKrestser. 1990. Immunoactive inhibin as marker of sertoli cell function following cytotoxic damage to the human testis. Hormone Res **34:**254–259.
89. Brauner, R, P Czernichow, P Cramer, G Schaison, and R Rappaport. 1983. Leydig cell function in children after direct testicular irradiation for acute lymphoblastic leukemia. NEJM **309:**25–28.
90. Castilo, L, A Craft, J Kernahan, R Evans, and A Aynsley-Green. 1990. Gonadal function after 12-Gy testicular irradiation in childhood acute lymphoblastic leukemia. Med Pediatr Oncol **18:**185–189.
91. Weber, AM, MD Walters, LR Schover, and A Mitchinson. 1995. Vaginal anatomy and sexual function. Obstet Gynecol **86:**946–949.
92. Bergmark, K, E Avall-Lundqvist, PW Dickman, L Henningsohn, and G Steineck. 1999. Vaginal changes and sexuality in women with a history of cervical cancer. NEJM **340:**1383–1389.
93. Flay, LD and JH Matthews. 1995. The effects of radiotherapy and surgery on the sexual function of women treated for cervical cancer. Int J Radiat Oncol Biol Phys **31:**399–404.
94. Incrocci, L, AK Slob, and PC Levendag. 2002. Sexual (dys)function after radiotherapy for prostate cancer: a review. Int J Radiat Oncol Biol Phys **52:**681–693.
95. Goldstein, I, MI Feldman, PJ Deckers, RK Babyan, and RJ Krane. 1984. Radiation-associated impotence, a clinical study of its mechanism. JAMA **251:**903–910.
96. Zelefsky, MJ and JF Eid. 1998. Elucidating the etiology of erectile dysfunction after definitive therapy for prostate cancer. Int J Radiat Oncol Biol Phys **40:**129–133.
97. Merrick, GS, KE WAllner, and WM Bulter. 2003. Management of sexual dysfunction after prostate brachytherapy. Oncology **17:**52–62.

98. Merrick, GS, WM Butler, KE Wallner, JH Lief, RL Anderson, BJ Smeiles, RW Galbreath, and ML Benson. 2002. The importance of radiation doses to the penile bulb vs. crura in the development of postbrachytherapy erecticle dysfunction. Int J Radiat Oncol Biol Phys **54:**1005–1062.
99. Fisch, BM, B Pickett, V Weinberg, and M Roach. 2001. Dose of radiation received by the bulb of the penis correlates with risk of impotence after three-dimensional conformal radiotherapy for prostate cancer. Urology **57:**955–959.
100. Merrick, GS, KE Wallner, and WM Bulter. 2003. Permanent interstitial brachytherapy for the management of carcinoma of the prostate gland. J Urol **169:**1643–1652.
101. Valicenti, RK, EA Bissonette, C Chen, and D Theodorescu. 2002. Longitudinal comparison of sexual function after 3-dimensional conformal radiation therapy or prostate brachytherapy. J Urol **168:**2499–2504.
102. Raina, R, A Agarwal, KK Goyal, C Jackson, J Ulchaker, K Angermeier, E Klein, J Ciezki, and CD Zippe. 2003. Long-term potency after iodine-125 radiotherapy for prostate cancer and role of sildenafil citrate. Urology **62:**1103–1108.
103. Sethi, A, N Mohideen, L Leybovich, and J Mulhall. 2003. Role if IMRT in reducing penile doses in dose escalation for prostate cancer. Int J Radiat Oncol Biol Phys **55:**970–978.
104. Libshitz, HI. 1994. Radiation changes in bone. Semin Roentgenol **29:**15–37.
105. Parmentier C, N Morardet, and M Tubiana. 1983. Late effects on human bone marrow after extended field radiotherapy. Int J Radiat Oncol Biol Phys **9:**1303–1311.
106. Sacks, E, ML Goris, E Glatstein, E Gilbert, and HS Kaplan. 1978. Bone marrow regeneration following large field ration. Influence of volume, age, dose and time. Cancer **42:**1057–1065.
107. Abe, H, M Nakamura, S Takahashi, S Maruoka, Y Ogawa, and K Sakamoto. 1992. Radiation induced insufficiency fractures of the pelvis: evaluation with 99mTc-methylene diphosphonate scintigraphy. J Roentgenol **158:**599–602.
108. Huh, SJ, B Kim, MK Kang, JE Lee, H Lim do, W Park, SS Shin, and YC Ahn. 2002. Pelvic insufficiency fracture after pelvic irradiation in uterine cervix cancer. Gynecol Oncol **86:**264–268.
109. Moreno, A, J Clemente, C Crespo, A Martinez, M Navarro, L Fernandez, J Minguell, G Vazquez, and FJ Andreu. 1999. Pelvic insufficiency fractures in patients with pelvic irradiation. Int J Radiat Oncol Biol Phys **44:**61–66.
110. Firat, S, K Murray, and B Erickson. 2003. High-dose whole abdominal and pelvic irradiation for treatment of ovarian carcinoma: long-term toxicity and outcomes. Int J Radiat Oncol Biol Phys **57:**201–207.
111. Phe, WC, PL Khong, and WY Ho. 1995 Insufficiency fractures of the sacrum and os pubis. Br J Hosp Med **54:**15–19.
112. Mumber, MP, KM Greven, and TM Haygood. 1997. Pelvic insufficiency fractures associated with radiation atrophy: clinical recognition and diagnostic evaluation. Skeletal Radiol **26:**94–99.
113. Ries, T. 1983. Detection of osteoporotic sacral fractures with radionuclides. Radiology **146:**783–785.
114. Grigsby, PW, HL Roberts, and CA Perez. 1995. Femoral neck fracture following groin irradiation. Int J Radiat Oncol Biol Phys **32:**63–67.
115. Ellis, RE. 1961. The distribution of active bone marrow in the adult. Phys Med Biol **5:**255–263.
116. Mauch, P, L Constine, J Greenberger, W Knospe, J Sullivan, JL Liesveld, and HJ Deeg. 1995. Hematopoietic stem cell transplant compartment: acute and late effects of radiation therapy and chemotherapy. Int J Radiat Oncol Biol Phys **31:**1319–1339.
117. Tai, P, A Hammond, JV Dyk, L Stitt, J Tonita, T Coad, and J Radwan. 2000. Pelvic fractures following irradiation of endometrial and vaginal cancers—a case series and review of the literature. Radiother Oncol **56:**23–28.
118. Seidenfeld, J, M Piper, C Flamm, V Hasselblad, JO Armitage, CL Bennett, MS Gordon, AE Lichtin, JL Wade, III, S Woolf, and N Aronson. 2001 Epoetin treatment of a anemia associated with cancer therapy: a systematic review and meta-analysis of controlled clinical trials. JNCI **93:**1204–1214.
119. Crawford, J, D Cella, and CS Cleeland. 2002. Relationship between changes in hemoglobin level and quality of life during chemotherapy in anemic cancer patients receiving epoetin alfa therapy. Cancer **95:**888–895.
120. Brixey, CJ, JC Roeske, AE Lujan, SD Yamada, J Rotmensch, and AJ Mundt. 2002. Impact of intensity-modulated radiotherapy on acute hematologic toxicity in women with gynecologic malignancies. Int J Radiat Oncol Biol Phys **54:**1388–1396.

7. RADIATION-INDUCED SKELETAL INJURY

MARK A. ENGLEMAN, MD
GAYLE WOLOSCHAK, Ph.D.
WILLIAM SMALL Jr., M.D.

The Robert H. Lurie Comprehensive Cancer Center of Northwestern University Medical School, Chicago, IL

INTRODUCTION

Irradiation of bone kills the cells that are responsible for bone maintenance and remodeling that renders the irradiated bone brittle and prone to injury. Though the incidence of bony injury has become increasingly uncommon with the use of megavoltage radiation and improved planning and radiation delivery techniques, even when careful attention is paid to radiation tolerance, bony injury can occur. Post-irradiation bony injuries include mandibular osteoradionecrosis (MORN), pelvic insufficiency fracture, hip fracture, fracture of long bones, rib fracture, and pediatric growth abnormalities. In this chapter, we will review the incidence, risk factors, techniques for risk reduction, and management of each of these bony radiation injuries.

A. MANDIBULAR OSTEORADIONECROSIS

Mandibular osteoradionecrosis is a hypocellular, hypovascular dissolution of bone following irradiation. The most vulnerable part of the mandible is the buccal cortex of the premolar, molar, and retromolar regions.[1] The molar and premolar regions are the most common sites of necrosis.[2,3]

There are three distinct types of MORN (Table 1[4]), but all begin similarly as erythema of overlying mucosa, which subsequently ulcerates to reveal the underlying necrotic bone.[5] The diagnosis of MORN includes an appropriate clinical picture supported by consistent bone scan, CT and/or MRI findings. Recurrent tumor should be ruled out.

Table 1. Subtypes of mandibular osteoradionecrosis

Type I—trauma-induced MORN which occurs when radiation or surgical wounding are coupled closely together
Type II—trauma-induced MORN which occurs years after radiation therapy. This is the most common type
Type III—spontaneous MORN which can occur anytime after radiotherapy without any obvious preceding surgical or traumatic event (6–24 months after radiotherapy)

Table 2. Risk factors for MORN

Presence of teeth[7]
Pre-irradiation dental morbidity
Volume of mandible irradiated
Radiation dose[7]
Fraction size
Tooth extraction
Male gender[9]
Use of orthovoltage equipment

The event that most commonly precipitates MORN is post-radiotherapy tooth extraction because of poor dentition. Early work at MD Anderson Cancer Center in the 1960s and 1970s demonstrated that those patients with teeth were at much higher risk for MORN than those without teeth.[6] Before it was realized that this risk could be reduced by appropriate dental care, all teeth in the anticipated radiation field were extracted. Current practice does not include total teeth extraction but rather meticulous dental care as outlined in Chapter 2 of this book.

Even with appropriate dental care, the risk of MORN is still greater in the dentulous patient than in the edentulous patient. In an early study, comparing these two groups, even with aggressive dental care, those with teeth were still more than twice as likely to develop mandibular necrosis than those with no teeth (24.2% vs. 11.9%).[7] In another study, 64.8% of MORN cases were related to either dental extraction or dental irritation.[8] In a third study of the patients who required extractions within 1 year of radiotherapy, 60% developed MORN.[6]

The radiation tolerance of the mandible is not simply a function of dose (Table 2). Factors including pre-irradiation morbidity, and volume of tissue irradiated are inseparable from dose when considering the risk of mandibular necrosis. The presence of more than one risk factor can have a synergistic effect on the risk of MORN. For example, in one study, factors predicting for an increased risk of necrosis included disease site related to the mandible, high dose (≥8000 cGy), and the presence of teeth. A patient with these features was almost 18 times more likely to develop mandibular necrosis than patients without these risk factors.[7]

Though radiation dose is not the only factor affecting the risk of MORN, it is one of the risk factors most readily controlled by the radiation oncologist. What then is the radiation dose tolerance of the mandible? Emami et al. estimated the TD 5/5 for the TMJ and mandible at 60 Gy and the TD 50/5 at 72 Gy, when treating the entire mandible using conventional fractionation. These values may be on the conservative side. Bedwinek et al. found that spontaneous mandibular necrosis did not occur with doses $\leq$60 Gy, it was 1.8% for doses between 60 and 70 Gy, and 9% with doses >70 Gy.[8] In the UCSF experience, MORN risk was 85% for dentulous patients receiving more than 75 Gy (50% for edentulous patients).[10] None of the patients who received <65 Gy to the mandible developed osteonecrosis. A recent RTOG IMRT protocol sets mandibular dose constraints at 70 Gy.[11]

MORN risk also varies with fraction size. There is evidence in the literature that the risk of MORN is substantially less in patients treated with hyperfractionated radiotherapy at 1.2–1.5 Gy per fraction.[12,13]

It is important to note that the mandible may receive more than the dose prescribed to tumor. In an analysis of the radiation plans of 18 patients treated with megavoltage EBRT for oropharyngeal cancers, parts of the mandible (most notably the retromolar region) received 101.3% ± 3.8% (range 90.2–109.1%).[14] Thus, parts of the mandible may receive almost 10% more than the prescribed dose.

Radiation tolerance is similar in patients receiving brachytherapy as a component of their radiation therapy. In the Stanford experience with base-of-tongue cancers, 41 patients received a combination of EBRT (median 50 Gy) followed by a low dose rate ^{192}Ir brachytherapy boost (median 26 Gy). Osteoradionecrosis occurred in 5% of patients. In another series of 12 patients with base-of-tongue carcinomas treated with 50 Gy EBRT (parallel opposed laterals) followed by neck dissection, and then 25–30 Gy interstitial brachytherapy (LDR ^{192}IR), a single patient (8.3%) developed osteoradionecrosis of the mandible.[15]

Though the timing of MORN is variable, most cases occur during the first year following radiotherapy (Table 3). The use of chemotherapy with radiotherapy can accelerate the onset of MORN. In a retrospective review of 830 patients who received radiation as component of their treatment for head and neck cancers, the time to onset of MORN was significantly shorter (9 months) for the combination treatment than for the radiotherapy alone (14 months).[9]

In summary, MORN continues to be a clinical problem especially when doses to the mandible significantly exceed 6000 cGy. If there are predisposing risk factors, e.g., poor dentition and poor likelihood of post-radiotherapy dental care, or a large volume of irradiated mandible, the risk of MORN will be increased for a given dose.

A1. Management

Prophylaxis to prevent toxicity is preferred. A dental evaluation prior to radiotherapy should be considered mandatory for all patients who are to receive head and neck irradiation. Ideally, the dentist should be experienced in the evaluation and management of these pre-irradiation patients. Unsalvageable teeth should be extracted. A minimum of 1 week–10 days should be allowed for healing prior to the initiation of radiotherapy. If the timing of the therapy allows, 2–3 weeks healing time is preferred.[5]

Many patients who have developed MORN have been successfully managed with conservative treatment. In our institution, the initial treatment for mandibular exposure/injury following irradiation consists of measures to keep the exposed mandible

Table 3. MORN timing, incidence, and correlation with dental extraction

Author	*N*	Site	Dose	MORN incidence	Time to MORN	Association with extraction
Grant[6]	176	Tonsil	60–110 Gy	37.5%	83% ≤1 year	Pre-XRT extraction 15%, post-XRT extraction 44%
Bedwinek[8]	381	OC, OP, NP	50–80 Gy	Overall: 14%	61% <1 year, 83% ≤2 years, 94% ≤3 years	65% of MORN cases associated with dental extraction
—			≤ 60 Gy	0%		
—			60–70 Gy	1.80%		
—			>70 Gy	9%		
Hoppe[16]	88	NP	65–70 Gy	2.3%	NS	
Morrish[10]		OC, OP, NP	50–75 Gy	Overall: 22%	Range: 1–72 months, 68% ≤1 year	All cases of osteonecrosis associated with dental extractions (9 cases) occurred with post-radiotherapy extractions
—			<65 Gy	0%		
—			>75 Gy (edentulous)	50%	Median: 10 months	Edentulous: 14%
—			>75 Gy (dentulous)	85%	Median: 22 months	Dentulous: 24%
Kaylie[15]	12	BOT	50 Gy EBRT + 25–30 Gy brachy	8.3%	NS	
Gibbs[17]	41	BOT	50 Gy EBRT + 26 Gy brachy	4.9%	>6 months	
Reuther[9]	830	Head and neck	40–90 Gy, Median: 60 Gy	Overall: 8.2%, male: 9.6%, female: 3.4%	Range: 2–122 months, median: 13 months	50% of MORN cases associated with dental extraction

clean and allow natural healing. We use saline and PERIDEX rinses and oral antibiotics if needed. Hyperbaric oxygen (HBO) is also considered. Management is in cooperation with an otolaryngologist/oral surgeon.

In the past, those who have not responded to, or who have progressed despite conservative therapy have had to undergo surgery. Patients who develop MORN late (>36 months) after radiotherapy, and those with more extensive MORN (including fracture and/or fistula) are more likely to fail conservative therapy and require surgery.[18]

Table 4. Prophylactic HBO results

Author	n	MORN (w/HBO)	MORN (w/o HBO)
Marx[20]	74	5.40%	30%
David[4]	24	4.20%	—
Vudiniabola[21]		3.40%	88%

HBO therapy is a potential adjunctive therapy that can be employed as a component of conservative therapy or in conjunction with surgery. Radiation-induced microvascular damage results in bony hypoxia, which can result in necrosis or fracture. Pressurized oxygen overcomes hypoxia from damaged microvasculature by "forcing" supra-normal levels of oxygen into tissues. In this non-hypoxic environment, it is more likely that damaged tissues will heal spontaneously. HBO therapy consists of breathing oxygen pressurized to 2.4 atm for approximately 60–90 minutes per session for ~15–40 sessions.[4] This is done in single- or multi-patient chambers.

In most of the available literature, HBO is beneficial in the treatment of MORN patients. In a review of 51 patients who received HBO as treatment for MORN, more than 90% experienced improvement or healing with HBO both when HBO was the only therapy, and when it was used in conjunction with surgery.[4] In a systematic review of the HBO literature for treatment of mandibular necrosis, 13 of 14 (93%) publications demonstrated a definite or probable benefit.[19]

Because dental extraction following radiotherapy is the strongest predictor of MORN, HBO can be given *prophylactically* to high-risk patients prior to post-radiotherapy dental extraction (Table 4). Marx et al. performed a randomized trial comparing prophylactic antibiotics versus prophylactic HBO in 74 patients requiring post-radiotherapy extraction.[20] In the antibiotic group, 11/37 (29.7%) developed MORN versus only 2/37 (5.4%) in the HBO group. In a review of 24 patients who received prophylactic HBO prior to post-radiotherapy extraction, only one (4.2%) experienced difficulties in healing.[4] In another case series MORN occurred in 3.4% prophylaxed with HBO versus 88% of those who did not receive HBO.[21] While the use of prophylactic HBO is still controversial, if it is available, it should certainly be considered in patients requiring post-radiotherapy extractions.

HBO therapy is not without risk of side effects. Potential complications include damage to the eardrums or sinuses, seizure (1.3 per 10,000 treatments), pneumothorax (rare), pulmonary oxygen toxicity (rare), and temporary visual refractive changes (rare).[22]

For further information on management, including information on pentoxyfylline and vitamin E, see Chapter 2 of this book.

B. LONG BONE FRACTURE

Long bone fracture as a complication following radiotherapy is most commonly seen following the higher doses used in the management of extremity sarcoma. Contemporary publications on limb-sparing treatment of soft tissue sarcoma of the extremities report a post-radiotherapy fracture incidence ranging from 4%[23] to 8.6%.[24] The most consistently important risk factor for fracture is periosteal excision (Table 5).

Table 5. Risk factors for long bone fracture

Periosteal excision (especially *extensive* periosteal excision)
Anterior thigh compartment tumor location
Close or positive margins

Alektiar et al. reported on 86 patients treated for soft tissue sarcoma of the knee or elbow at Memorial Sloan-Kettering Cancer Center.[24] Forty-six of the 86 patients reviewed (53%) received radiotherapy as a component of their therapy. The majority (82%) of patients who received radiation received a median of 45 Gy with LDR brachytherapy via catheters placed at surgery; 18% received a 20 Gy brachytherapy boost following 45 Gy EBRT. The overall actuarial 5-year fracture rate was 3%. The actuarial 5-year fracture rate was 3% in the group that received radiotherapy versus 5% in the group that did not; this difference was not statistically significant ($P = 0.5$).

Periosteal excision, which is sometimes necessary for margin clearance, can substantially increase the risk of fracture following radiotherapy. For example, Lin et al. reported on 205 consecutive patients whose lower extremity sarcoma was managed by limb-sparing surgery and radiation therapy at Memorial Sloan-Kettering Cancer Center.[25] Twenty-six percent of the patients had undergone periosteal excision. Nine of the 205 patients (4.4%) suffered from femoral fracture following treatment; all 9 patients had undergone periosteal excision. This represented a 5-year incidence of 29% for those who had undergone periosteal excision by Kaplan–Meier survivorship analysis. Periosteal excision was the only independent risk factor for fracture.

Helmstedter et al. reported on 285 patients who were treated with surgery and radiation therapy for soft tissue tumors.[26] Seven percent experienced post-therapy fractures after a mean of 40.5 months. Risk factors for fracture included anterior thigh compartment primary site, extensive periosteal stripping, and a marginal or intralesional margin of resection. The authors recommend consideration of prophylactic femoral rodding for high-risk sarcoma patients at the time of surgical resection.[26]

If a patient presents with a long bone fracture following extremity radiotherapy, an orthopedic surgeon should be consulted immediately. After tumor recurrence with resultant pathologic fracture is ruled out, management of the fracture should be by the orthopedic surgeon.

In summary, long bone fracture is a relatively uncommon complication following irradiation. Patients with multiple risk factors for post-radiotherapy fracture are at much higher risk, and, where possible, treatment can be tailored to minimize post-treatment morbidity should fracture arise (e.g., prophylactic femoral rodding as described above).

C. FEMORAL HEAD AND NECK

The radiation tolerance of the femoral head and neck is substantially lower than the radiation tolerance of long bones. This complication is increasingly rare as routine pelvic fields include blocking of the femoral neck and most of the femoral heads (Figure 1). If the inguinal nodes must be treated, the femoral head and neck will unavoidably receive a substantial radiation dose, and care must be taken not to exceed the radiation tolerance of these structures.

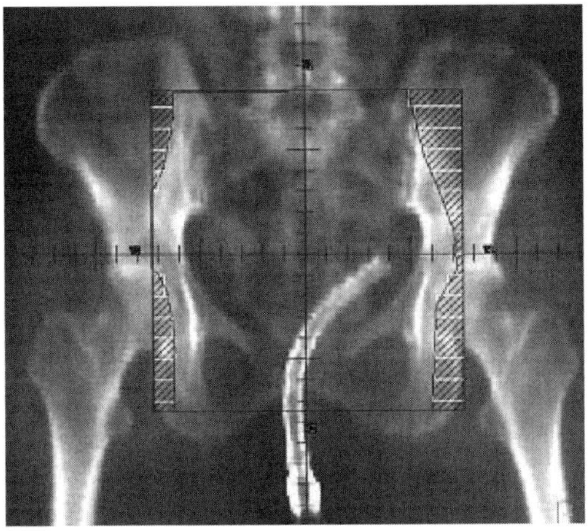

Figure 1. Pelvic field with femoral heads blocked.

Grigsby et al. reported on 207 patients who received groin irradiation as a component of pelvic irradiation for advanced or recurrent cancers of the vagina, vulva cervix, and endometrium.[27] Most of the patients' groins were irradiated as part of the primary photon field, prescribed to midplane; 71 patients received groin boosts, most with high-energy photons. The incidence of femoral neck fracture was 4.8%; 40% of those patients with femoral neck fracture had fractures bilaterally. The actuarial cumulative incidence of fracture was 11% at 5 years, and 15% at 10 years (the authors describe these actuarial incidences as "excessive"). Mean doses were 52 Gy in those patients with fractures, and 47.6 Gy in those without. Irradiation dose was not a significant predictor of fracture, though there were no fractures with femoral neck doses below 42 Gy. Cigarette use correlated with the likelihood of femoral neck fracture ($P = 0.027$); there was also a correlation with radiologically confirmed pre-irradiation osteoporosis which approached statistical significance ($P = 0.068$). With an absence of fractures below 42 Gy, these data would suggest that the TD 5/5 of the femoral neck is between 42 and 52 Gy.

C1. Therapy

Again, the best "therapy" for femoral head and neck fractures is prevention. Unless the femoral head/neck must be in the treatment field to encompass the PTV, they should be blocked. It is acceptable to include the most medial aspect of the femoral heads in order to adequately cover the pelvic lymph nodes at risk. If the femoral heads or necks must be treated, careful attention should be paid to keeping doses to these sensitive structures as low as possible.

Surgical repair of femoral head/neck fractures following radiotherapy may require special mechanical reinforcement due to the poor quality of bone following irradiation. In a retrospective study of 71 total hip replacements for complications following pelvic irradiation, the authors found a higher than typical post-replacement failure rate.[28] When

Table 6. Risk factors for osteoporotic fracture[32] and osteonecrosis

Low body weight (<58 kg)	Systemic lupus erythematous
Smoking tobacco 1st degree relative with low-trauma fracture Personal history of low-trauma fracture	Rheumatoid arthritis Steroid use

standard cemented components were used, 52% suffered acetabular loosening. When acetabular reinforcement rings were used, the rate of aseptic acetabular loosening was reduced to 19%.

D. PELVIS

Almost any part of the bony pelvis can fracture following pelvic irradiation, and fractures have been observed following irradiation for almost all pelvic disease sites including prostate,[29] endometrium, cervix,[30] and rectum.[31]

Insufficiency fracture occurs as a result of normal stresses on weakened brittle bone.[30] Risk factors for pelvic insufficiency fracture following irradiation are similar to the risk factors for osteoporotic fracture and osteonecrosis (Table 6). These risk factors appear to increase the risk of osteoradionecrosis when they are present as comorbid conditions as well.[30]

The most common presenting complaint in patients with radiation-induced pelvic insufficiency fractures is pain. The incidence of symptomatic pelvic insufficiency fractures following pelvic radiotherapy ranges from 2.7% to 17%, though there is evidence to suggest that the incidence (including asymptomatic fractures) may be much higher.

At the lower end of this range, the incidence of severe radionecrosis in patients who underwent pelvic radiotherapy (45 Gy EBRT + Brachytherapy) at Royal Marsden hospital for carcinoma of the cervix was 2.7%.[30] Erickson et al. found a somewhat higher rate of symptomatic pelvic ischemic damage and/or fracture of 5.9% in the Medical College of Wisconsin experience.[33] They found that 101 of 1700 patients developed ischemic damage and/or fracture. Ninety percent of these 101 patients were symptomatic. The median radiation dose was 45 Gy to the whole pelvis and 55.8 Gy to a reduced field. Median follow-up was 50 months, and median time until injury was 13 months. Seventy-three percent had multiple sites of injury on imaging. Symptoms resolved after a median of 20 months. More than 90% had at least partial symptomatic relief, and 57% enjoyed complete symptomatic relief.

In contrast, Ogino et al. found a significantly higher incidence of pelvic insufficiency fracture of 17%.[34] The authors reported on 335 women treated with radiation therapy alone for advanced cervical cancer. Patients received 45–50 Gy EBRT and a total of 25–30 Gy high dose rate intracavitary brachytherapy. Radiation was delivered as 4 daily fractions (1.8–2 Gy) and 1 weekly HDR treatment (5–6 Gy). A total of 57 of the 335 (17%) patients were found to have had pelvic insufficiency fracture. Eighty-two percent of those patients with fractures were asymptomatic. One hundred percent of the fractures involved the sacrum. Both body weight ≤49 kg and >3 deliveries were significant predictors of fracture.

In a paper that detailed the natural history of pelvic fracture following radiotherapy, Blomlie et al. documented a higher-than-expected rate of pelvic insufficiency fracture.[35] Eighteen women who were to receive pelvic radiotherapy for IIB or IIIB cervical carcinoma were followed with serial MRIs, before, during, and after treatment. The patient population included both pre- and postmenopausal patients. Patients received ~46 Gy EBRT + ~44 Gy intracavitary brachytherapy, and underwent a total of 12 MRI scans. Eighty-nine percent of the women had MRI evidence of pelvic insufficiency fracture and almost all had more than 1 fracture. The diagnosis of fracture was confirmed by CT, bone scan, or both. Postmenopausal women were more likely to suffer fracture and had more fractures per patient than premenopausal women. The most common fracture sites were the lateral sacrum (14/18) and medial ilium (10/18). No fractures were seen outside of the radiation field. Most of the fractures were identified between 3 and 18 months following radiotherapy. The majority of lesions (79%) subsided and 11 of 41 (27%) disappeared completely. Of the total patient population, 59% complained of pelvic pain during the observation period. Symptomatic patients had a mean of 4 fractures, while asymptomatic patients had a mean of 1.8 fractures. All patients had resolution of their pain during the study period.

The likelihood of fracture is much higher in symptomatic than in asymptomatic patients. In a retrospective review by Abe et al., 80 patients who received pelvic radiotherapy for endometrial cancer were evaluated with bone scan.[36] Of the 25 patients with pelvic pain, 21 (84%) were found to have insufficiency fracture(s), while only 6 of 55 (11%) asymptomatic patients were found to have insufficiency fracture(s).

In the patient with bony pelvic pain following radiotherapy, it is important to distinguish between bony metastases and pelvic insufficiency fractures. In a review of 8 cases of pelvic insufficiency fracture, all patients presented with pain and bone scan abnormalities in the pelvis only; no other bone scan abnormalities were identified.[37] Sixty-three percent of these patients were initially diagnosed with bone metastases. Cervical and endometrial cancers rarely metastasize to the skeleton (~15%), so in a patient with pain and isolated pelvic bone scan findings, the diagnosis of insufficiency fracture should be in the differential. If, on follow-up scan, the lesion progresses, or there are lesions outside of the radiation field, bone metastases are more likely. If, however, the lesion(s) is resolving, the most likely etiology is post-radiotherapy insufficiency fracture. We have observed cases where a patient with pelvic pain and a corresponding radiographic abnormality was initially diagnosed with pelvic metastasis and were subsequently found have been suffering from pelvic insufficiency fracture. This type of case exemplifies the importance of patients maintaining good follow-up with their radiation oncologist.

D1. Therapy

Radiation oncologists who treat pelvic malignancies should attempt to ensure that their patients have had the current standard screening for osteoporosis and appropriate therapy if necessary. When insufficiency fractures do occur, they almost always resolve with conservative therapy including analgesics and physical therapy. Symptoms typically improve within a month and resolve within 12 months.[38] Bisphosphonates may help promote healing and decrease the risk of subsequent fractures. Our current recommendations for insufficiency fractures are orthopedic consultation, appropriate analgesia and therapy for any pre-morbid osteoporosis.

E. RIB FRACTURES

Rib fractures are a long recognized late complication of breast and chest wall irradiation. In a review of the literature, Pierce et al. found that the incidence of rib fractures following breast irradiation ranged from 0% to almost 20%,[39] though when restricting the review to studies using "modern techniques", the incidence was 1–3%. In other contemporary series, the incidence of rib fracture following breast-conserving therapy is well below 1%.[40]

Risk factors for post-irradiation rib fracture include high radiation dose, chemotherapy, and large fraction size (Table 7).

Pierce et al. reported on 1624 patients who were treated at the Joint Center for Radiation Therapy with breast-conserving therapy including conservative surgery and radiation therapy.[39] All patients were treated with megavoltage radiation, though some were treated with 4 MV photons, and some were treated with 6 or 8 MV photons. With a median tumor dose of 64.8 Gy (median 46 Gy whole breast + boost), the incidence of rib fracture was 1.8%. Seventy-three percent had radiographic confirmation of fracture. Of women with rib fractures, 94% had more than 1 fracture, and the 4th, 5th, or 6th rib was involved in 88% of women. Median time to fracture was 12 months. The incidence of rib fracture was related to both photon energy and dose. Fracture was more common in women who were treated with 4 MV (2.2%) versus 6 or 8 MV (0.4%) ($P = 0.005$). Women who received <50 Gy *whole breast dose* had an incidence of 1.5% versus 5.3% for those who received 50 Gy or more ($P = 0.0001$). The use of chemotherapy, though not whether it was given before or after radiotherapy, was also found to be a risk factor for rib fracture. For those patients who received less than 50 Gy to the whole breast, those who were treated with chemotherapy had a risk of rib fracture of 2.3% versus 0.5% for those who did not ($P = 0.01$). The authors found that the site of fractures corresponded to dosimetric hot spots; the size and magnitude of these hot spots decreased with increasing machine energy. All of the fractures healed without intervention.

Chemotherapy as a risk factor for rib fracture was delineated in greater detail in a paper by Markiewicz et al. They reported on 1053 early stage breast patients who received radiotherapy as a component of breast-conserving therapy.[41] Patients were treated with a median whole breast dose of 46 Gy followed by an electron or brachytherapy boost of median dose of 16.6 Gy. With a median follow-up of 6.7 years, the incidence of rib fracture in those who also received chemotherapy was 1.7% versus 0.5% for those who

Table 7. Risk factors for rib fracture following radiotherapy

Photon energy <6 MV
Whole breast dose >50 Gy
Chemotherapy
Dosimetric hot spots
Comprehensive nodal irradiation
Large fraction size

did not; this difference was not statistically significant ($P = 0.12$). There was a difference, though, in the subset of patients who received nodal irradiation and chemotherapy; their incidence of rib fracture was 2.2% versus 0% in patients who received nodal irradiation without chemotherapy ($P = 0.02$). The use of *concurrent* chemotherapy did not significantly affect rib fracture incidence, though other authors have found an increase in the rib fracture incidence with the use of concurrent chemotherapy.[42] The use of hormonal therapy did not alter the risk of rib fracture.

As would be expected in a late toxicity like rib fracture, its incidence increases with increasing fraction size. Overgaard reported on 231 patients who received post-mastectomy radiation.[43] Thirty-six percent of the patients were treated to 50.8 Gy in 12 twice-weekly fractions (4.2 Gy/fraction), 35% were treated to 46.7 Gy in 12 twice-weekly fractions (3.8 Gy/fraction), and 29% patients were treated to 51.3 Gy in 22 daily fractions (2.33 Gy/fraction). Those treated with the larger fraction size had a significantly higher incidence of rib fracture: 48% in the 4.2 Gy group, 19% in the 3.8 Gy group, and 6% in the 2.33 Gy group.

E1. Management

As with all of the other sites discussed in this chapter, after confirming fracture, recurrent tumor must be ruled out.[43] The vast majority of rib fractures will heal without intervention.[39] Analgesics may be given as needed.

F. PEDIATRIC GROWTH ABNORMALITIES

The primary skeletal toxicity following pediatric irradiation is growth abnormality. Growth abnormalities can be broadly grouped into loss of stature and problems associated with asymmetric growth. The human skeleton grows from birth until late puberty. The growth of the long bones takes place in the epiphyseal (growth) plate. As with several other stem-cell based systems (skin, gut, mucosa, etc.) which contain rapidly dividing cells, cells from the proliferative zone of the growth plate are especially sensitive to radiation injury. Following irradiation of pediatric patients, bone growth retardation occurs beginning at doses as low as 10 Gy, but doses above 15 Gy result in larger and more lasting deficits in stature.[44]

Willman et al. reported on the Stanford experience with growth retardation following irradiation.[45] They demonstrated that doses ≥ 33 Gy to sub-total/total lymphoid fields resulted in a loss of final attained stature of 7–8% (13 cm). Children who received lesser doses, or radiation to smaller fields, did not experience as severe loss of stature.

Hogeboom et al. reported on the National Wilms Tumor Study Group's (NWTSG) experience with stature loss following childhood irradiation.[44] Over the last 30 years, the NWTSG has reduced the recommended radiation dosage in successive protocols, from as much as 40 Gy in NWTS 1 to as little as 10 Gy in NWTS 4. The authors reviewed data on 7500 children who were registered with the NWTSG between 1969 and 1974; 2778 were evaluable and 1323 of these received radiation. They noted that prior data, which indicated that the degree of radiation effect on bone was dependent on age at administration, modality/photon source, and field size, were confirmed by their results. They found that radiation to the flank was a significant predictor of reduction

Table 8. Height deficit following irradiation for Wilms tumor[44]

Group	<15 Gy	≥15 Gy	<1-year old and >10 Gy
Height deficit (cm) versus unirradiated counterparts	4 cm @ 16-years old, but 0 cm by 18-years old	4–7 cm by ≥ 15-years old	7 cm by ≥15-years old; 7.7 cm predicted adult height deficit

in stature, which was more pronounced in larger (e.g., abdominopelvic) fields, and in children who received higher doses (Table 8). Younger children were especially sensitive to radiation; irradiation doses of 10 Gy or more resulted in greater stature deficits than seen in older children who received significantly greater dose. Children irradiated during puberty were not at increased risk of radiation-induced stature loss when compared to children irradiated at other ages.

The effects of chemotherapy + radiotherapy on stature loss were mixed: cyclophosphamide did not affect stature, while stature deficit was greater in those children who received doxorubicin.

While loss of adult height results from bilaterally symmetric treatment fields, or to fields that treat included vertebral bodies homogeneously, asymmetric fields can result in differential growth. Treating one femur can result in marked asymmetry of the length of the legs. Treating only 1/2 of a vertebral body can result in a growth differential between the irradiated and unirradiated parts of even a single vertebral body resulting in scoliosis. The incidence and severity of scoliosis vary with bone dose and dose inhomogeneity.[46]

Chen et al. reported on 6 patients treated for childhood tumors (3 Wilms' tumors, 2 neuroblastomas, and 1 lymphoma) who later developed post-radiation spinal deformities.[47] The mean radiation dose was 35.7 Gy. The deformities consisted of kyphoscoliosis which were concave toward the irradiated side. The kyphotic component was more severe than the scoliotic component. All cases were managed surgically.

In addition to observing the above described dose constraints, portal design can significantly influence the likelihood of growth abnormalities. As noted above the epiphyseal plate is the most radiosensitive area of bone, and the site, which if irradiated, is most likely to result in growth abnormalities. Each long bone contains both a proximal and a distal epiphyseal plate. Bone growth occurs differentially between these two growth centers. For example, 70% of the femoral growth occurs at the *distal* growth plate, while 60% of the tibial growth occurs at the *proximal* growth plate.[48] Knee portals for Ewing's sarcoma encompassing both the distal femur and proximal tibia resulted in the most prominent extremity growth asymmetry.[49,50] Additionally, radiation fields that split growth plates or vertebral bodies can result in differential growth within the bone and may result in deformity. Thus, if a growth plate must be included in a radiation field, the entire growth plate should be irradiated.[51] Therefore, if a vertebral body is to be irradiated, the entire vertebral body should be in the field with enough margin to give a homogenous dose to the entire vertebral body.[51]

G. OTHER PEDIATRIC SKELETAL TOXICITIES

As with adults, pediatric patients can suffer from long bone fracture following radiotherapy. In a review of 93 consecutive Ewing's sarcoma patients, 15% experienced fracture. Fracture occurred most commonly in the femur, and was more common in patients with tumors of the proximal 1/3 of the femur.[52]

In addition to loss of stature and asymmetric growth abnormalities, slipped capital femoral epiphysis (>25 Gy)[53] and avascular necrosis (>30 Gy)[54] also occur following hip irradiation. Significant craniofacial growth abnormalities can also occur following WBRT. In one study, abnormalities were more common/more severe at 24 Gy versus 18 Gy.[55]

G1. Management

The primary management of pediatric growth abnormalities following irradiation is surgery.[47] To avoid this invasive therapy, careful field design is essential in minimizing the extent of the abnormalities.

Though there are no human data regarding radioprotectants in this setting, there is a growing body of intriguing animal literature regarding the use of Amifostine to minimize growth abnormalities. In rat and rabbit models, the use of Amifostine prior to irradiation results in a significant reduction in extremity,[56] craniofacial,[57] and growth plate[58,59] growth abnormalities as well as improvements in bone density.[60] The magnitude of the reduction appears to correlate with the dose of Amifostine.[58]

REFERENCES

1. Bras, J, HK de Jonge, and JP van Merkesteyn. 1990. Osteoradionecrosis of the mandible: pathogenesis. Am J Otolaryngol **11:**244–250.
2. Thorn, JJ, HS Hansen, L Specht, and L Bastholt. 2000. Osteoradionecrosis of the jaws: clinical characteristics and relation to the field of irradiation. J Oral Maxillofac Surg **58:**1088–1093.
3. Hermans, R, E Fossion, E Ioannides, W Van den Bogaert, I Ghekiere, and AL Baert. 1996. CT findings in osteoradionecrosis of the mandible. Skeletal Radiol **25:**31–36.
4. David, LA, GK Sandor, AW Evans, et al. 2001. Hyperbaric oxygen therapy and mandibular osteoradionecrosis: a retrospective study and analysis of treatment outcomes. J Can Dent Assoc **67:**384.
5. Cooper, JS, K Fu, J Maerks, et al. 1994. Late effects of radiation therapy in the head and neck region. Int J Radiat Oncol Biol Phys **31:**1141–1164.
6. Grant, B and G Fletcher. 1966. Analysis of complications following megavoltage therapy for squamous cell carcinomas of the tonsillar area. Am J Roentgenol **96(1):**28–36.
7. Murray, CG, J Herson, TE Daly, et al. 1980. Radiation necrosis of the mandible: a 10 year study. Part I. Factors influencing the onset of necrosis. Int J Radiat Oncol Biol Phys **6:**543–548.
8. Bedwinek, JM, LJ Shukovsky, GH Fletcher, et al. 1976. Osteonecrosis in patients treated with definitive radiotherapy for squamous cell carcinomas of the oral cavity and naso- and oropharynx. Radiology **119:**665–667.
9. Reuther, T, T Schuster, U Mende, et al. 2003. Osteoradionecrosis of the jaws as a side effect of radiotherapy of head and neck tumour patients—a report of a thirty year retrospective review. Int J Oral Maxillofac Surg **32:**289–295.
10. Morrish, RB, E Chan, S Silverman, et al. 1981. Osteonecrosis in patients irradiated for head and neck carcinoma. Cancer **47:**1980–1983.
11. Radiation Therapy Oncology Group RTOG 0225. 2003. A phase II Study of Intensity Modulated Radiation Therapy (IMRT) +/− Chemotherapy for Nasopharyngeal Cancer, http://www.rtog.org/members/protocols/0225/0225.pdf
12. Dische, S, M Saunders, A Barrett, A Harvey, O Gibson, and M Parmar. 1997. A randomized multicentre trial of CHART versus conventional radiotherapy in head and neck cancer. Radiother Oncol **44:**123–136.

13. Glanzmann, E and KW Gratz. 1995. Radionecrosis of the mandible: a retrospective analysis of the incidence and risk factors. Radiother Oncol **36:**94–100.
14. Jereczek-Fossa, BA, G Catalano, C Bocci, et al. 2003. Analysis of mandibular dose distribution in radiotherapy (RT) for oropharyngeal cancer: dosimetric and clinical results in 18 patients. Radiother Oncol **66(1):**49–56.
15. Kaylie, DM, KR Stevens, MY Kang, et al. 2000. External beam radiation followed by planned neck dissection and brachytherapy for base of tongue squamous cell carcinoma. Laryngoscope **110(10):**1633–1636.
16. Hoppe, RT, DR Goffinet, and MA Bagshaw. 1976. Carcinoma of the nasopharynx—eighteen years experience with megavoltage radiation therapy. Cancer **37:**2605–2612.
17. Gibbs, IC, QT Le, RD Shah, et al. 2003. Long term outcomes after external beam irradiation and brachytherapy boost for base-of-tongue cancers. Int J Radiat Oncol Biol Phys **57(2):**489–494.
18. Notani, K, Y Yamazaki, H Kitada, et al. 2003. Management of mandibular osteoradionecrosis and the method of radiotherapy. Head Neck **25(3):**181–186.
19. Feldmeier, JJ and NB Hampson. 2002. A systematic review of the literature reporting the application of hyperbaric oxygen prevention and treatment of delayed radiation injuries: an evidence based approach. Undersea Hyperb Med **29(1):**4–30.
20. Marx, RE, RP Johnson, and SN Kline. 1985. Prevention of osteoradionecrosis: a randomized prospective clinical trial of hyperbaric oxygen versus penicillin. J Am Dent Assoc **111(1):**49–54.
21. Vudiniabola, S, C Pirone, J Williamson, and AN Goss. 1999. Hyperbaric oxygen in the prevention of osteoradionecrosis of the jaws. Aust Dent J **44(4):**243–247.
22. Porter, BR and JE Brian, Jr. 1999. Hyperbaric oxygen therapy and osteoradionecrosis. Iowa Dent J **85(3):**23–27.
23. Alektiar, KM, MJ Zelefsky, and MF Brennan. 2000. Morbidity of adjuvant brachytherapy in soft tissue sarcoma of the extremity and superficial trunk. Int J Radiat Oncol Biol Phys **47(5):**1273–1279.
24. Alektiar, KM, AB McKee, JM Jacobs, et al. 2002. Outcome of primary soft tissue sarcoma of the knee and elbow. Int J Radiat Oncol Biol Phys **54(1):**163–169.
25. Lin, PP, KD Schupak, PJ Boland, et al. 1998. Pathologic femoral fracture after periosteal excision and radiation for the treatment of soft tissue sarcoma. Cancer **82(12):**2356–2365.
26. Helmstedter, CS, M Goebel, R Zlotecki, et al. 2001. Pathologic fractures after surgery and radiation for soft tissue tumors. Clin Orthop **389:**165–172.
27. Grigsby, PW, HL Roberts, and CA Perez. 1995. Femoral neck fracture following groin irradiation. Int J Radiat Oncol Biol Phys **32(1):**63–67.
28. Massin, P and J Duparc. 1995. Total hip replacement in irradiated hips. A retrospective study of 71 cases. J Bone Joint Surg Br **77(6):**847–852.
29. Csuka, M, B Brewer, K Lynch, et al. 1987. Osteonecrosis, fractures, and protrusio acetabuli secondary to X-irradiation therapy for prostatic carcinoma. J Rheumatol **14(1):**165–170.
30. Bliss, P, CA Parsons, PR Blake, et al. 1996. Incidence and possible etiological factors in the development of pelvic insufficiency fractures following radical radiotherapy. Br J Radiol **69:**548–554.
31. Holm, T, T Singnomklao, LE Rutqvist, et al. 1996. Adjuvant preoperative radiotherapy in patients with rectal carcinoma. Adverse effects during long term follow-up of 2 randomized trials. Cancer **78(5):**968–976.
32. Eastell, R. 1998. Drug therapy: treatment of postmenopausal osteoporosis. N Engl J Med **338:**736–746.
33. Erickson, BA, KJ Murray, SJ Erickson, et al. 2000. Radiation-induced pelvic bone complications: an underestimated sequelae of pelvic irradiation. Int J Radiat Oncol Biol Phys **48(3, Suppl 1):**126.
34. Ogino, I, N Okamoto, O Yoshimi, et al. 2003. Pelvic insufficiency fractures in postmenopausal woman with advanced cervical cancer treated by radiotherapy. Radiother Oncol **68:**61–67.
35. Blomlie, V, EK Rofstad, and K Talle. 1996. Incidence of radiation-induced insufficiency fractures of the female pelvis: evaluation with MR imaging. Am J Roentgenol **167:**1205–1210.
36. Abe, H, M Nakamura, S Takahashi, et al. 1992. Radiation-induced insufficiency fractures of the pelvis: evaluation with 99 m Tc-methylene diphosphonate scintigraphy. Am J Roentgenol **158:**599–602.
37. Moreno, A, J Clemente, C Crespo, et al. 1999. Pelvic insufficiency fractures in patients with pelvic irradiation. Int J Radiat Oncol Biol Phys **44:**61–66.
38. Konski, A and M Sowers. 1996. Pelvic fractures following irradiation for endometrial carcinoma. Int J Radiat Oncol Biol Phys **35** 361–367.
39. Pierce, SM, A Recht, TI Lingos, A Abner, et al. 1992. Long-term radiation complications following conservative surgery (CS) and radiation therapy (RT) in patients with early stage breast cancer. Int J Radiat Oncol Biol Phys **23(5):**915–923.

40. Meric, F, TA Buchholz, NQ Mirza, et al. 2002. Long-term complications associated with breast-conservation surgery and radiotherapy. Ann Surg Oncol **9(6)**:543–549.
41. Markiewicz, DA, DJ Schultz, JA Haas, et al. 1996. The effects of sequence and the type of chemotherapy and radiation therapy on cosmesis and complications after breast conservation therapy. Int J Radiat Oncol Biol Phys **35(4)**:661–668.
42. Ray, G, VJ Fish, JB Marmor, et al. 1984. Impact of adjuvant chemotherapy on cosmesis and complications in stages I and II carcinoma of the breast treated by biopsy and radiation therapy. Int J Radiat Oncol Biol Phys **10**:837–841.
43. Overgaard, M. 1988. Spontaneous radiation-induced rib fractures in breast cancer patients treated with postmastectomy irradiation. A clinical radiobiological analysis of the influence of fraction size and dose-response relationships on late bone damage. Acta Oncol **27(2)**:117–122.
44. Hogeboom, CJ, SC Grosser, KA Guthrie, et al. 2001. Stature loss following treatment for Wilms tumor. Med Pediatr Oncol **36**:295–304.
45. Willman, K, R Cox, and S Donaldson. 1994. Radiation induced height impairment in pediatric hodgkins disease. Int J Radiat Oncol Biol Phys **28**:85–92.
46. Riseborough, E, S Grabias, and R Burton. 1976. Skeletal alterations following irradiation for Wilms' tumor. Bone Joint Surg **58**:526–536.
47. Chen, SH, PQ Chen, TJ Huang, et al. 2003. Surgical correction of postradiation spinal deformity. Chang Gung Med J **26(3)**:160–169.
48. Anderson, M, W Green, and M Messner. 1963. Predictions of growth in the lower extremities. J Bone Joint Surg **45A**:1–14.
49. Gonzales, D and K Breuer. 1983. Clinical data from irradiated growing long bones in children. Int J Radiat Oncol Biol Phys **9**:671–677.
50. Jentzsch, K, H Binder, H Cramer, et al. 1981. Leg function after radiotherapy for ewing's sarcoma. Cancer **47**:1267–1278.
51. Eifel, PJ, SS Donaldson, and PR Thomas. 1995. Response of growing bone to irradiation: a proposed late effects scoring system. Int J Radiat Oncol Biol Phys **30,31(5)**:1301–1307.
52. Wagner, LM, MD Neel, AS Pappo, et al. 2001. Fractures in pediatric Ewing sarcoma. J Pediatr Hematol Oncol **23(9)**:568–571.
53. Silverman, C, P Thomas, W McAlister, et al. 1981. Slipped capital femoral epiphysis in irradiated children: dose volume and age relationships. Int J Radiat Oncol Biol Phys **7**:1357–1363.
54. Libshitz, H and B Edeikin. 1981. Radiotherapy changes of the pediatric hip. Am J Roentgenol **137**:585–588.
55. Sonis, A, N Tarbell, and R Valachovic. 1990. Dentofacial development in long-term survivors of acute lymphoblastic leukemia. A comparison of 3 treatment modalities. Cancer **66**:2645–2652.
56. Spadaro, JA, MR Baesl, AC Conta, et al. 2003. Effects of irradiation on the appositional and longitudinal growth of the Tibia and Fibula of the rat with and without radioprotectant. J Pediatr Orthop **23**:35–40.
57. Forrest, CR, DA O'Donovan, I Yeung, et al. 2002. Efficacy of radioprotection in the prevention of radiation-induced craniofacial bone growth inhibition. Plast Reconstr Surg **109(4)**:1311–1323.
58. Damron, TA, JA Spadaro, B Margulies, et al. 2000. Dose response of amifostine in protection of growth plate function from irradiation effects. Int J Cancer **90(2)**:73–79.
59. Damron, TA, BS Margulies, JA Strauss, et al. 2003. Sequential histomorphometric analysis of the growth plate following irradiation with and without radioprotection. J Bone Joint Surg Am **85-A(7)**:1302–1313.
60. Margulies, B, H Morgan, M Allen, et al. 2003. Transiently increased bone density after irradiation and the radioprotectant drug amifostine in a rat model. Am J Clin Oncol **26(4)**:e106–e114.

8. SKIN CHANGES

GLORIA WOOD, RN, BSN

H. Lee Moffitt Cancer Center, Tampa, FL

LINDA CASEY, MS, ARNP, AOCN

James A. Haley VA Medical Center, Tampa, FL

ANDY TROTTI, MD

H. Lee Moffitt Cancer Center, Tampa, FL

Radiation therapy has a direct effect on the skin. The effects of radiation can be dramatic. Providers are challenged to classify and minimize both acute and late effects and to manage the complications of treatment. Strategies to manage radiation skin reactions are ongoing topics of research and have led to a variety of clinical management models. Managing skin reactions can help alleviate distress caused by these symptoms and improve quality-of-life during and following radiation therapy. In this chapter, we will describe our institutional approach to skin management during radiation therapy.

A. NORMAL SKIN RESPONSE TO RADIATION

The skin-sparing capabilities of megavoltage, high-energy equipment, and increasingly sophisticated treatment planning methods have reduced the incidence of severe skin complications. However, certain acute and late side effects of radiation occur and, in some instances, are expected and unavoidable as the radiation must enter, exit, or be deposited near the skin to reach the target volume. Skin cells, because they originate from a rapidly reproducing differentiated stem cell, are relatively radiosensitive. Skin reactions occur as a result of inflammatory response and the depletion of actively proliferating cells in a renewing cell population. Archambeau et al.[1] describe the early and late changes as dependent on the dose and are a reflection of changes in the cellular components of the epidermis, dermis, and vasculature.

Normal skin response to radiation depends on numerous patient- and treatment-related factors. Radiation factors include the beam type and energy, use of tangent fields, use of tissue equivalent (bolus) material, weekly dose rate, accelerated fractionation, and field size. Patient factors include skin folds in the treatment volume, nutritional status, comorbidities, and the use of irritants to irradiated skin.[2] Individual differences in radiosensitivity and concurrent chemotherapy also influence skin tissue response to irradiation.[24]

There is a dose-dependent loss of cells from irradiation in the epidermis, dermis, and microvasculature endothelium.[3] Dose above the tolerance of the tissue may eventually result in necrosis. Acute skin reactions are a reflection of inflammatory response and the inability of dermal and epidermal cells to keep up with the accelerated loss caused by radiation.

Skin changes from radiation are apparent within days of the first exposure. Acute effects of radiation are those that occur during and within 6 weeks of exposure while late effects occur a few months to years after exposure to radiation. Acute effects of radiation are usually considered temporary, as the normal cells are often capable of repair. Late radiation effects are usually permanent and may become more severe as time passes. The severity of acute and late effects is dependent on the dose of radiation, time over which the total dose was delivered and the volume of tissue radiated. The presence and severity of acute radiation skin reactions may predict late effects of radiation. Late skin effects such as tissue fibrosis or necrosis can occur independent of acute reactions. Side effects of radiation on the skin, both acute and late, are local and confined to the actual tissue irradiated.

B. ACUTE SKIN EFFECTS

Acute skin reactions associated with radiation include erythema, dry desquamation, hyperpigmentation, and moist desquamation (Table 1).[14] All patients do not experience all acute skin reactions. However, there may be a combination of reactions occurring

Table 1. Acute effects of radiation on skin

Tissue response	Onset/Duration	Clinical presentation
Erythema	Onset within 4–14 days of first treatment (dose 10–30 Gy), peaks at 4–5 weeks. Resolves 2–6 weeks after last treatment	Faint to brisk redness that outlines treatment field. Intensifies as treatment continues. Increased skin temperature. Slight edema
Dry desquamation	As early as 3rd–4th week (40 Gy), but typically by 5th–6th; earlier with accelerated RT or chemotherapy. Resolves 3–4 weeks after completion of treatment	Dryness, flaking, and peeling often accompanied by itching, a layer of dry, dead, dark skin can accumulate over part or all of the treatment field and will eventually slough off. Mild pain
Hyperpigmentation	As early as 2–3 weeks of standard fractionated radiation therapy, depending on baseline skin pigmentation. Usually resolves 3 months–1 year following completion of treatment; occasionally chronic	Tanned appearance
Moist desquamation	Following 40–50 Gy or with trauma/excess friction, bolus material, or chemotherapy. Recovery usually 2–6 weeks after completion of treatment	Bright erythema, sloughing skin, exposed dermis, serous exudates and mucus oozing from skin surface. Moderate pain

simultaneously in the radiation treatment field. There are a number of factors influencing the onset, duration, and intensity of acute skin reactions. These include

- Skin folds in the neck, or behind ear lobe. Skin folds provide a warm, moist environment, and friction with movement, all of which contribute to increased risk for acute reactions and skin breakdown.
- Some types of skin tolerate radiation better than others. The scalp has the greatest tolerance followed in decreasing order by the face, neck, trunk, ears, groin, and extremities.[4]
- Beam type: electrons generally increase skin reactions and photons are generally deposited below the skin resulting in fewer acute skin reactions.
- The use of tissue equivalent materials, e.g., bolus, in close proximity to the skin will increase the severity of the skin reaction.
- Age, skin integrity at initiation of treatment, nutritional status, and comorbidities also influence skin response.
- Previous radiation therapy to the same field, prior or concurrent chemotherapy increase skin reactions.
- Patient compliance with daily skin care recommendations may diminish severity of skin response.

Acute skin reactions can cause discomfort and varying degrees of somatic pain. If the reaction progresses to moist desquamation, pain may increase and the risk of superficial skin infection increases. Regular routine skin assessment is essential in minimizing and managing skin reactions.

B1. Assessment of Acute Skin Effects

An evaluation of the skin should be performed before initiation of treatment to identify factors that may increase the skin reaction. The purpose of a skin assessment is to establish a baseline assessment for future comparison and to determine the severity of skin alteration. The frequency of assessments vary with the patient's condition and needs; however, a visual examination of the skin within the treatment fields (including exit sites) should be conducted once a week during treatment and at all regular follow-up examinations. Skin should be assessed for color, drainage, odor, dryness, and the presence of sloughing, necrosis, or infection. Patients should be questioned about the presence of pain or pruritus.[22]

There are several grading systems for acute radiation skin reactions. The most recent is the 2003 version of the Common Terminology Criteria for Adverse Events version 3.0 (CTCAE).[11] Table 2 summarizes grading of acute skin reactions using this evaluation scale. The Oncology Nursing Society's Radiation Oncology Documentation tool[5] is another instrument to assist health professionals to objectively monitor patients and accurately document skin reactions (Table 3).

B2. Management of Acute Skin Reactions

Patient education regarding anticipated skin reactions (acute and late), time frame for occurrence, onset and duration, as well as self care guidelines, promotes optimal

Table 2. Acute radiation scoring criteria (CTCAE v3.0)

	Grade				
Adverse event	1	2	3	4	5
Rash: dermatitis associated with radiation	Faint erythema or dry desquamation	Moderate to brisk erythema; patchy moist desquamation, mostly confined to skin folds and creases; moderate edema	Moist desquamation other than skin folds and creases; bleeding induced by minor trauma or abrasion	Skin necrosis or ulceration of full thickness dermis; spontaneous bleeding from involved site	Death
Hyperpigmentation	Slight or localized	Marked or generalized	—	—	—
Hypopigmentation	Slight or localized	Marked or generalized	—	—	—
Pruritus/Itching	Mild or localized	Intense or widespread	Intense or widespread, interfering with ADL	—	—
Alopecia	Thinning or patchy	Complete	—	—	—

outcomes. Table 4 provides frequent skin care recommendations for patients as well as the rationale for the recommendations. Instructions for skin care after radiation is also included.[10,20,33]

There are many preventive and interventional skin care regimens in use; however, there is a paucity of scientific data to support most practice interventions. Goals of management include minimizing symptoms, promoting healing, and prevention of infection. Historically, clinical dogma suggests that no products (such as topical emollients) be applied to skin in the treatment field just before treatment. The belief is that the product

Table 3. ONS skin assessment scoring criteria

Skin integrity	
0	No changes noted
1	Faint or dull erythema, follicular reaction, itching
2	Bright erythema, tender to touch
3	Dry desquamation with or without erythema
4	Small to moderate amount of wet desquamation
5	Confluent moist desquamation: edema
6	Ulceration, hemorrhage, or necrosis
Drainage	
0	None
1	Small to moderate amount of clear serous fluid: no odor noted
2	Moderate to large amount of serous fluid: no odor present
3	Moderate to large amount of serosanguineous fluid
4	Moderate to large amount of seropurulent fluid: foul odor present

Table 4. Patient instructions for skin care during and after radiation therapy

While receiving radiation therapy, the skin in the treatment area may become dry, reddened, tanned, and sensitive. Skin changes are usually gradual and become noticeable after 2 or 3 treatments, becoming more obvious as treatment continues. Care must be taken to protect the skin and prevent trauma. The following guidelines pertain only to the skin within the radiation treatment field.
During treatment
Shower or bathe using lukewarm water. Gently wash the area using fingertips. Rinse well and pat dry with soft cloth
Avoid harsh soap. If it is necessary to use a cleaning solution, use baking soda and water (1/2 box to one tub of water) or a creamy mild soap made for sensitive skin
Do not apply any ointment, cream, lotion, deodorant, perfume, cologne, powder, cosmetics, or home remedy to the skin unless specifically instructed to do so. Kitchen cornstarch (unscented) may be used in place of deodorant or to decrease itching. Apply lightly to dry skin using a powder puff or cotton ball
If instructed, apply a recommended mild, water-soluble lubricant to reduce itching and discomfort. Apply 2–3 times/day
Avoid shaving if possible. Use an electric razor if shaving is necessary
Avoid extreme temperatures to skin in the treatment area. Do not use water bottles, heating pads, sun lamps, ice bags, etc.
Avoid tight-fitting clothing made of irritating fabric. Clothes made of cotton or cotton blends are preferred over wool and polyester. If skin becomes irritated from clothing, change to a mild detergent or different fitting garments
Avoid exposing skin to sun. Use wide-brimmed hats, long sleeves, and gloves to prevent exposure. Always apply a sunscreen with an SPF of 15 or higher before sun exposure, even under lightweight clothing
Do not apply tape or adhesive bandages to skin in the radiation treatment field
Drink at least 3 qt of fluid each day
After treatment
Continue following the above guidelines for 2–3 weeks after the completion of treatment
Apply an unscented hydrophilic emollient (lotion or cream) 2–3 times each day for 1–2 months after treatment and then daily. Application to damp (not wet) skin after bathing will help seal in moisturizers
Always avoid exposing previously irradiated skin to the sun. When this is not possible, use a sunscreen with an SPF of 15 or greater

will act as a bolus and enhance the skin reaction. Burch et al.[6] investigated what occurs on the skin surface when deodorants, powders, and creams are applied in the treatment area prior to radiation treatments. Results indicated essentially no difference in surface dose of radiation. Skin reactions were not measured as the study used a phantom rather than humans. Because of the lack of definitive data regarding the efficacy of skin care products and regimens, most skin care guidelines are institution-specific and based on habit, anecdotal experience, and provider preference. In our opinion, a thin layer (less than 2 mm) of skin product should not be of concern for enhancing skin reactions due to a "bolus effect". Excess product may need to be removed to avoid interference with set-up procedures or devices. Table 5 summarizes suggested skin care guidelines for acute skin reactions.[16,17,18,21,26,27,28,29]

B3. Late Skin Effects

Late radiation changes are progressive and may begin to appear 10 weeks after radiation.[1,7] Reactions may progress slowly and subclinically from months to years following treatment. Not all patients will have noticeable late effects, and those who do will experience them in varying degrees. Several factors may increase the risk and severity

Table 5. Management of acute radiation skin reactions

Reaction	Agent/class	Application	Rationale	Comments
Normal skin	Mild cleanser and moisturizer	Daily and PRN	Promotes healthy skin and prevents infection. Helps decrease incidence of folliculitis. Prevents dryness	Avoid cleansers, perfumes, and deodorants as they contain chemicals and heavy metal ions that may irritate skin and may enhance skin reactions
Erythema	Cleanser and moisturizer	BID to TID	Prevents dryness and reduces discomfort in treatment field	Good skin care can help minimize skin reaction
Dry desquamation	Lubricants—water-soluble, petrolatum-based products	Increase frequency to BID to TID + PRN	Decrease itching to increase comfort, stimulates epithelialization, and reduces the risk of skin cracking and fissure formation	Discontinue use if moist desquamation occurs
	Topical steroids—mild	Application is usually 0.25% BID	Anti-inflammatory and anti-pruritic action. Often used when there is a risk for mechanical trauma from scratching or when sleep disruption occurs as a result of pruritus/scratching	Use is controversial as topical steroids may result in further thinning of the epidermis causing the skin to be more susceptible to infection
Moist desquamation	Lubricants—petrolatum or lanolin based	Keep area coated at all times	Protects area from air which diminishes pain. Provides moist healing environment	May be messy and need cleaning and reapplication
	Silvadene	Apply every 6 hours. May alternate with lubricants	Seals and dries area. Helps prevent infection	Messy to use. May traumatize new skin when cleaning
	Hydrogel primary wound dressings	Remove film from one side and place hydrogel portion on the wound or skin. Cover with non-adherent dressing such as Telfa and secure with paper tape placed outside of the radiation treatment field. May be used following mild astringent soaks	Composed of 98% water and 2% cellulose fiber. Maintains moist environment, protects newly formed epithelial cells from trauma, and increases comfort by covering exposed nerve endings. Mildly absorbent	Expensive. Difficult to secure. Must not be allowed to dry. Dressing can be removed and reapplied for routine soaks and cleaning. Must be removed during radiation treatment

Table 5. *Continued*

Wound cleansers and epithelial stimulants	Cleanse wound with gentle spray BID or TID. Apply liberal amount of gel to denuded area and cover with non-adherent dressing such as Telfa. Secure with paper tape placed outside of the radiation treatment field or flexible netting	Cleanser aids in debridement and maintenance of wound bed pH. Does not harm proliferating fibroblasts. Wound gel maintains moist environment and stimulates epithelialization. Promotes comfort by covering exposed nerve endings	Expensive. Difficult to secure. Gel must be applied liberally to avoid drying between dressing changes. Must be removed during radiation treatment
Occlusive hydrocolloid dressings	Cleanse wound. Choose dressing size that provides 1.25-in margin around wound. Apply as directed on package. Dressing can remain in place for up to 7 days. Removal—use great care to prevent harm to new skin. If necessary, small amounts of sterile saline may be used to aid in removal	Maintains moist environment. Promotes rapid epithelialization and aids in debridement. Isolates wound against bacterial contamination. Promotes comfort by covering exposed nerve endings and preventing friction. Absorbent	Cost-effective. Do not use if infection is present. May produce amalodoro yellow-brown fluid that may be mistaken as an infection. If this occurs, remove dressing, cleanse wound, and apply new dressing, if needed. Should not be used during treatment as daily removal disturbs wound bed.

of late effects. These include the dose and volume of tissue irradiated with higher total doses delivered to larger volumes increasing the risk. Tissues altered prior to radiation (surgery for example) are more prone to late radiation skin effects. Late effects of the skin may limit the total dose that can be delivered to a target in a re-irradiated setting. In turn, this can affect the chance to cure. This is an area of more intense research in recent years. Traditional dose limitations are being challenged and the long-term sequelae of increasing radiation doses provide new data regarding maximum safe doses. Late skin reactions associated with radiation therapy include photosensitivity, xerosis (dry skin), pigmentation changes, atrophy, fibrosis, telangiectasia, ulceration, and necrosis (Table 6).[31] They are more severe when daily fractions are 250–300 cGy or higher. Treatment using daily fractions of 180–200 cGy markedly reduces the risk of late skin effects.[1,25]

B4. Assessment and Management of Late Skin Effects

Because late effects of radiation therapy cannot be altered once present, management is aimed at symptom relief, prevention of infection, avoidance of skin breakdown, and promotion of healing. Fortunately, late reactions are infrequent and vary in severity. The

Table 6. Late effects of radiation on skin

Tissue response	Onset/Duration	Clinical presentation	Physiological rationale
Photosensitivity	Begins during treatment and is lifelong	Enhanced erythema over skin exposed to UV radiation from sun and tanning beds/booths	Destruction of melanocytes in the irradiated dermis and slower melanin production following irradiation reduce the skin's ability to protect itself from UV rays
Hyperpigmentation	Refer to Table 1		
Hypopigmentation	May begin anytime following resolution of hyperpigmentation. Permanent	Lack of skin color	Radiation doses necessary to eradicate cancer may permanently destroy melanocytes, which results in the skin's inability to form pigment
Atrophy	Following epidermal regrowth. Permanent	Thin and fragile epidermis	Newly formed epidermis is thinner. The epidermis thickens over time, but never attains its pre-irradiation thickness
Fibrosis	Usually begins 4–6 months following completion of treatment. May worsen over time	Dense, hard, uneven skin texture. If extensive, may cause considerable induration	Fibroblasts, responsible for producing collagen, demonstrate uneven cellular division resulting in faulty collagen remodeling. Fibrotic tissue results, giving the skin an uneven texture
Telangiectasia	May appear within 1 year and can worsen up to 8 years post-radiation. Permanent	Purple-red, spider-like appearance of blood vessels in skin	Dose and fraction size-dependent. Basement membrane thickening results in a decreased permeability of material through capillary walls. With capillary occlusion, there are fewer functioning small vessels and a decreased capacity for capillary regeneration. This results in increased pressure of blood flow through remaining undamaged superficial structures
Ulceration and necrosis	Rare. May occur up to 20 year following treatment. Usually occurs as a result of inflammation and trauma to previously irradiated tissue	Painful ulcers with red, raised edges and a shaggy, necrotic base. Usually shows little or no tendency to epithelialize or contract. Despite local treatment, ulcers tend to deepen and become more painful	Although the mechanism is not clear, late ulceration and necrosis occur as a result of connective tissue damage. Electron microscopic studies suggest that permanent damage to fibroblasts and their precursor cells prevent stem cell replication, angiogenesis, and wound contraction. Occasionally, sustained vascular occlusion and tissue ischemia may be responsible for ulceration and necrosis

Adapted from Perez CA, Brady LW, Dow KH, Hilderly LJ, Margolin SG, et al. 1997. In: Sitton E, McDonald A, Groenwald, SL, Frogge, MH, Goodman, M and Yarbro CH, eds. Cancer Nursing: Principles and Practice, 4th ed. Sudbury, MA, Jones and Bartlett, 1997, p 775.

Table 7. Late skin effects grading criteria (CTCAE v3.0)

Adverse event	Grade 1	Grade 2	Grade 3	Grade 4
Photosensitivity	Painless erythema	Painful erythema	Erythema with desquamation	Life threatening; disabling
Atrophy, subcutaneous fat	Detectable	Marked	—	—
Induration/fibrosis skin and subcutaneous tissue	Increased density on palpation	Moderate impairment of function not interfering with ADL; marked increase in density and firmness on palpation with or without minimal retraction	Dysfunction interfering with ADL; very marked density, retraction, or fixation	—
Hyper/ Hypopigmentation	Slight or localized	Marked or general	—	—
Telangiectasia	Few	Moderate number	Many and confluent	—
Dry skin (xerosis)	Asymptomatic	Symptomatic, not interfering with ADL	Symptomatic, interfering with ADL	
Ulceration	—	Superficial ulceration <2 cm size; local wound care; medical intervention indicated	Ulceration ≥2 cm size; operative debridement, primary closure or other invasive intervention indicated (e.g., hyperbaric oxygen)	Life-threatening consequences; major invasive intervention indicated (e.g., complete resection, tissue reconstruction, flap or grafting)

CTCAE offers an objective grading system for late radiation skin reactions (Table 7). Severe late effects of the skin are not usually painful unless associated with skin breakdown or necrosis. Care is individualized based on patient assessment and type of reaction. Each patient needs an individualized plan to improve skin texture and elasticity as well as to reduce risks for trauma. Table 8 outlines methods to maintain skin texture and elasticity as well as reduce risk for trauma. If skin breakdown or necrosis occurs, a local recurrence of cancer should be ruled out. Referral to a chronic wound care specialist can facilitate expert management and alleviate symptoms.

Pentoxifylline has been used to assist with healing of soft tissue necrosis. Pentoxifylline appears to accelerate healing of soft tissue necrosis and may have some effect in fibrosis.[9,12] It produces dose-related Rheologic effects, lowers blood viscosity, improves erythrocyte flexibility, and increases tissue oxygenation. In our institution, pentoxifylline 400 mg (controlled release) every 8 hours combined with 400 i.u. of vitamin E three times daily (or 1000 i.u. qd) is given for a minimum of 3 months and is continued for at least 1 month post-healing. Hyperbaric oxygen therapy has also been used to manage soft tissue

Table 8. Patient instructions for management of late skin reactions

Skin texture and elasticity
• Apply moisturizing lotion that includes vitamin E or aloe vera gel (not alone as it may be drying) to the treatment field at least once a day
• Avoid exposure to the sun or generously apply an appropriate sunscreen and repeat during sun exposure (minimum of 15 SPF)
• Initiate physical therapy with gentle massage or myofascial release to increase elasticity and to reduce fibrosis and scar formation
Reduce risk for trauma
• Avoid activities that increase risk of skin break or bruising
• Avoid scratching, the use of adhesive tape, and other activities that increase skin friction
• Avoid temperature extremes including hot water bottles, heating pads, ice packs and the use of sun lamps
• Avoid activities that increase risk of lymphedema
• Immediately report to the physician any skin changes or injury

From Higgs and Amdur in Watkins-Bruner, D., Moore-Higgs, G., and Haas, M. 2001. *Outcomes in Radiation Therapy: Multidisciplinary Management.*

necrosis. It provides 100% systemic oxygen to increase angiogenesis, reduce local tissue edema, and improve response to infection.[10]

C. SUMMARY

The response of skin to irradiation is highly complex and is dependent on many radiation-related, patient-related, and treatment-related factors. No standardized treatment of skin reactions related to radiation exists at this time. Ongoing research studying acute and late skin effects works to minimize reactions and improve patient quality-of-life. However, research with strong methodology is needed to determine if any management strategy is superior.

REFERENCES

1. Archambeau, JO, R Pezner, and T Wasserman. 1995. Pathophysiology of irradiated skin and breast. Int J Rad Oncol Biol Phys **31:**1171–1185.
2. Sitton, E. 1992. Early and late radiation-induced skin alterations: part I. Mechanisms of skin changes. Oncol Nurs Forum **19:**801–807.
3. Sitton, E. 1997. Managing side effects of skin changes and fatigue. In: Dow, KH, Bucholtz, JD, Iwamoto, R, Fieler, V, and Hilderly, L, eds. Nursing Care in Radiation Oncology Philadelphia: W. B. Saunders, pp. 79–100.
4. Dutreix, J. 1986. Human skin: early and late reactions in relation to dose and its time distribution. Br J Radiol **19(Suppl)**:22–28.
5. Oncology Nursing Society. 1994. Radiation Therapy Patient Care Record: A tool for Documenting Nursing Care. Pittsburgh: Oncology Nursing Press. 1–23.
6. Burch, SE, SA Parker, AM Vann, and JC Arazie. 1997. Measurement of 6 MV x-ray surface dose when topical agents are applied prior to external beam irradiation. Int J Rad Oncol Biol Phys **38:**447–451.
7. Panizzon, RG and H Goldschmidt. 1991. Radiation reactions and sequelae. In: Goldschmidt, H and Panizzon, RG, eds. Modern Dermatologic Radiation Therapy. New York: Springer-Verlag, pp. 25–36.
8. Futran, ND, A Trotti, and C Gwede. 1997. Pentoxifylline in the treatment of radiation-related soft tissue injury: preliminary observations. Laryngscope **107(3)**:391–395.
9. King, G, J Scheetz, RF Jacob, and JW Martin. 1989. Electrotherapy and hyperbaric oxygen: promising treatments for postradiation complications. J Prosthet Dent **62(3):**331–334.
10. Bord, MA, ND McCray, and S Shaffer. 1991. Alteration in comfort: pruritus. In: McNalley, JC, Somerville, ET, Miaskowski, C, and Rostad, M, eds. Guidelines for Oncology Nursing Practice. Philadelphia: W. B. Saunders, pp. 143–147.

11. Cancer Therapy Evaluation Program, Common Terminology Criteria for Adverse Events, Version 3.0, DCTD, NCI, NIH, DHHS March 31, 2003 (http://ctep.cancer.gov/reporting/ CTC.html), published: June 10, 2003.
12. Delanian, S. 1998. Striking regression of radiation-induced fibrosis by a combination of pentoxifylline and tocopherol. Br Radiol **71:**848, 892–894.
13. Dow, KH and LJ Hilderly. 1992. Nursing Care in Radiation Oncology. Philadelphia: Saunders.
14. Goodman, M, LJ Hilderly, and S Purl. 1997. Integumentary and mucous membrane alterations. In: Groenwald, SL, Goodman, M, and Yarbro, CH, eds. Cancer Nursing Principles and Practice, 4th ed. Boston: Jones and Bartlett, pp. 768–822.
15. Haisfield-Wolfe, ME and C Rund. 2000. A Nursing protocol for the management of perineal-rectal skin alterations. Clin J Oncol Nurs **4(1)**:15–21.
16. Hassey, K and C Rose. 1982. Altered skin integrity in patients receiving radiation. Oncol Nurs Forum **9:**44–50.
17. Hutchinson, JJ and M McGuckin. 1990. Occlusive dressings: a microbiologic and clinical review. Am J Infect Control **18:**257–268.
18. Maher, KE. 2000. Radiation therapy: toxicities and management. In: Yarbro, CH, Frogge, MH, Goodman, M, and Groenwald, SL, eds. Cancer Nursing Principles and Practice, 5th ed. Boston: Jones and Bartlett, pp. 323–351.
19. Margolin, SG, JC Breneman, and DL Denman, P LaChapelle, L Wechbach, and B Aron. 1990. Management of radiation-induced moist desquamation using hydrocolloid dressings. Cancer Nurs **13:**71–80.
20. Maienza, J. 1988. Alternatives to cornstarch for itchiness. Oncol Nurs **15:**199–200.
21. McDonald, A. 1992. Altered protective mechanisms. In: Dow KH and Hilderly LJ, eds. Nursing Care in Radiation Oncology. Philadelphia: Saunders, pp. 96–125.
22. McNally, JC and RA Strohl. 1991. Skin integrity, impairment of, related to radiation therapy. In: McNalley, JC, Somerville, ET, Miaskowski, C, and Rostad, M, eds. Guidelines for Oncology Nursing Practice. Philadelphia: W. B. Saunders, pp. 236–240.
23. Oncology Nursing Society. 1998. Manual for Radiation Oncology Nursing Practice and Education. Pittsburg, PA: Oncology Nursing Society. 1–290.
24. O'Rourke, M. 1987. Enhanced cutaneous effects in combined modality treatment. Oncol Nurs Forum **14(6):**31–35.
25. Perez, CA and LW Brady. 1992. Principles and Practice of Radiation Oncology. 2nd ed. Philadelphia: Lippincott. 155–204
26. Ratliff, C. 1990. Impaired skin integrity related to radiation therapy. J Enterostomal Ther **17:**193–198.
27. Reeves, D. 1999. Alopecia. In: Yarbro, CH, Frogge, MH, and Goodman, M, eds. Cancer Symptom Management Boston: Jones and Bartlett, pp. 275–284.
28. Seiz, AM and CH Yarbro. 1999. Pruritus. In: Yarbro, CH, Frogge, MH, and Goodman, M, eds. Cancer Symptom Management Boston: Jones and Bartlett, pp. 328–343.
29. Shell, J, F Stanutz, and J Grimm. 1986. Comparison of moisture vapor permeable (MVP) dressing to conventional dressings for management of radiation skin reactions. Oncol Nurs Forum **13:**11–16.
30. Sitton, E. 1992. Early and late radiation induced skin alterations, Part II: nursing care of irradiated skin. Oncol Nurs Forum **19(6)**: 907–912.
31. Strohl, R. 1988. The nursing role in radiation therapy oncology. Symptom management of acute and chronic reactions. Oncol Nurs Forum **15(4):**429–434.
32. Watkins-Bruner, D, G Moore-Higgs, and M Haas. 2001. Outcomes in Radiation Therapy: Multidisciplinary Management. Massachusetts: Jones and Bartlett. 493–518.
33. Witt, ME, A Lynch, and J Lydon 1990. Enhancing skin comfort during radiation therapy. Oncol Nurs Forum **17:**276–277.

INDEX